AF329460

XV Congrès International de Médecine

Lisbonne—19-26 Avril 1906

Section I

ANATOMIE

1.er FASCICULE

LISBONNE
IMPRIMERIE ADOLPHO DE MENDONÇA
1906

XV Congrès International de Médecine

LISBONNE, 19 26 AVRIL 1906

I

XV Congrès International de Médecine

LISBONNE, 19-26 AVRIL 1906

Section I

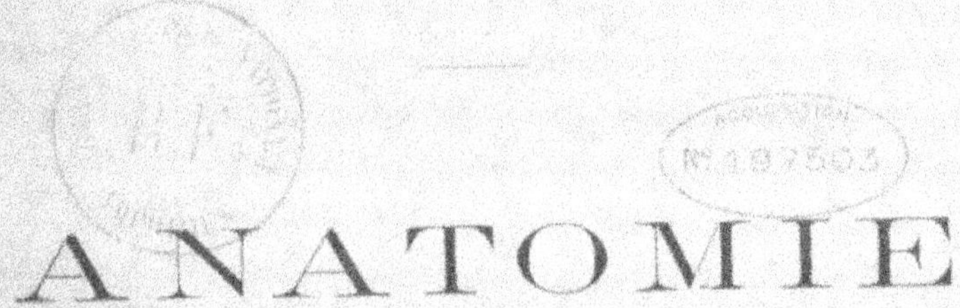

ANATOMIE

(Anatomie descriptive et comparée, Anthropologie,
Embryologie, Histologie)

LISBONNE

IMPRIMERIE ADOLPHO DE MENDONÇA

1906

Organisation de la section

Rapports officiels

1. — Nomenclature histologique, cytologique et embryologique (étendue à toute la
    série animale). — Bases d'une classification.
    Rapporteurs : MM. Nathan Loewenthal, Lausanne; Karl Benda, Berlin.
2. — Définition, structure et composition du protoplasme.
    Rapporteur : M. Gustav Mann, Oxford.
3. — Origine, nature et classification des pigments.
    Rapporteur : M. Marck Athias, Lisbonne.
4. — Phénomènes histologiques de la sécrétion, particulièrement dans les glandules
    à sécrétion interne.
    Rapporteurs : Hennegay, Paris; Swale Vincent, Winnipeg.
5. — Structure des éléments musculaires en général, et spécialement des éléments
    cardiaques.
    Rapporteur : N.
6. — Classification, origine et rôle probable des leucocytes, MASTZELLEN et PLAS-
    MAZELLEN.
    Rapporteurs : MM. Guglielmo Romiti et Francesco Pardi, Pise;
        Artur Pappenheim, Hamburg; G. L. Gulland, Edimbourg.
7. — Métamérisation embryonnaire; son importance au point de vue de l'anatomie
    comparée.
    Rapporteur : Prof. Roule, Toulouse.

Sujets recommandés

1. — Métamorphoses internes.
2. — Altérations cellulaires dans les tissus normaux.
3. — Modifications produites dans les tissus par les radiations lumineuses.
4. — Connexions de la cellule nerveuse.
5. — Etat actuel de la question de la spermatogénèse.
6. — Evolution et involution du thymus.

SECTION D'ANATOMIE

(Anatomie descriptive et comparée, Anthropologie, Embryologie, Histologie)

Rapports officiels

THÈME 4. — PHÉNOMÈNES HISTOLOGIQUES DE LA SÉCRÉTION, PARTICULIÈREMENT DANS LES GLANDULES A SÉCRÉTION INTERNE

(Some points in connection with the Histological Phenomena of Secretion, especially Internal Secretion)

Par M. SWALE VINCENT (Winnipeg)

Prof. of Physiology in the University of Manitoba

Contents

1. Introductory.
2. Histological phenomena of the secretion of the suprarenal capsule — cortex and medulla.
3. Histological phenomena of the secretion of the thyroid gland.
4. The relationship between thyroid and parathyroid.
5. The histological changes in the pancreas during secretion, etc., the relation between the islets of Langerhans, and the secreting acini of the pancreas.

1. Introductory

So far as I am aware no new facts of importance have recently come to light, bearing upon the histological changes occurring during the act of secretion in glands like the salivary and the pancreas. Although new methods have been employed, as, for example, the employment of secretin, instead of pilocarpine to provoke the secretion, yet as regards the cytological details of the changes involved in the actual secretions — the discharge of the zimogen granules and the growth from the base of the cell of the chromatophilous substance — nothing new was observed ([1]

---

[1] Dale, *Phil. Trans.*, 1906, p. 29.

XV C. I. M. — ANATOMIE

The question as to the effects of such secretion on the mutual relationship of secreting tubules and «islets» in the pancreas, will be dealt with later.

I shall not describe in any great detail the histological changes which have been supposed to accompany the internal secretion of the «ductless glands», because in my opinion the significance of many of the appearances which have been described is very doubtful and in some cases it may even be alleged with some reason that we are or should be uncertain as to the fact of secretion at all.

2. *Histological phenomena of the secretion of the suprarenal capsule — cortex and medulla*

In the present section a brief account will be given of some of the papers describing changes or histological details in the cells of the suprarenal capsule. In regard to the medulla of the gland, there are good reasons for belief that it is in fact a secreting gland, though it would be rash to assert that the question has passed out of the realm of discussion. As pointed out elsewhere[1] the direct physiological evidence for such secretion is very meagre.

Carlier[2] described the suprarenal body of a hibernating hedgehog, and called attention to the granular nature of the medullary cells. He says: «Granules similar to those in the cells may be seen mingled with the red blood corpuscles in the venous sinuses, either separated or run together into little irregular clusters, they are undoubtedly derived from the cells and in some cases indeed may be actually seen in process of passing through the cell wall towards the sinuses. The small lymph channels which are present here may also contain similar granules, no doubt derived from the same source. These granules closely resemble both in appearance and in staining reactions the well-known zymogen granules present in the cells of the pancreas and some other glands, and I think it very probable that they may be granules of some kind of ferment produced by the cells of the medulla of the suprarenal, which are secreted into the blood-vessels and possibly into the lymph vessels also, there to act upon and render innocuous certain poisonous products of metabolism which we have every reason to believe exist in the circulating bloods.

This it will be seen is a theory compounded of the internal secretion and auto-intoxication (antitoxic) theories.

Canalis [1] appears to have been the first to describe granules in the cells of the medulla. This was confirmed by Pfaundler [2].

Hultgren and Andersson [3] consider that the particles of secretion pass through the walls of the blood-vessels.

Srdénko [4] mentions finely granular masses in the blood-spaces, and the granules have the same microchemical reactions as the cells of the medulla.

Lydia Félicine [5] describes in the rabbit, cat, dog, fieldmouse, and other animals, sharply defined spaces between the medullary cells which she regards as intercellular canals. These communicate with blood-spaces and sometimes not only the medullary vessels, but also the lacunæ and the intercellular spaces are filled with darkly-staining fine particles. But the authoress cannot be sure that these are in fact particles of the secreted substance, though she concludes that «die Marksubstanz der Nebenniere ist eine Drüse mit innerer Sekretion.»

The particles described by Canalis and Pfaundler were probably, according to Ciaccio [6], centrosomes. The last-named author is strongly inclined to the view that, while the cortex destroys the toxic products of metabolisme, the medulla elaborates a substance essential to the economy. Ciaccio also describes [7] pericellular canaliculi which he considers are intimately related to the processes of secretion. In a later communication [8] the same author describes specific granules in the medullary cells and these of two kinds, the one kind having a special affinity for the salts of chromic acid — the chromaffin granules, the other having a special affinity for perchloride of iron. This author believes that the cortex provides not only a secretion common to all the layers, but also a liquid secretion from the zona media and a granular secretion from the zona interna.

[1] [illegible] R. Accad. di Med. di Torino, 1888.
[2] Sitz. d. kais. Akad. d. Wiss., 1892.
[3] Skand. Archiv f. Physiol. Bd. IX, 1899.
[4] Anat. Anz. XVIII Bd., S. 500, 1900.
[5] Anat. Anz. XXII, 1903. Sep. Abdruck f. nähr. Anat. Bd. 63, 1903.
[6] Anat. Anz. XXIII Bd., S. 452, 1903.
[7] Anat. Anz. XXII Bd., 1903.
[8] Anat. Anz. XXIV Bd., 1914.

Gottschau [1], Diamare [2], Giacomini [3], and Biedl and Wiesel [4] all believe that the suprarenal medulla is an internally secreting gland.

Da Costa [5] looks upon the cortical cell as representing a special type of cell, — an epithelial cell specially set apart to elaborate an adipose substance.

3. *Histological phenomena of the secretion of the thyroid gland*

So far as I am aware there have been no very recent investigations upon the process of secretion of the thyroid colloid material. It is very probable that the colloid arises as a secretion from the epithelial cells lining the vesicle. The epithelium consists of cells having all the characters of true glandular cells, and according to many authors the secretion is formed as specific granules in the reticular protoplasm. According to this view, details of the process of secretion are given by Langendorff [6], Hürthle [7], and Schmid [8].

4. *The relationship between thyroid & parathyroid*

In the course of a recent investigation conducted in conjunction with W. A. Jolly [9], on microscopic examination of parathyroids left *in situ* after removal of the thyroid, we have been struck by the conspicuous alteration in structure which these exhibit [10]. This presented itself to us at first as a difficulty in recognising whether small structures which had been left behind were thyroid or parathyroid. Later, we became convinced that

[1] Biol. Centralb. Bd III. 1883

[2] [illegible], Vol. XX B 4, 1900, S. 318. Arch. Zool. Vol. 13, Fasc. 3°, 1898.

[3] Intr. dei Processi secretori della R. Accad. dei Fisiocritici in Siena, etc. [illegible] [illegible] della R. Accad. dei Fisiocritici in Siena 1898. Monitore Zool. Ital. Anno XIII N. 6. Firenze, 1902.

[4] Arch. f. d. ges. Physiol. Bd XCI 1902.

[5] Segnatelo de Medicina Contemp., Lisboa — 1905.

[6] Arch. f. Anat. u. Physiol. 1889 Suppl. B. S. 332.

[7] Arch. f. d. ges. Physiol. 56, 1894.

[8] Arch. f. mikr. Anat. Bd 47, 1896.

[9] Journ. of Physiol. Vol. XXXII. The illustrations were drawn for us for this paper by Mr. Thomas Lewis, University College, London.

[10] We have as yet noticed these changes only in cats.

these were in fact intermediate in structure between the two. We are now compelled to adopt the view that parathyroid tissue when left behind approximates in appearance to ordinary thyroid tissue, so that the final product in some cases cannot be distinguished from it (¹). Figs. 1, 2, 3, and 4 show normal parathyroid, two intermediate stages, and normal thyroid. Fig. 1 represents a portion of normal parathyroid embedded in the thyroid of a cat.

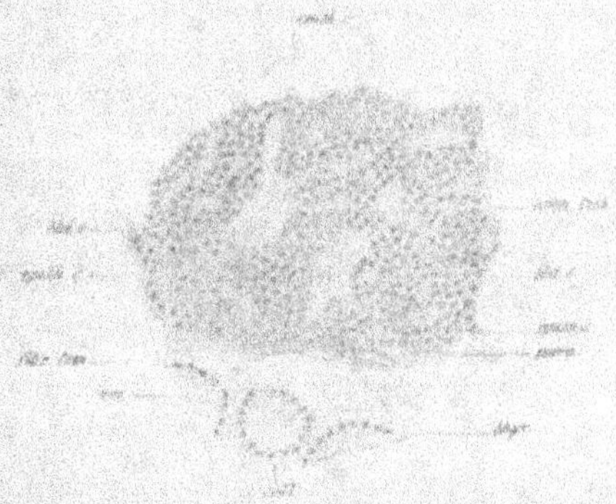

Lettering common to the four figures: *bld. v.*, blood vessels; *coll.*, colloid; *col. epith. c.*, columnar epithelial cells; *conn. tiss.*, richly vascular interstitial tissue; *d.*, debris of cells; *epith. c.*, solid columns of epithelial cells; *fibr. tiss.*, fibrous boundary between thyroid and parathyroid; *para.*, parathyroid; *prim. ves.*, irregular or cleft-like openings, being the first stage in the development of thyroid vesicles; *thyr.*, thyroid; *ves.*, vesicles.

Figure 1 shows a small portion of parathyroid of a cat embedded in thyroid tissue. It is seen to consist for the most part of solid columns of epithelial cells with streams of vascular connective tissue. A thyroid vesicle and portions of two others are shown in the lower part of the figure, separated from the parathyroid by a fibrous tissue capsule. As seen under a magnifying power of 500 diam.

(¹) It is remarkable, however, that under these circumstances the parathyroid, so far as we have seen, does not hypertrophy.

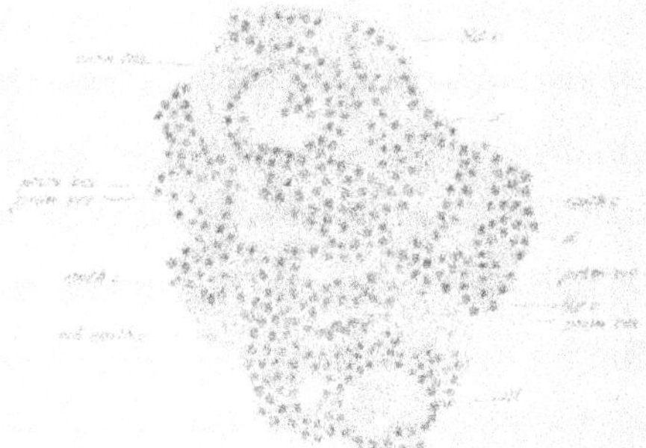

Figure 2 represents a section of a portion of parathyroid of a cat which had been left behind after removal of both thyroid lobes, examined several weeks later. There are to be seen in various parts of the section numerous irregular or cleft-like spaces with regular boundaries of epithelial cells, which are sometimes of a columnar form. These spaces may either be empty or may contain cellular débris or colloid material. This, in fact, represents the first stage of transition from parathyroid to thyroid. As seen under a magnifying power of 630 diams.

It is seen to be composed of solid columns of epithelial cells with richly vascular interstitial tissue; a portion of thyroid tissue appears below. Fig. 2 represents the first stage of the development towards thyroid tissue. There are to be seen in different parts of the section numerous cleft-like or irregular spaces, round which he epithelial cells regularly arranged. These are in some places

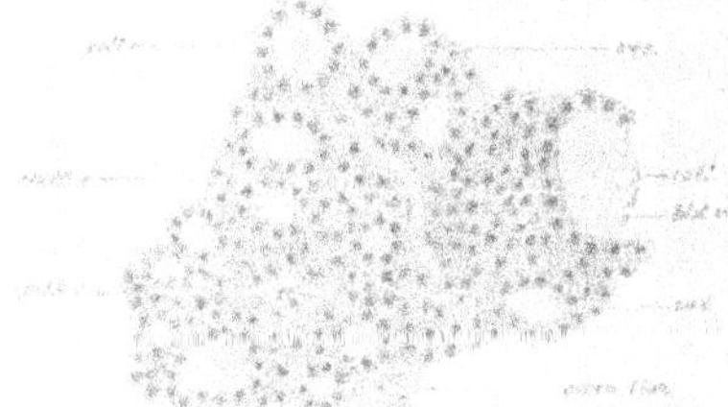

Figure 3 represents a further stage in the development of parathyroid into thyroid. The vesicles are tending to become fully formed, but a large part of the section is still occupied by solid columns of cells. The vesicles are for the most part small, and some are still irregular in shape. As seen under a magnifying power of 630 diams.

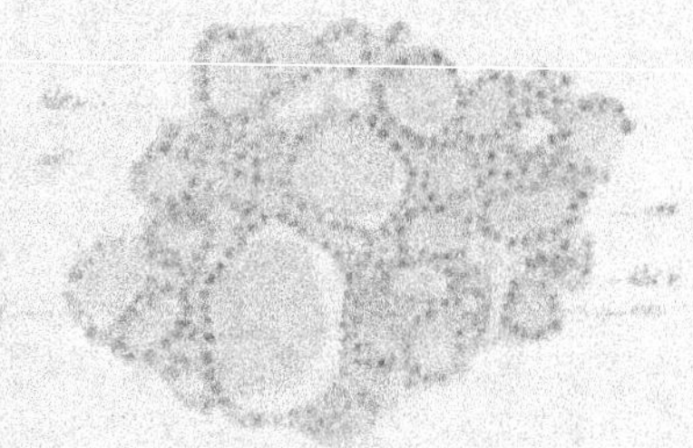

Figure 4 represents a section of the normal thyroid of a rat. The vesicles are larger,
and the intervesicular tissue less in amount than in the preceding figure.

columnar. The space is either empty or occupied by débris of cells,
or even, in parts, by colloid material. Fig. 3 shows a later stage
of the process. A large part of the section still consists of solid
masses of cells, but there are numerous small rounded vesicles,
as in normal thyroid, many of which contain colloid. In Fig. 4
will be seen part of a section of the normal thyroid of a cat.
It will be noted that the intervesicular material is here considerably
less in amount than that in Fig. 3.

This histological change accompanies, we think, a functional
alteration which takes place in the parathyroids when the thyroid
is absent. The parathyroids are then capable of physiologically
replacing the thyroid, and when one or more were left *in situ* we
have had no cases which terminated fatally. But it must be borne
in mind that in many of our experiments no such replacement
has been necessary in order to enable the animals to survive.
We have described a number of cases where survival followed
the removal of all thyroid and parathyroid tissue and in the case
of one cat the degeneration which occurred (instead of modification
on the lines above described) was not followed by death. We have
no direct evidence that parathyroids after thyroidectomy increase
in size, but it is possible that some of the bodies found *post
mortem* in the neck, which we supposed had developed from
shreds of thyroid left behind at the operation, may in reality have
been originally parathyroid which had undergone a complete transformation into thyroid tissue. Where two parathyroids had been
left behind at the operation, we found on examining them later
that they seldom presented the same degree of modification, one,
as a rule, remaining ordinary parathyroid, while the second cor-

responded to one or other of the intermediate stages figured. Occasionally both gave evidence of some transformation, which, however, had not usually proceeded with equal rapidity on the two sides.

We have also observed an earlier stage of modification than that depicted in Fig. 2. This is indicated by pale (slightly stained) patches in the section. These we interpret as areas of cellular degeneration, preliminary to the actual formation of the clefts above described. We cannot offer at present any further details as to how this preliminary disintegration takes place.

If it be true, as we believe, that parathyroid tissue may thus develope into thyroid, it is most natural to suppose that the parathyroids are embryonic thyroids. It is accordingly of interest to note that this was the earliest view with regard to them; their discoverer Sandström, indeed, saying in so many words that they are embryonic structures destined to form thyroid tissue. In the same year that Sandström's memoir was written, Baber [1], unaware of Sandström's work, in his second memoir upon the thyroid gland devotes a special section to what he calls «undeveloped portions». The structure as he describes it, and a very excellent drawing which he gives, show conclusively that he was dealing with the parathyroids. While taking the same view as Sandström with regard to the embryonic nature of the parathyroids, Baber could find no direct evidence that they undergo further development. Horsley [2], who was also unacquainted with Sandström's discovery, reinvestigated the «embryonic tissue» described by Baber and expressed a doubt whether it ever developed in thyroid. The observations of Sandström, Baber, and Horsley fell into almost complete oblivion till 1891, when Gley [3] rediscovered the parathyroids. This author states that parathyroids left behind in the rabbit after removal of the thyroid undergo a more or less complete transformation into thyroid tissue. This view, subsequently abandoned by Gley himself, has been recently revived by Kishi, who definitely states, as did the older observers, that the parathyroids are not separate and independent organs, but are embryonic thyroids. From morphological and developmental reasons

[1] Phil. Trans., Vol. [illegible], p. [illegible].
[2] Lancet II, p. [illegible], 1885.
[3] Soc. de Biol. et Notgen, T. [illegible], [illegible].

(¹) we should hesitate to adopt this view in its entirety. The thyroid is developed as a median invagination of the floor of the pharynx between the first and second branchial arches (²). The parathyroids, on the other hand, arise as thickenings of the epithelium on the dorsal aspect of the third and fourth visceral clefts. However this may be, there can be no doubt, from the detailed evidence above given, that parathyroid tissue, under certain conditions, develops in the direction of thyroid tissue, and our present evidence would indicate that a functional replacement also takes place (³).

Kohn (⁴) lays great stress on the statement that the parathyroids are «selbständige Organe eigener Art», and have only a secondary relation to the thyroid. In order to emphasize their independence of the thyroid, he proposes instead of the historic name «glandulæ parathyroideæ», the term «Epithelkörperchen» which had been used by Maurer (⁵) for many years for similar organs in Amphibia. Under the more general name of «Epithelkörper» (*Corpora glandulæformia*) Kohn includes along with the parathyroids the glandular part of the pituitary body, the cortex of the suprarenal capsule, and the islets of Langerhans in the pancreas. Some evidence (⁶) has been recently adduced which tends to show that these islets are in reality not structures *sui generis*, but functionally and morphologically part and parcel of the pancreas. If this be confirmed, analogy might lend some little support to the views of the earlier observers as to the relationship between thyroid and parathyroid (⁷).

There are, moreover, other reasons which lead one to conclude that thyroid and parathyroid are not separate and independent organs. In the human parathyroid it is not rare to find colloid vesicles in all respects resembling those of the thyroid. In fact, it would seem that there is after all no fundamental distinction between the essential histological constituents of the two tissues. The intervesicular cells of the thyroid are almost identical with

(¹) See Kohn, *loc. cit.*, where full references will be found.

(²) According to the the most recent account (Verdun, *C. R. Soc. Biol.*, 1899, *Thèse Toulouse*, 1898) the thyroid of man and mammals is derived exclusively from the median anlage and the post branchial body degenerates.

(³) See Vincent and Jolly, *loc. cit.*

(⁴) *Loc. cit.*

(⁵) *Morph. Jahrb.*, Bd XIII, 1897.

(⁶) *Phil. Trans.*, 1901.

(⁷) Several observers, foremost among whom are Diamare and Rennie, hold the opposite view as to the islets of Langerhans. This subject will be dealt with later on.

the parathyroid cells, and such differences in arrangement as exist
may be the direct result of the formation of the colloid substance.
Further it is not rare in my own experience to find structures even
in normal animals about which it is difficult to say whether they
are thyroids or parathyroids. In many thyroids there are solid
masses of cells, not, however, so distinctly marked off as the
proper parathyroids, which are practically identical in structure
with the latter bodies. The internal parathyroid is frequently in
direct continuity with the thyroid at one part and it is impossible
to draw any strict line of demarcation between the two.

5. *The histological changes in the pancreas during secretion, etc.: the relation between «islets» and secreting acini.*

A question analogous to that just discussed in regard to
thyroid and parathyroid arises also in the case of the «islets» of
Langerhans» and the zymogenous tubules of the pancreas.

The structures now usually termed «islets of Langerhans»
were first described by the author of that name in 1869 [1]. Since
then they have been very frequently described and their nature
has been the subject of much discussion. The earlier observers
for the most part did not hesitate in considering the structures
to be permanent and distinct from the secreting acini [2]. But
Lewaschew [3] in 1886 described what he thought was a continuity between alveoli and islets and found cells intermediate in
character between those of the islets and those of the secreting
acini. He looked upon the islets as groups of alveolar cells altered
by fatigue [4].

Laguesse [5] also from embryological considerations regards

[1] [illegible] *Arch. f. Hist.* [illegible] Inaug. Diss. Berlin, 1869.
[2] [illegible]
[3] *Arch. f. mikr. Anat.*, Bd. 26, S. 453, 1886.
[4] [illegible]
[5] [illegible]

the islets as phases in the functional history of the secreting-tubules.[1]

Dale [2] considers that the islets of Langerhans are the result of a transformation, temporary or permanent, of the ordinary secreting tissue of the pancreas. His observations are the outcome of an investigation of the histological changes produced in the pancreas by the activity called forth by «secretin». [3] His results are as follows:—

1. The islets of Langerhans are not independent structures of separate origin to the rest of the pancreas, but are formed by certain definite changes in the arrangement and properties of the cells of the ordinary secreting tissue. The changes are of such a kind as to assimilate all the cells to those forming the epithelium of the ductules and the centro-acinary cells, thus bringing about a reversion to embryonic type. The lumina disappear in this process, and all the cells are brought into more intimate relation with the blood capillaries. Such changes have been observed both in mammals and amphibia.

2. In the pancreas of the toad some evidence was found of cell-multiplication in the islets, and of reconstruction of alveoli from them. Such evidence is at present wanting in the case of mammals.

3. The change from the secreting to the "islet" condition is greatly accelerated both in mammals and in amphibia by exhaustion of the gland by means of secretin. True exhaustion of the mammalian gland was not found possible unless the animal was also bled. This suggests that secretin stimulates both anabolic and katabolic activity of the pancreatic cells, and that anabolism must be otherwise depressed if the exhaustion effect is to be produced.

4. The proportion of islet tissue to secreting tissue is also increased by prolonged fasting. In other words, disappearance of the stored material of the secretory cells, whether by discharge into the duct, to produce the secretion, or by absorption into the blood and lymph, when the nutrition of the body fails, is attended by increased formation of islets from secretory alveoli.

5. Occlusion of the duct causes a disappearance of most of the pancreatic tissue in the course of a few weeks. That which escapes destruction assumes a form resembling the islets, but the already existing islets exhibit no special immunity from the destructive effects of the operation.

There can be no doubt that the *appearances* described by Dale can be readily observed. I have, during the last year, confirmed these in the dog, both after injection of secretin and after the animal has fasted for some days. The changes are in my experience much more marked in the latter case than in the former. But the precise interpretation of these appearances is a matter of

---

[1] For further references see infra. Phil. Trans. 1905.
[2] Loc. cit.
[3] Bayliss & Starling. Journ. of Physiol. Vol. 28 & 29. 1902 & 1903.

considerable difficulty. It seems clear that one can induce by the
above methods a transformation of secreting tubules into structures which at any rate bear a striking resemblance to the islets of
Langerhans; but whether these newly formed structures are in
fact identical in their nature with the islets of the normal gland
is not easy to determine. In them one can clearly see the vestiges
of the alveolar arrangement. The lumen has disappeared, but the
double row of nuclei remains and in some cases one can map
out the areas of the original acini. The question as to transitions
from one structure to the other and as to intermediate forms of
cells presents great difficulties. The possibility exists that the original islets of Langerhans remain unaltered, and that the exhausted tubules, though strongly resembling them, bear no relation to
them.

It is moreover difficult to reconcile the view of Dale with
some of the facts of comparative anatomy. Thus Rennie (¹) states:
«The conditions observed in various Teleostei force the conclusion that here «islets» and pancreas are distinct organs. In certain
genera, e. g. Lophius, Pholis, Zoarces, Syngnathus, the «islet» tissue has no more intimate relation to pancreas than to neighbour-
ing organs.» In many of these fishes there is, according to Rennie, an encapsuled islet («principal islet») of relatively large size
and of constant occurrence, whose relation to the pancreatic tissue is frequently extremely slight. This author believes that the islets are blood-glands which have entered into a secondary relation with the pancreas. This has been brought about in Teleostei
mainly by the tendency of the diffuse pancreas to envelope or in-
vade other tissues. He finds no evidence of transitional forms to
support the view that the islets undergo metamorphosis into zymogenous tissue, and suggests: «The reported changes of zymogenous elements to islet tissue are possibly degenerative or regressive to the «cellular process» condition of the embryo».

The relations of the «principal islet» to the pancreas in *Zoarces viviparus*, as shown in Rennie's drawing, is very suggestive
that here at any rate we have to deal with an organ quite distinct from the pancreas. In this species the islet is surrounded by
a fairly thick capsule, and it is difficult to conceive how there
could be any kind of transition forms or how such a mass of cells
could function as a secreting constituent of the pancreas.

(¹) Quart. Journ. Micr. Sci., Vol. 65, Part III, Nov. 1914.

Diamare [1] has for some years maintained that the islets are epithelial organs *sui generis* and discredits the views of Laguesse, Dale and others as to transitions between acini and islets. He is further opposed to the view that the secreting alveoli may under certain circumstances become converted into islets. His experimental work has led him to conclude that the internal secretion of the islets is intimately connected with the sugar metabolism of the body.

It is of course possible that, as Laguesse teaches, the islet is formed from the solid embryonic pancreas, before this becomes tubular, and that in some animals this islet tissue may remain as a solid mass of cells distinct from the pancreas, and having no functional relationship to it, while in others it may be more intimately attached to the tubular tissue and may even be converted into acini and back again into islet according to the state of functional activity of the pancreas.

Further researches in the direction both of comparative anatomy and physiology are needed before we can draw any positive conclusions as to the morphological and physiological significance of the islets of Langerhans.

THÈME I. — CLASSIFICATION. ORIGINE ET RÔLE PROBABLE DES LEUCO-
CYTES. — MASTZELLEN ET PLASMAZELLEN

(Clasmatocytes et Mastzellen)

Par MM. les Prof. GUGLIELMO ROMITI et FRANCESCO PARDI (Pisa)

Quoique remontant à une époque relativement récente la découverte, faite par RANVIER, de certains éléments qu'il a nommés *clasmatocytes* dans l'aponévrose fémorale de *Rana esculenta* et dans le mésentère de *Molge cristata*, ainsi que dans l'épiploon des mammifères, la littérature de la question est déjà riche en travaux intéressants. Mais l'accord parmi les auteurs est loin d'être

---

[1] Mem. I. *Internat. Monatschr. f. Anat. u. Phys.*, B. XXVI, Hef. 7, 1899, tav. I-III ; *Anat. Anz.* XV b., 1899 ; *Res. Congr. Zool. di Napoli*, 1910 ; *Monitore Zoologico*, 1911 ; Diamare V., sud Kulabko A., *Centralbl. f. Physiol.*, B. XVIII, Wien 1904 ; *Riv.* B. XIX, Nr. 4, 1905 ; Mem. II. *Internat. Monatschr. f. Anat. u. Physiol.* B. XXVII, 1911.

complet soit pour ce qui concerne l'origine et la signification de ces éléments, soit pour ce qui a trait à leur morphologie.

Dans un travail sur les cellules vasoformatrices et sur l'origine intra-cellulaire des érythrocytes, l'un de nous s'est occupé de la question des clasmatocytes du grand épiploon de mammifères jeunes; il a émis alors quelques vues qui se rapprochent par plusieurs points de celles posées par SCHWARZ dans un travail récent.

Reprendre la question, rassembler la bibliographie, s'efforcer d'éclaircir les controverses existant entre les différents observateurs et apporter une contribution personnelle à la connaissance des clasmatocytes sont des choses intéressantes à plusieurs points de vue, et surtout à cause de l'importance que les pathologistes, parmi lesquels il suffit de rappeler MARCHAND, SCHREIBER et NEUMANN, MAXIMOW, SCHWARZ, plus encore que les anatomistes, donnent à ces singuliers éléments.

Dans une autre occasion nous aurons à résumer largement la bibliographie, et examiner les divergences qui existent à propos des *clasmatocytes*; ici nous ne voulons que rendre compte, d'une façon sommaire, des résultats auxquels nos études nous ont amenés.

Nos observations ont été pratiquées sur le mésentère des Amphibiens urodèles (*Molge cristata*, *Salamandrina perspicillata*, *Spelerpes fuscus*) et sur le grand épiploon de jeunes Mammifères (*Lepus cuniculus*, *Canis familiaris*, *Felis domestica*, *Homo*).

Les études faites sur le mésentère des Amphibiens urodèles nous ont conduits aux conclusions suivantes:

1.° C'est seulement dans le mésentère de *Molge cristata*, parmi toutes les espèces animales observées par nous, que nous avons trouvé de très nombreux *clasmatocytes*, tels que RANVIER les a décrits. Ce sont des éléments de dimensions colossales, supérieures peut-être, à celles des *chromoblastes*, pourvus de prolongements moniliformes alternativement gonflés et rétrécis, qui ne s'anastomosent jamais avec ceux des éléments identiques voisins; le corps cellulaire et les prolongements sont remplis de granulations qui se colorent *métachromatiquement* en rouge-violet par les couleurs basiques d'aniline telles que le violet de méthyle 5 B, le bleu polychrome d'UNNA, la thionine.

2.° Dans le mésentère de *Salamandrina perspicillata* et de *Spelerpes fuscus* on ne trouve que de rares *Mastzellen*, qui sont, par contre, très abondantes dans celui de *Molge cristata*.

3.° Ainsi que l'ont démontré JOLLY, SCHREIBER et NEUMANN

et SCHWARZ, les clasmatocytes des Amphibiens urodèles doivent être considérés comme une modalité de *Mastzellen*, desquelles ils ne diffèrent que par la forme; ils en possèdent tous les caractères les plus importants, et notamment la même réaction histo-chimique des granulations; cette conviction est encore soutenue par deux faits:

a) l'existence, dans le mésentère de *Molge cristata* où les *Mastzellen* et les *clasmatocytes* sont si nombreux, de formes inter-médiaires entre les deux sortes d'éléments;

b) l'absence de *clasmatocytes* dans le mésentère de *Salamandrina perspicillata* et de *Spelerpes fuscus*, espèces animales chez lesquelles les *Mastzellen* sont excessivement rares.

L'étude du grand épiploon des Mammifères à la dernière période fœtale et aux premières périodes post-fœtales, nous a montré:

1.º que les éléments fusiformes ou ramifiés du grand épiploon de *Lepus cuniculus* que RANVIER a appelés *clasmatocytes*, correspondants à ceux des Amphibiens urodèles et anoures, doivent être regardés comme étant des éléments de nature différente, car s'il est vrai que ces éléments se colorent d'une manière homogène à la façon des clasmatocytes des Amphibiens, par la méthode de RANVIER (acide osmique à 1 %, violet de méthyle 5 B), il est également vrai que par des méthodes de technique plus adéquates (coloration régressive par la thionine, bleu polychrome et même par le violet de méthyle 5 B, après fixation au liquide de ZENKER ou à l'alcool) on ne réussit pas à mettre en évidence dans le pro-toplasma des premiers les granulations *métachromatiques* si caractéristiques des seconds;

2.º que tandis que chez les Amphibiens urodèles on peut assurer qu'il y a parfaite identité des *clasmatocytes* et des *Mastzellen* (la différence de forme et d'aspect n'ayant que peu de valeur vis-à-vis de l'importance que possède la présence des granulations douées d'une même réaction histochimique, WESTPHAL), pour les Mammifères on ne peut en dire autant; nous admettons avec JOLLY que les *clasmatocytes* des Mammifères sont des éléments bien distincts des *Mastzellen* et avec SCHWARZ que les *clasmatocytes* de *Lepus cuniculus* et de l'homme ne sont que des formes modifiées des primitives cellules migratrices mononucléaires (einkernige Wanderzellen); ceci est démontré par le fait de l'existence de formes de transition entre celles-ci et ceux-là.

THÈME — **NOMENCLATURE HISTOLOGIQUE, CYTOLOGIQUE ET EMBRYOLOGIQUE (ÉTENDUE A TOUTE LA SÉRIE ANIMALE) BASES D'UNE CLASSIFICATION**

(Contribution à l'étude de l'unification de la nomenclature histologique et histophysiologique)

Par M. le Prof. NATHAN LOEWENTHAL (Lausanne)

Professeur d'histologie à la Faculté de Médecine de Lausanne

Éléments figurés des Tissus. Geformte Bestandteile der Gewebe.

Parties plastiques élémentaires	*Plastische Elementarteile*
Granulations histogènes	Histogene Granula
Microsomes	Mikrosomen
Plasmosomes	Plasmosomen
Caryosomes	Karyosomen
Fibrilles	Fibrillen (Mitochondrien)
Inclusions figurées	*Geformte Einschlüsse*
(Granulations deutos ou paraplasmiques)	(Deutos. paraplasmatische Granula)
Éléments anatomiques (Unités histologiques)	*Biotomische Einheiten*
Cellules	Zellen
Fibrocytes, Fibres cellules	Faserzellen
» simples	» einfache
» composées	» zusammengesetzte
Syncytium	
à cellules confluentes	mit angelöteten Zellen
» anastomotiques (agrégats cellulaires)	mit anastomosirenden Zellen (Zellenkonglomerate)

Cellule   Zelle

Configuration	*Gestaltung*
Globuleuse	Kugelförmige
Ovoïde	Ovoïde
Ellipsoïde	Ellipsoidische
Cylindrique	Zylindrische
Prismatique	Prismatische
Conique	Konische
Pyramidale	Pyramidenförmige
Fusiforme	Spindelförmige
En bâtonnet	Stäbchenförmige
En massue	Keulenförmige

Caliciforme	Becherförmige
Cyathiforme	
Cubique	Kubische
Polyédrique	Polyedrische
Discoïde	Scheibenförmige
Ovalaire	Ovale
Elliptique	Elliptische
Polygonale	Polygonale
Rubanée	Bandförmige
Ramifiée	Verzweigte
Étoilée	Sternförmige
En araignée	Spinnenförmige
Cellule à pied	Fusszelle
Cellule à ailes	Flügelzelle

PARTIES CONSTITUANTES DES CELLULES — BESTANDTEILE DER ZELLEN

ENVELOPPE — UMHÜLLUNG

Couche cortico-plasmique	Kortikale Grenzschicht, Rindenschicht
Membranes d'enveloppe	Hüllen
a) amibites	strukturlose,
b) striées ou poreuses	gestreifte oder mit Poren versehene;
c) doublées de noyaux ou de revêtement cellulaire	mit kernhaltiger oder zelliger Unterlage.
Capsules	Kapsein
Plateaux cuticulaires	Kutikularsäume
a) non ciliés	wimperlose
homogènes	homogene
striés	gestreifte
(bordure à brosse)	(Bürstensaum)
b) ciliés	bewimperte

CORPS CELLULAIRE — ZELLLEIB

Syn. *Bioplasma — Protoplasma, Cytoplasma*

Mitoplasma	Mitom (*Flemming*)
Spongioplasma	
Granulations histogènes	Histogene Granula
Plasmosomes	Plastosomen
Hyaloplasma	Enchylema
Filaments basaux (ergastoplastiques?)	Basalfäden
Appareil réticulaire	Fadennetzapparat
Canalicules trophiques	Trophospongien
Granulations deuto- ou paraplasmiques	Deuto- s. paraplasmatische Granula.
protéiques	albuminoide
glycogéniques	Glycogensubstanz.

N. F. R. — ANATOMIE

— mucinogènes	schleimbildende
— colloïdes	kolloide
— vitellines (lécithes)	Dotterplättchen
— dites chromophiles	s. g. chromophile (*Altmann'sche Granula*)
— nucléoïdes	nucleoïde
— de kératohyaline	Keratohyalin
— d'éléidine	Eleïdin
— pigmentaires	Pigmentkörnchen
— cristalloïdes	Kristalloïde
Gouttelettes graisseuses	Fetttröpfchen
— huileuses colorées	gefärbte Oeltröpfchen
Vacuoles	Vakuolen
Noyaux accessoires	Nebenkörne, Paranuclei
Corps vitellin (*Balbiani*)	Dotterkern
Centrosoma	
Syn. Corpuscule polaire	Polkörperchen
Corpuscule central	Centralkörperchen
— simple	einfaches
— double (Diplosoma)	doppeltes
— multiples (?)	mehrzählige Centralkörperchen, Mikrocentrum
Hyalome polaire	Homogene Centralschicht
Astrocœle	
Zone granulo-radiaire	Granuloradiäre Schicht
Exoplasma	
Mésoplasma	
Endoplasma	
Unissant (ou anneau) perinucléaire	perinucleäre Sichel

Structures protoplasmiques   Plasmastrukturen

a) striée, fibrillaire	Streifige, fibrilläre
b) réticulée (réseaux de plastine)	Netzstruktur (Plastinnetze)
c) aréolaire	Wabenstruktur

NOYAU, ZELLKERN, NUCLEUS.

Configuration   Gestaltung

Regulière	Regelmässige
— arrondie	Runde
— ovalaire	Ovale
— en bâtonnet	Stäbchenförmige
Irregulière	Unregelmässige
Irregulière lobée	Gelappte
— bosselée (noyaux bourgeons)	
— nante	Höckerige (Sprossende Kerne)

... en boudin	Wurstförmige
Noyaux troués	Topfkernige
Cellules uni- bi- plurinucléées	Ein- zwei- mehrkernige Zellen

Situation	*Lage*
Centrale	Mittelständige
Excentrique	Excentrische
Marginale	Randständige
Basale	
Apicale	
Proximorale	
Oppositocale	
... chromatique	Exosomatische

Structure	*Struktur*
Couche marginale	Kerngrenzschicht
Membrane nucléaire	Kernmembran
Réticule nucléaire	Kerngerüst (-netz)
... chromatique	Chromatinnetz
	Nucleospongium
Caryomitome	Karyomitom
Filaments nucléaires	Kernfäden, Kernfadenwerk
... chromatiques	Chromatische Kernfäden
Segments chromatiques	Chromatische Segmente
Nodosités claires	Netzknoten
Chromosomes	Chromosomen
Caryosomes	Karyosomen
Filaments de linine	Lininfäden
Granules de chromatine	Chromatogranula
Nucléo-Caryo-plasma	Karyochylema

NUCLÉOLE — KERNKÖRPERCHEN — NUCLEOLUS

Configuration	*Gestaltung*
Régulière	Regelmäßige
Irrégulière	Unregelmäßige
(Amiboïsme nucléolaire	Kernkörperchen — Amöboismus)

Nombre	*Zahl*
Noyaux uni- plurinucléolés	mono- polynukleoläre Kerne

Situation	*Lage*
Centrale	Mittelständige
Excentrique	Excentrische
Pariétale	Wandständige

Nucléoles dispersés	Zerstreute Kernkörperchen
conglomérés	Zusammengeballte
Composition	*Beschaffenheit*
Nucléoles plasmatiques	Plasmatische Nucleolen
chromatiques	Chromatische
composés	Zusammengesetzte Nucleolen
Stroma nucléaire	Grundsubstanz
Partie chromatique	Chromatischer Anteil
Nucléoles cyanophiles	Cyanophile
érythrophiles	Erythrophile
Couche cyanophile marginale	Cyanophile Randschicht
Zone hyaline périnucléaire	Heller perinukleärer Raum
hyaline périnucléolaire	perinukleolärer Raum
Couronne granulaire	Körnchenkreis (Kranz)

Division nucléaire et cellulaire. Kern- und Zelltheilung

Division autonucléaire	Kernteilung
Division nucléo-cellulaire par étranglement	Kern-Zellteilung durch Einschnürung
Synon. Scission simple	Halbirung
Division directe	Directe Teilung
Amitotique	Amitotische
Akinétique	Akinetische
symétrique	symmetrische
asymétrique. fragmentation	unsymmetrische (Fragmentirung)
Parcellage. Synon. Par plaque nu-	Durch Spaltung (vermittelst Kern, resp.
cléaire ou cellulaire	Zellplatte)
symétrique	symmetrische
asymétrique	unsymmetrische
Scission caryo-métabolique	Karyo-metabolische Teilung
(Synon. Fragmentation indirecte)	(Indirekte Fragmentirung)
Division cinétique (Synon. Caryocinéti-	Kinetische (karyokinetische, mitotische,
que, mitotique, caryolytique)	karyolytische)

Phases	*Phasen*
Prophases	Prophase
Peloton continue	Knäuel
Aster chromatique (Monaster)	Mutterstern
Metakinèse	Metakinese
Mitoschisis	Fadenspaltung
Plaque équatoriale	(equatorialplatte)
Diaster chromatique	Tochtersterne
Dispersion Dispatem	Tochterknäuel
Telophases	Endphasen
Encroûne noyau-pelotte	Kern-Fäden-Passement
Repos nucléaire	Kern-Periode

Anses chromatiques alternées	Verirrte Chromatinschleifen
Peloton dense	Dichter Knäuel
lâche	Lockerer Knäuel
Pycnose	
Couronne (chromatique)	Kranzform
Tonnelet chromatique	Tonnenform
Astrosphères	Astrosphären
Sphères limites polaires	Polzentren
Sphères attractives	Attraktionssphären
Amphiaster (*Fol*)	
Rayons polaires	Polstrahlung
Fuseau de direction	Richtungsspindel
Fuseau nucléaire	Kernspindel
central	Zentralspindel
Plaque cellulaire de segmentation	Zellteilungsplatte (Zellplatte, Zwischen platte)
Corpuscules intermédiaires	Zwischenkörperchen

Caryoses multipolaires — Multipolare Zellteilungen

Triastériques	Triaster
Tétrastériques	Tetraster
Polyastériques	Polyaster

Transformations cellulaires — Zellumbildungen

Progressives	Progressive
Régressives	Regressive

Transform. progressives   *Progressive Umbildungen*

Accroissement	Wachstum
Différenciation	Differenzierung
cellulaire	Zelldiff —
nucléaire	Kern —
Reconstruction nucléaire	Kernrekonstruktion
Noyaux chromata partites	Chromatopartite Kerne
chromata axialés	Chromatomodelirte —

Transformations régressives   *Regressive Umbildungen*

Destructives	Destruktive
Formatives (plastiques)	Plastische
Destructives	—Destruktive
du corps cellulaire	*des Zellleibes*
Dégénérescence graisseuse	Fettige Entartung
granuleuse et grana bengraisseux	Granulöse —
hyaline	Hyaline

" muqueuse	Schleimige
" pigmentaire	Pigmentatrophie
du noyau	des Kernes
Atrophie hyaline simple	Hyaline Atrophie
Fentes périnucléaires	Perinukleäre Spalträume
Régression chromatolytique	Chromatolytische Entartung
" formatives	Plastische
Kératinisation	Verhornung
Formation de l'émail	Schmelzbildung

SUBSTANCES INTERCELLULAIRES	INTERZELLULARSUBSTANZEN
Cimentaires	Kittsubstanzen
Fondamentales:	Grundsubstanzen:
" liquides	Flüssige
" gélatineuses	Gallertartige
" solides	Feste
Substances fondamentales solides	Feste Grundsubstanzen
" chondrinogène	Chondrinogene.
" fibreuse, fibro-élastique	Faserige, faserig-elastische
" lamelleuse canaliculé	Röhrchenlamellen.

AGENCEMENT DES CELLULES	ANORDNUNG DER ZELLEN
Cellules libres	Freie Zellen
Trames cellulaires continues	Kontinuirliche Zellschichten
Cellules endolacunaires	Endolakunäre Zellen
" endocavitaires	Endokaviöre
" encapsulées	Eingekapselte
" intra-réticulaires	Intraretikuläre

CONNEXIONS DES CELLULES	VERBINDUNG DER ZELLEN
— De continuité	— Per continuitatem
" ponticules plasmiques	Zellbrückenverbindung
" anastomotiques	Anastomotische
" pandendritiques	Netzverbindung
— De contiguïté	— Per contiguitatem
" par de la substance cémentaire	Kittsubstanzverbindung
	Kittleisten
" péridendritique	Peridendritische
" interdendritique	Interdendritische

CELLULES COMME PARTIES INTÉGRANTES DES TISSUS	ZELLEN ALS BESTANDTEILE DER GEWEBE
Nommer … cellules sexuelles	Geschlechtszellen, Stammzellen
Cellules ne formant pas de tissus con- tinus ou stables	Zellen, die weder kontinuirliche noch dauernde Gewebe bilden.

Cellules migratrices	Wanderzellen
» géantes	Riesenzellen
» déciduales	Deciduazellen
» du corps jaune	Luteinzellen
Éléments figurés du sang et de la lymphe	Geformte Bestandteile des Blutes und der Lymphe

Tissus holocytaires non isoblastiques — *Holocytäre, nicht isoblastische Gewebe*

Épithélium et dérivés	Epithel und Derivate
Tissu nerveux primaire	Primäres Nervengewebe
Tissu musculaire primaire	Primäres Muskelgewebe

Tissus isoplastiques — *Isoplastische Gewebe*

Tissu conjonctif	Bindegewebe
» osseux	Knochengewebe
» cartilagineux	Knorpelgewebe
— Tissus d'origine mixte	— Gewebe gemischten Ursprungs
Tissu lymphadénoïde (?)	Lymphadenoides Gewebe (?)
Muscles striés	Gestreifte Muskeln
Nerfs	Nerven
Glandes composées	Drüsen
Formations cornées d'origine mixte	Horngebilde gemischten Ursprungs
Tissus archiblastiques	Archiblastische Gewebe
» parablastiques	Parablastische "
» mésenchymateux	Mesenchymgewebe "

Cellules sexuelles — Gonocytes — Geschlechtszellen

OVULE. PHASES HISTOGÉNÉTIQUES — EIZELLE. HISTOGENETISCHE REIHEN

Ooblastes	Ooblasten
Oogonies	Oogonien
Oocytes	Oocyten
Oocytes de 1er ordre (primordiaux)	» Uroocyten
» de 2e ordre (ou de transition)	» Uebergangsoocyten
» de 3e ordre (oocytes mûrs)	» Reife Oocyten
Ovules tubaires (œufs)	Oviducteier

OOCYTES. ŒUFS — OOCYTEN. EIER

Enveloppes — *Hüllen*

— primaires	— primäre
Zone pellucide	Zona pellucida
Zone radiaire	» radiata
Membrane vitelline (Ovolemme)	Dotterhaut (Oolemma)
Micropyle	Mikropyle
Bâtonnets de la zone pellucide	Zona-Stäbchen
— secondaires	— sekundäre
(Gauche) enveloppe albumineuse	Albuminschicht

Coquille	Schale (Kalkschale)
Membrane coquillère	Schalenhaut
feuillet externe, feuillet interne, chambre à air	äusseres Blatt, inneres Blatt, Luftkammer
Albumine d'œuf (albumen)	Eiweiss
Chalazes	Chalazen (Nagelschnüre)
Membrane parolemnière	Lederhülle
Couche (enveloppe) gélatineuse	Gallertschicht (Gallerthülle)

Vitellus — *Dotter*

Couche strao-vitelline	Gestreifte Dotterschicht
Couche globo-vitelline	Dotterkugelschicht
C. granulo-vitelline interne	innere granulierte Dotterschicht

Inclusions vitellines — *Dottereinschlüsse*
(vitellus nutritif) — (Nahrungsdotter, *Heubert*)

Granulations vitellines	Dotterkörpchen
Sphères vitellines	Dotterkugeln
Plaquettes vitellines	Dotterplättchen
Globes vitellins	Dotterschollen
Vitellus blanc	Weisser Dotter
Vitellus jaune	Gelber Dotter
Granulations pigmentaires	Pigmentkörnchen
Cristalloïdes	Krystalloïde
Noyau (corps vitellin de Balbiani)	Dotterkern
— disque germinatif (cicatricule)	— Keimscheibe (Hahnentritt)
Vitellus formatif	Bildungsdotter
Noyau de Pander	Panderscher Kern
Latebra	

Vésicule germinative — *Keimbläschen*

Membrane	Kernmembran
Tache (s) germinative (s)	Kernflecke
— pariétales	— wandständige
Filaments nucléaires pinnulés	Gefiederte Kernfäden
Nucléoles nucléaires	Kernsaftion
Zone exonucléaire	Aeussere Kernzone
Couronne nucléolaire	Kernkörperchenkranz
Zone intra-granuleuse centrale	Centrale Körnerfadenzone
Granulations nucléoliformes	Nucleolenähnliche Granula
Granulations karyoplasmatiques	Karyophreinatische Granula

Œufs alécithes (?)	dotterfreie (?)
oligolécithes	dotterarme
polylécithes	dotterreiche
centrolécithes	mit mittelständigem Nahrungsdotter
télolécithes	mit polständigem

Oeufs holoblastiques	Holoblastische Eier
à segmentation égale	mit äqualer Furchung
à segmentation inégale	mit inäqualer
pôle animal	animaler Pol
pigmenté	Pigmentpol
végétatif	vegetativer Pol
Oeufs méroblastiques	Meroblastische Eier
à segmentation discoïdale	mit discoïdaler Furchung
à segmentation superficielle	mit superficialer
pôle formatif	Bildungspol
pôle nutritif	Dotterpol

SPERMATOZOIDE   SPERMATOZOON

Syn. Spermatozoïdes, zoospermes   *Samenfäden, Spermien*

Segment céphalique (tête)	Kopf
intermédiaire	Mittelstück
caudal (queue)	Schwanz
Segment céphalique	Kopf
partie terminale	Endteil
acrosoma	Akrosoma
bouton de la pointe	Endknopf
coiffe céphalique	
capuchon céphalique	Kopfkappe
perforatorium	
pointe céphalique	Kopfspitze
dard	Spies
partie principale	Hauptteil
portion hyaline (Hyalosoma)	innerer Teil
portion réfringente (Vitreosoma)	vitröser
stries céphaliques	Querbänder
Segment intermédiaire	Mittelstück
col (filament unitif)	Collum
bouton cervical (centro-soma?)	Halskopf
bâtonnet axile	axiles Stäbchen
Filament spiralé (gaîne spiralée)	Spiralfaden (Spiralschicht)
Coussinet cervical	Halspolster
Segment caudal	Schwanz
partie principale	Hauptteil
terminale	Endteil
filament axile	Axenfaden
enveloppe plasmatique (manteau caudal)	Plasmahülle (Schwanzmantel)
membrane ondulante	Wellenmembran
filament spiralé	Spiralfaden
filament terminal	Endfaden
Dimorphisme des spermatozoïdes	Dimorphismus der Samenkörperchen

Spermatogonies	Spermatogonien
Spermatocytes	Spermatocyten
Spermatides	Spermatiden
Spermatocystes (La Valette St. Georges)	Spermatocysten
Ovules mâles	männliche Eier

Maturation et fécondation de l'œuf. Reifung und Befruchtung

Maturation — Reifung

Migration polaire de la vésicule germinative	Polwanderung des Keimbläschens
Désorganisation de la vés. germ.	Entbildung d. Keimbl.
Chromosomes de maturation	Reifungschromosomen
1er fuseau de maturation	1. Reifungsspindel
Expulsion du 1er globule polaire	Ausstossung des 1. Polkörperchens
Rétraction du vitellus (espace périvitellin)	Zurückziehung des Dotters (perivitelliner Raum)
2e fuseau de maturation	2. Richtungsspindel
Expulsion du 2e globule polaire (division de réduction)	Ausstossung des 2. Polkörperchens (Reduktionsteilung)
Rétraction du vitellus	Zurückziehung des Dotters
Pronucleus femelle (Syn. Caryomérite femelle)	Weiblicher Vorkern (Eikern, weibl. Karyomerit)
Ovocentre (?)	Ovocentrum

Fécondation — Befruchtung

Cône d'attraction	Empfängnishügel
» d'imprégnation	Imprägnationshügel
Voie de la pénétration	Penetrationsbahn, Spermastrasse
Trainée pigmentaire	Pigmentstrasse
Désorganisation du spermatozoïde	Entbildung des Spermatozoon
Pronucleus mâle (Synon. Caryomérite mâle)	Männlicher Vorkern, Spermakern (männlicher Karyomerit)
Spermocentre	Spermocentrum
Aster mâle	Spermastrahlung
Accolement des caryomérites	Berührung der Karyomeriten
Conjugaison des caryomérites	Verschmelzung der Karyomeriten
Noyau de segmentation	Furchungskern

Ebauches embryologiques et histogénétiques générales. Allgemeine embryologisch-histogenetische Anlagen

Segmentation de l'œuf (Fractionnement)	Furchung
Plans de segmentation	Furchungsebenen
» méridional	meridionale
» horizontal (équatorial)	horizontale (äquatoriale)
Sillons méridionaux	Meridionalfurchen

,, équatoriaux	Aequatorialfurchen
Sphères de segmentation (Syn. Blasto-	
mères)	Furchungskugeln, Blastomeren
Blastomères animales (Micramères)	Animale ...
Blastomères végétatives (Macramères)	Vegetative, Megasphären
Morula	Maulbeerstadium
Blastula	
Vésicule blastodermique	Keimblase (v. *Baer*)
Blastoderme primitif	Urkeimblatt
Amas vitellin (?)	Zellhaufen
Syn. Bourrelet entodermique (?)	Entodermwulst (?)
Cavité de segmentation	Furchungshöhle
Liquide de segmentation	Urinpher
Gastrula	
Blastopore (Anus de *Rusconi*)	Urmund
Archentéron	Urdarmhöhle
Feuillets blastodermiques (*Pander*)	Keimblätter
Ectoderme (Épiblaste)	Ektoderm (Epiblast)
Entoderme (Endoblaste)	Entoderm (Entoblast)
Mésoderme primitif (Mésoblaste primitif)	Primäres Mesoderm (Mesoblast)
Feuillet pariétal	Parietales Blatt
,, viscéral	Viscerales ,,
Cavité cœlomique	Cölom
Mésoderme secondaire	Sekundäres Mesoderm
Mésenchyme	Mesenchym
Aire embryonnaire	Fruchthof (Embryonalschild)
Ligne primitive	Primitivstreifen
Sillon primitif	Primitivrinne
Sillon en croissant	Sichelrinne
Renflement du croissant	Sichelknopf
Nœud de *Hensen*	*Hensen*'scher Knoten
	Kopffortsatz
Aire transparente	Area pellucida (heller Hof)
Aire opaque (vasculaire)	Area opaca (Gefässhof)
Bourrelet germinal	Keimwall
Îlots de *Wolff* (sanguins)	Blutinseln
Sinus terminal	Randsinus
Replis médullaires	Medullarwülste
Gouttière médullaire	Medullarrinne
Tube médullaire (neural)	Medullarrohr
Crête ganglionnaire	Ganglienleiste
Canal neurentérique	Canalis neurentericus
Corde dorsale	Rückensaite (Chorda dorsalis)
Tige sous-cordale	Subchordaler Strang
Somites. Syn. Protovertèbres	Somiten, Urwirbelplatten
Myotomes (Myomères)	Myotomen, Muskelsegmente
Myocœle	Myocöl
Sclérotome	Sklerotom
Région intermédiaire du mésoderme	Mittelplatten

Lames latérales mésodermiques	Seitenplatten
feuillet pariétal	Parietales Blatt
sac. somatopleure	Somatopleura
cutané	Hautplatte
musculo-cutané	
feuillet viscéral	Viscerales Blatt
splanchnopleure	Splanchnopleura
fibro-intestinal	Harnfaserplatte
Cavité cœlomique	Cölom
Feuillet vasculaire	Gefässblatt
Zone somitique (rachidienne) de l'aire embryonnaire	Stammzone
Zone pariétale	Parietalzone
Capuchon céphalique (repli amniotique antérieur)	Kopffalte
Capuchon caudal (repli amniotique postérieur)	Schwanzfalte
Vésicules cérébrales primitives	primitive Hirnblasen
antérieure	vordere
moyenne	mittlere
postérieure	hintere
Vésicule cérébrale antérieure	vordere Hirnblase
prosencéphale propr. dit	Telencephalon
vésicules hémisphériques	Hemisphärenhirn
diencéphale (cerveau intermédiaire)	Diencephalon, Zwischenhirn
thalamencéphale	Thalamencephalon
diverticule épiphysaire	Epiphysäre Ausstülpung
infundibulaire	Infundibulum
vésicules optiques (oculaires)	Augenblasen
cupule rétinienne	Augenbecher
pédicule optique	Augenstiel
fente oculaire	Augenspalte
Vésicule cérébrale moyenne	Mittlere Hirnblase
mésencéphale	Mesencephalon
(lobes optiques)	(Lobi optici)
Vésicule cérébrale postérieure (rhombencéphale)	Hintere Hirnblase (Rhombencephalon)
Cerveau postérieur (vésicule cérébelleuse)	Metencephalon (Kleinhirnbläschen)
Arrière-cerveau	Nachhirn
Syn. Myélencéphale	Myelencephalon
Fossette cristallinienne	Linsengrübchen
Vésicule	Linsenbläschen
Fossette auditive	Gehörgrübchen
Vésicule auditive	Gehörbläschen
Fossette olfactive	Riechgrübchen
Diverticule de *Jacobson*	*Jacobson'sches Grübchen*
Gouttière intestinale primitive	Primitive Darmrinne
Intestin céphalique (Procentéron primitif)	Kopfdarm

Arcs viscéraux	Visceralbogen
Fentes viscérales	Visceralspalten
Intestin moyen	Mitteldarm
Vésicule vitelline (ombilicale)	Dotterblase
Conduit vitellin	Dottergang, Ductus omphalo-mesentericus
Intestin postérieur	Hinterdarm
Mésentère antérieur	Mesenterium commune
postérieur	*
Vésicule allantoïdienne	Allantois
Ouraque	Urachus
Dépression buccale (Stomodaeum)	Mundbucht
Poche de *Rathke* (hypophysaire)	*Rathke*'sche Tasche
Poche de *Seessel*	*Seessel*'sche Tasche
Membrane obturante	Membrana obturatoria
pharyngée	Rachenhaut
Intestin caudal	Schwanzdarm
Intestin post-anal	postanaler Darm
Membrane cloacale	Kloakenmembran
Membrane anale	Aftermembran
Proctodeum	
Anus secondaire	After (secundärer)
Conduits hépatiques primitifs	Lebergänge
Bourgeon hépatique	Leberwulst
Ebauches pancréatiques	Pankreas-Anlagen
supérieure (dorsale)	dorsale ,,
inférieure (ventrale) (hépato-pancréatique)	ventrale ,,
Septum transversum	
Pronéphros (Rein céphalique)	Vorniere
Néphrostomes	Nierentrichter
Mésonephros (Rein primitif)	Urniere
Corps de *Wolff*	*Wolff*'scher Körper
Canal ,,	,, Gang
Métanephros	
Rein définitif	bleibende Niere
Ligament inguinal du rein primitif	Leistenband der Urniere
Portion sexuelle du corps de *Wolff*	Geschlechtsteil der Urniere
,, rénale	Nierenteil
Epithélium germinatif	Keimepithel (*Waldeyer*)
Eminence génitale	Geschlechtswulst
Glande génitale	Geschlechtsdrüse
Canal de *Müller*	*Müller*'scher Gang
Sinus urogénital	Sinus uro-genitalis
Tubercule génital	Geschlechtshöcker
Replis génitaux	Geschlechtsfalten
,, internes	,, innere
,, externes	,, äussere (Geschlechts-wülste)

gouttière urogénitale	Geschlechtsrinne
syn. sillon génital	
Cavité naso-pharyngienne primitive	Primitive Rachenhöhle
Bourgeon frontal	Stirnfortsatz
Bourgeon nasal interne	innerer Nasenfortsatz
" nasal externe	äusserer "
" maxillaire supérieur	Oberkieferfortsatz
Sillon naso-oculaire (= lacrymal)	Augennasenrinne
" nasal	Nasenrinne
Arc maxillaire inférieur (mandibulaire)	Unterkieferbogen (Mandibularbogen)
Cartilage de *Meckel*	*Meckel'scher* Knorpel
Crête dentaire	Zahnleiste
Germes dentaires	Schmelzkeim
Organe de l'émail (syn. adamantin)	
Arc hyoïdien	Zungenbeinanlagen
Cartilage de *Reichert*	*Reichert'scher* Knorpel
III- IVe(?) arcs viscéraux	Dritter-fünfter (sechster) Visceralbogen
Ire fente viscérale (pharyngo-nodale)	Erste Visceralspalte
IIe-IVe fentes viscérales	Zweite-vierte "
Diverticule thyroïdien médian	Mediane Schilddrüsenanlage
Conduit thyréoglosse	Ductus thyreoglossus
Ebauches thyroïdiennes latérales	laterale Schilddrüsenanlagen
Ebauches thymiques (latérales)	Thymusanlagen
Sillon pulmonaire	Lungenrinne
Conduits broncho-pulmonaires primitifs	Primitive Lungenschläuche
Ebauches cardiaques latérales	Laterale Herzanlagen
Ebauche cardiaque médiane (impaire)	Unpaare (mediane) Herzanlage
Tube cardiaque	Herzschlauch
" endothélial	Endothelrohr
" musculaire	Muskelrohr
Mésocardium dorsal	Dorsales Mesokardium
" ventral	Ventrales "
Tube cardiaque en S	S-förmiger Herzschlauch
Segment veineux	Venöse Abteilung
canal auriculaire	Ohrkanal
Segment artériel	Arterielle Abteilung
Freins *Halleri*	
Bulbe aortique	Aortenbulbus
Aortes primitives	Primitive Aorten
Arcs aortiques	Aortenbogen
Artères vitellines (omphalo-mésentériques)	Dotterarterien
Artères ombilicales	Nabelarterien
Veines vitellines (omphalo-mésentériques)	Dottervenen
Veines ombilicales	Nabelvenen
Veines cardinales	Kardinalvenen
Veines jugulaires	Jugularvenen
Canaux de *Cuvier*	*Cuvier'sche* Gänge

Sinus terminus	
Crête de Wolff	Wolff'sche Leiste
Palettes terminales	Extremitätenplatten
(s. ou digitales)	

Membranes fœtales. Annexes fœtales	Embryonalhüllen
Prochorion	
Chorion amniogène	Amniogenes Chorion
Amnios	Amnion (Schafhaut)
Séreuse de v. Baer	Serosa
Chorion allantoïdien	
Chorion villeux	Ch. frondosum
Chorion lisse	Ch. laeve
Magma reticulare	
Caduque réfléchie (capsulaire)	Decidua reflexa s. capsularis
Cordon ombilical	Nabelschnur
Placenta	Mutterkuchen
„ fœtal	Placenta fœtalis
„ maternel	„ uterina
Caduque sérotine (basale)	Decidua basalis (serotina)

Tissus. Systèmes. Gewebe. Systeme

EPITHÉLIUM. EPITHEL.

Plat (lamelleux, pavimenteux)	Plattes
Cubique	Kubisches
Polyédrique	Polyedrisches
Cylindrique (prismatique)	Zylindrisches (prismatisches)
„ pyramidal	Pyramidenförmiges
„ conique	Konisches
„ en bâtonnet	Stäbchenförmiges
„ en pilier	Säulenförmiges
„ en massue	Keulenförmiges
„ fusiforme	Spindelförmiges
„ en pointe	Stiftförmiges
„ à pied	Fusszellen
„ à onglet	Benagelte Zellen
Cylindrique à plateau	Besäumtes Zylinderepithel
„ à plateau strié	Gestreifter Saum
„ à ... non strié	Ungestreifter
„ à cils vibratiles	Flimmerepithel
„ à cils simples (flagellifor-	Einfache Cilien
mes)	
„ à cils agrégés	zusammengeklebte
„ à cils denticulés (bacillifor-	Stäbchencilien
mes)	
Plateau sous-cilié (basal)	Basalsaum

Granulations cilio-basales (Ciliosomes)	Ciliosomen
Zone cilio-radiculaire	Wurzelzone
Epithélium caliciforme	Becherzellen
à calice marginal	mit randständigem Becher
à calice profond	mit tiefem Becher
à base sans prolongements	mit fortsätziger Basis
à base muni lui frange	mit bestielter Basis
à prolongement nucléo-	mit kernhaltigem Fortsatze
Pore	Porus
Thèque	Theca
Epithélium crénelé	Riffzellen
Epithélium de transition	Uebergangsepithel
Epithélium pavimenteux à alvéoles	Mit Alveolen versehenes Pflasterepithel
trapezoïdal	trapezoïdales
Epithélium festonné	Ausgeschnittenes
digité	Mit fingerförmigen Fortsätzen versehenes
dendroïde	Verzweigtes

ÉPITHÉLIUM DE REVÊTEMENT

d'origine ecto- ou entodermique

DECKEPITHEL

(ecto- oder entodermalen Ursprungs)

Epithélium pavimenteux	Pflasterepithel
simple	einfaches
stratifié	geschichtetes
Couches:	Schichten:
cellules cylindriques (germinatives, basales)	Zylinderzellen (basale, Keimschicht)
cellules polyédriques (épineuses)	Polyedrische (Riffzellen)
aplaties (lamelleuses)	Platte Zellen
non cuticulées	Ohne Kutikularsaum
à plateau cuticulaire	Mit
Epith. pavimenteux à transformation cornée	Verhorntes Epithel
Epithél. cylindrique	Zylindrisches Deckepithel
simple	einfaches
pavimenté	pflasterförmiges
cilié	Flimmerepithel
à plateau	mit Kutikularsaum
à plusieurs rangées de noyaux	mehrreihiges
Epithél. cylindr.	Geschichtetes Zylinderepithel
cilié	Flimmerepithel
Couches:	Schichten:
basale	Basalschicht
intermédiaire	Zwischen
polymorphe	
cylindrique superficielle	Oberflächliche Zylinderzellschicht

Epithélium mixte stratifié	Uebergangsepithel (gemischtes)
Couches	Schichten
basale	Basalschicht
intermédiaire (polymorphe)	Zwischenschicht
superficielle (de transition)	Oberflächliches Uebergangsepithel

ÉPITHÉLIUM DE REVÊTEMENT — **DECKEPITHEL**

mésodermique (coelomique) — *mesodermalen Ursprungs (Cölomepithel)*

Epithélium de l'éminence uro-génitale	Epithel des urogenitalen Wulstes
Epithélium cilié péritonéal	Peritoneales Flimmerepithel

Épithélium sensoriel — *Sinnesepithel*

(Neuro-epithélium)	(Neuroepithel)
des épithéliums de revêtement	in Deckepithelien
des organes de sens propres	in besonderen Sinnesorganen

Épithélium de soutènement — *Stützepithel*

des organes des sens	der Sinnesorgane
(cellules de soutènement)	Stützzellen
des centres nerveux	des centralen Nervensystems
Névroglie (d'origine épendymaire)	Neuroglia (ependymalen Ursprungs)

Épithélium du cristallin — *Linsenepithel*

Épithélium de l'organe adamantin — *Schmelzorgan*

Épithélium des formations cornées — *Horngebilde*

Épithélium glandulaire — *Drüsenepithel*

Cellules sébacées (sébocrines)	Sebokrine Zellen (fettabsondernde)
à noyau central	mit mittelständigem Kern
à noyau excentrique ou pariétal	mit excentrisch gelegenem oder wandständigem Kern
Cellules mucipares (mucocrines)	Mukokrine (Schleimzellen)
Cellules zymocrines (séreuses)	Zymokrine Zellen (seröse)
Cellules pancréatiques	Pankreaszellen
Cellules à bâtonnets	Stäbchenepithel

Autres parties constituantes des épithéliums — *Andere Bestandteile der Epithelien*

Cellules migratrices	Wanderzellen
Cellules pigmentaires ramifiées	verästelte Pigmentzellen
Terminaisons nerveuses	Nervenendigungen
Réseaux terminaux intra-épithéliaux	Endnetze (intra-epitheliale)
(Plexus terminaux)	(Endgeflechte)

terminaisons libres	freie Endigungen
boutons terminaux	Endknöpfe
plaques terminales	Endplatten
calices sous-épithéliaux	subepitheliale Kelche
ménisques et cellules tactiles	Tastscheiben und Tastzellen
arborisations terminales	Endbäumchen (Tetatendrien?)
péricellulaires	perizelluläre
adcellulaires	adzelluläre
Plexus sous-épithélial	subepithelialer Plexus
sous-basal	subbasaler
fondamental (dans le chorion)	Grundplexus (im chorion)

Dérivés épithéliaux hétéroplastiques — *Heteroplastische Epithel-Derivate*

Epithélium des lames médullaires	Epithel der Medullarplatten
Cellules des glandes carotidien et coc-	Zellen d. Carotiden und Steissknötchens
cygien	
Myozimes (?)	Myozimen (?)
Corde dorsale	Chorda dorsalis

Cellules épithélioïdes — *Epitheloide Zellen*

(Origine ?)	(Herkunft ?)
Cellules dites interstitielles	S. gen. interstitielle Zellen
de l'ovaire	des Eierstockes
du testicule	des Hodens
Cellules du corps jaune (lutéiniennes)	Luteinzellen
déciduales	Deciduazellen

Endothélium — *Endothel*

des membranes séreuses	der serösen Häute
vasculaire sanguin	Blutgefässenbothel
vasculaire lymphatique	Lymphgefässendothel
du système lymphatique lacunaire	der lymphatischen Spalträume

GLANDES EN GÉNÉRAL — DRÜSEN IM ALLGEMEINEN

Cryptes — *Krypten*

pseudo-épithéliales	pseudo-epitheliale
(lymphadénoïdes)	lymphadenoide Krypten
glandulaires	drüsige Krypten

Glandes — *Drüsen*

exocrines	exokrine
à ...	...
closes	geschlossene

Types glandulaires simples :	einfache Drüsenformen :
tubuleux	tubulöse, röhrenförmige
acineux × vésiculeux × alvéolaire	azinöse, bläschenförmige, alveolare
utriculaire	sackförmige
Types composés :	zusammengesetzte Formen
tubulo-acineux	tubulo-azinöse × alveolare
tubulo-utriculaire	tubulo-utrikuläre
infundibulo-acineux	infundibulo-azinöse
utriculo-acineux	utriculo-azinöse

CATÉGORIES DE GLANDES SELON LEUR COMPLEXITÉ	DRÜSENKATEGORIEN JE NACH DER KOMPLEXITÄT
Glandes simples	*Einfache Drüsen*
Glandes agminées	*Agglomerierte (agglomeratae)*
.. digitées ou ramifiées	.. fingerförmig geteilte, verzweigte
.. en grappe simple	.. traubenförmige
.. à confluent central	.. mit gemeinschaftlichen Central-raum
Glandes subcomposées	*Halbzusammengesetzte (subcompositae)*
Glandes composées	*Zusammengesetzte (compositae)*
Modes d'embouchures des glandes :	*Mündungsweise der Drüsen :*

pore excréteur	Porus
rigole interépithéliale	interepitheliale Rinne
fossette (ou entonnoir)	Grübchen (Trichter)
goulot terminal	Endkals
conduit excréteur	Ausführgang
.. indivis	.. ungeteilter
.. ramifié	.. verzweigter
conduit terminal	Endgang
branches extraglandulaires (lobaires)	lobäre Äste
.. interlobaires	interlobäre
.. interlobulaires	interlobuläre
.. intralobulaires	intralobuläre
portions intercalaires	Schaltstücke

VARIÉTÉS DE GLANDES	DRÜSENARTEN
Glandes acineuses (vésiculeuses)	*Acinöse Drüsen (bläschenförmige)*
simples	einfache :
fond de l'acinus	Fundus (Grund)
sommet	apikale Region
rigole excrétrice	Exkretorische Rinne
pore excréteur	Porus
agminées ou groupe simple	gehäufte, einfach traubenförmig
acini (vésicules)	Acini, Bläschen

latéraux	seitenständige
terminaux	terminale
canal excréteur	Ausführgang
portion interalvéolaire (conduit alvéolaire)	Alveolargang
portion terminale (conduit ex- cret. propr. dit)	Endgang

Infundibula urinosa — *Infundibulo-artige*

Acineuses déhiscentes — *Acinöse dehiscente*

Glandes tubuleuses — *Tubulöse Drüsen*

Simples (et droites)	Einfache
fond	Fundus
corps	Drüsenkörper
canal	Lumen
pôre excréteur	Porus
Glomérulées	Knäueldrüsen
glomérule	Knäuel
conduit excréteur	Ausführgang
portion principale	Hauptteil
portion interépithéliale	Zwischenepithelialer Teil
Agminées tubuleuses digitées	gehäufte, geteilte
tubes sécréteurs	Secernirende Tubuli
collet	Halsteil
fossette ou entonnoir	Gröbchen, Trichter
Agminées à conduit central	Gehäufte mit gemeinsch. Zentralraum
conduit excréteur	Ausführgang
confluent	Zentralraum
tubes sécréteurs	secernirende Tubuli
Agminées composées à conduits con- tro-lobulaires ramifiés	gehäufte, zusammengesetze, mit ver- zweigten Zentralräumen
Composées à système intermédiaire de canaux excréteurs-réticuleux	zusammengesetzte mit intermediärem netzförmigem Gangsystem
Agminées composées à glomérules vas- culaires et à émonctoire commun	gehäufte, zusammengesetzte, mit Ge- fäss-Knäueln und gemeinschaftl- chem Emunctorium
Composées trabéculaires	zusammengesetzte netzförmige.

Glandes alvéolaires — *Cirienlaire Drüsen (Sackchendrüsen)*

Simples	Einfache
fond	Fundus (Grund)
corps	Drüsenkorper
sommet	Apicale Region
col	Hals
pore	Porus
Agminées, simples ou divisées	Gehäufte, einfache oder geteilte

Acineuses, divisées, divisées	gehäufte, geteilte
corps de sac glandulaires	Drüsensäckchen
cols	Hals
conduit excréteur	Ausführgang
Biato-acineuses composées	gehäufte-zusammenges. Säckchendr.
Lobules	Läppchen.
Utricules glandulaires	Drüsensäckchen
Conduits primaires	Ausführgänge
Conduits collecteurs	Sammelgänge
Acinées - Composées à confluents centro-lobulaires.	gehäufte - zusammengesetzte mit gemeinschaftlichen Zentralräumen.
Lobules	Läppchen
Utricules	Drüsensäckchen
Confluents centro-lobulaires	lobuläre Zentralräume
confluent excréteur	gemeinschaftlicher Zentralgang
conduit excréteur	Ausführgang
Glandes utriculo-acineuses (acinées)	utriculo-acinöse Drüsen (gehäufte)

Glandes tubulo-acineuses et tubulo-utriculaires — *Tubulo-acinöse und tubulo-utriculäre Drüsen*

Simples	Einfache
pore excréteur (Mündung)	Porus
conduit alvéolair	Alveolargang
dilatations ampullaires	ampulläre Ausstülpungen
axiales	axiale
collatérales	kollaterale
Acinées - subcomposées, composées	gehäufte - halbzusammengesetzte, zusammengesetzte
eurytubulaires	eurytubuläre
sténoalvéolaires ou utriculaires	steno-alveoläre oder utrikuläre
Variété intermédiaire: sténoalvéolaire à canaux intralobulaires dilatés	Varietät: steno-alveoläre mit erweiterten Alveolargängen

Glandes hétérophores (mixtes) — *Heterogene (gemischte) Drüsen*

par rapport au type structural	in betreff des Drüsentypus
Glandes tubulo-acineuses, partie eurytubulaires, partie sténo-alvéolaires (ou sacculaires)	tubulo-acinöse teils eurytubuläre teils steno-alveoläre Drüsen
Glandes partie utriculaires, partie sténo-alvéolaires	teils säckchenförmige, teils steno-alveoläre Drüsen
par rapport à la nature de l'épithélium et de la sécrétion	in betreff der Beschaffenheit des Epithels
Glandes séro-muqueuses	teils seröse, teils Schleimdrüsen
séro-schéuses	teils seröse, teils Eiweißdrüsen
séro-colloïdes	teils seröse, teils Colloiddrüsen

Glandes closes (à sécrétion interne) — *Geschlossene Drüsen*

acineuses	acinöse (alveoläre)
atypiques	atypische

Structure fine des glandes	*Feinerer Drüsenbau*
Enveloppes et tissu conjonctif inter-stitiel	Hüllen und interstitielles Bindegewebe
Enveloppe conjonctive lâche	lockere Bindegewebshülle
Membrane fibreuse (capsule)	fibröse Häute (Kapseln)
(Albuginée)	(Albuginea)
Travées interstitielles	bindegewebige Septa
„ interlobaires	interlobäre „
„ interlobulaires	interlobuläre „
„ interlobulaires	interacinöse „
s. interacineuses	s. interacinöse „
s. interacineuses	s. interacinöse „
cellules adipeuses	Fettzellen
cellules plasmatiques	Plasmazellen
	Mastzellen
lymphocytes	Lymphocyten
tissu lymphatique noueux	lymphadenoides Gewebe
cellules épithéliales interstitielles	epitheloide, s. g. interstitielle Zellen
cellules pigmentaires	Pigmentzellen
cellules musculaires lisses	glatte Muskelzellen
fibres musculaires lisses	glatte Muskelfasern
fibres ou travées	Gitterfasern
cellules étoilées (?)	Sternzellen

Parties glandulaires	*Drüsenteile*
Membrane propre	Membrana propria
Cellules en panier	Korbzellen
Cellules intra-épithéliales	intra-epitheliale Zellen
Epithélium sécrétoire	secernierendes Epithel
„ homoemorphe	homoemorphes „
„ hétéromorphe	heteromorphes „
Capillaires (canalicules) sécrétoires	Sekretkapillaren
„ intercellulaires	„ zwischenzellige
„ intracellulaires	„ binnenzellige

Conduits excréteurs	*Ausführgänge*
membrane propre	Membrana propria
épithélium	Epithel
cylindrique simple	einfaches Zylinderepithel
„ à deux ou plusieurs rangées de noyaux	zwei-, mehrreihiges „
cellules caliciformes	Becherzellen
épithélium vibratile bâtonnets	Stäbchenepithel
cilié	Flimmerepithel
cubique	kubisches
plat	plattes

pavimenteux stratifié	geschichtetes Plattenepithel
tunique adventice	Tunica adventitia
follicules lymphadénoïdes	Lymphfollikel
couche musculaire lisse	glatte Muskelschicht

Conduits excréteurs terminaux de certaines glandes	*Terminale Ausführgänge von einigen Drüsen*

tunique fibro-élastique	faserig-elastische Schicht
tunique musculaire	Muskelschicht
couche sous-muqueuse	Submucosa
tunique muqueuse	Mucosa
cryptes épithéliaux	Epithel Krypten
glandules accessoires	accessorische Drüschen

Vaisseaux sanguins	*Drüsengefässe*

Vaisseaux du hile	Hilusgefässe
Vaisseaux superficiels	oberflächliche Gefässe
» capsulaires	kapsuläre »
» sous-capsulaires	subkapsuläre »
» profonds	tiefe Gefässe
» interlobaires	interlobäre »
» interlobulaires	interlobuläre »
» intralobulaires	intralobuläre »
Réseaux capillaires	Kapillarnetze
péri-tubuleux, acineux ou sacculaires	peri-tubulöse, acinöse, s. utriculäre
glomérules vasculaires	Gefässknäuel
Réseaux capillaires péricellulaires	pericelluläre Kapillarnetze
Vaisseaux de la substance corticale	Gefässe der Rindenschicht
» de la subst. médullaire	» der Markschicht
	Gefässe der Ausführgänge

Vaisseaux lymphatiques	*Lymphatische Gefässe*

Lymphatiques superficiels	oberflächliche »
» profonds	tiefe »
Fentes lymphatiques	Lymphspalten

Nerfs	*Drüsennerven*

Nerfs des travées conjonctives	Septa-Nerven
» interlobaires	interlobäre »
» interlobulaires	interlobuläre »
Ganglions nerveux	Nervenganglien
Plexus interalvéolaire	inter-alveolärer Plexus
Plexus périacineux	periacinöser Plexus
Cellules nerveuses interstitielles	interstitielle Nervenzellen
Fibres perforantes	durchbohrende Fasern

Fibres hypolemmales	hypolemmale Fasern
Terminaisons nerveuses:	Nervenendigungen:
» plexus intercellulaire	perizelluläres Geflecht
» arborisations terminales	Endbäumchen
(terminaisons adcellulaires)	(adzelluläre Nervenendigungen)
Plexus nerveux des canaux excréteurs	Nervenplexus der Ausführgänge

TISSU NERVEUX. NERVENGEWEBE

Éléments constitutifs:	*Bestandteile:*
Cellules nerveuses (Neurocytes)	Nervenzellen (Neurocyten)
Fibres nerveuses	Nervenfasern
Tissu interstitiel (organe de soutiennement)	interstitielles Gewebe (Stützgewebe)
Tissu enveloppant	umhüllendes Gewebe

CELLULES NERVEUSES DE L'AXE CÉRÉBRO-SPINAL · NERVENZELLEN DES ZENTRALNERVENSYSTEM

Neurocytes (sans membrane d'enveloppe)	hüllenlose Neurocyten
pyramidaux	pyramidenförmige
piriformes	birnenförmige
en cloche, en mitre	glocken-, mützenförmige
multipolaires	multipolare
fusiformes	spindelförmige
globuleux (cellules-grains)	kugelige (Körnerzellen)

Corps cellulaire	*Zellleib*
Neurofibrilles	Neurofibrillen
Touffes chromophiles	chromophile Körnerhäufchen
	Körnerschollen
Substance tigroïde (?)	Tigroidsubstanz (?)
Amas pigmentaires	Pigmenthäufchen

Prolongements dendritiques	*Dendritenfortsätze*
protoplasmiques	protoplasmatische
base	Basalteil, Wurzel
ramifications	Verzweigungen
buissons ou arbres dendritiques	Feldendrisen
	knäuelförmiges
en bouquet	büschelförmiges
prolongements dendritiques lisses	glatte Dendritenfortsätze
dorsaux	dorsale
basaux	basale
apicaux	apikale
latéraux	Seitenfortsätze

prolongements péritropes

oppositotropes

homotropes

en bois de cerf   Geweihartige.

Prolongement nerveux; Sys. cylindra-   *Nervenfortsatz. Axencylinderfortsatz.*
*   xile, de Deiters, neurite, axone*   *Deiters'scher Neuraxon, Neurit.*

cône d'implantation   Ursprungskegel.
rétrécissement intermédiaire (collet)   intermediäre Einschnürung
filament neuraxile   neuraxiler Faden
branches collatérales   Kollateralen
prolongements nerveux axiles (type de   axile Neuriten (Deiters'scher Typus)
    Deiters)
prolong. nerveux arborescents (type de   Dendroneuriten (Golgi'scher Typus)
    Golgi)
prolongements cellulaires atypiques   atypische Zellfortsätze
Noyau   Kern
Nucléole principal   Haupt-Nucleolus
Nucléoles accessoires   accessorische Nucleolus

Cellules ganglionnaires cérébro-spinales   *Cerebro-spinale Ganglienzellen*

Membrane d'enveloppe   *Hülle*

revêtement cellulaire de la membrane   Zelllager der Hülle
noyaux   Kerne
couche protoplasmique   protoplasmatische Schicht.

Corps cellulaire   *Zellleib*

Zone exoplasmique   exoplasmatische Zone
Zone fibrillaire   fibrilläre Zone
Apparato reticolare
Zone endoplasmique   endoplasmatische Zone
Touffes chromophiles   chromophile Büschel
Granulations nucléaires   nucleare Granula
Centrosoma
amas pigmentaires   Pigmenthäufchen
canalicules trophiques (?)   Trophospongien
Cellules ganglionnaires chromophiles   chromophile Ganglienzellen

Noyau   *Kern*
Nucléole principal   *Haupt-Nucleolus*
Nucléoles accessoires   *accessorische Nucleolen*

Prolongements nerveux   *Fortsätze*
cylindraxile   Nervenfortsatz
en T ou Y   T oder Y förmiger
cellules pseudo-unipolaires   pseudounipolare Zellen
Zone d'origine du prolongement nerv.   Ursprungszone des Neuriten

région amyélinique ..	myelinfreie Region
branches collatérales (?)	Kollateralen
Cellules à prolongement nerveux tri-partite	Zellen mit dreiteiligem Fortsatze
Cellules d'association	Associationszellen
Prolongements dendritiques (proplasmiques)	Dendriten
.. intra-capsulaires	intralemmale
.. extra-capsulaires	extralemmale
Terminaisons péricellulaires	pericelluläre Teledendrien

Cellules ganglionnaires bipolaires (des vertébrés supérieurs) — *Bipolare Ganglien-Zellen (höhere Vertebraten)*

Cellules ganglionnaires bipolaires (des poissons osseux) — *Bipolare Ganglienzellen (Knochen-Fische)*

membrane d'enveloppe	Hülle
gaine de myéline	Myelinscheide
cuticule interne	innere Kutikula
région polaire de la cellule	Polargend der Zelle
région nucléogène ..	kernhaltige Region
prolongements nerveux polaires	polare Nervenfortsätze

Cellules nerveuses sympathiques (mammifères) — *Sympathische Nervenzellen (Säugthiere)*

Cellules des ganglions sympathiques centraux	Zellen des Grenzstranges
» membrane nucléée	kernhaltige Hülle
» prolongements nerveux	Neuriten
» branches collatérales (?)	Kollateralen
» prolongements dendritiques	Dendriten
Amas pigmentaires	Pigmenthäufchen
Type moteur (?)	motorischer Typus
» sensitif (?)	sensitiver
Cellules des ganglions sympathiques périphériques (viscéraux)	Zellen der peripherischen sympathischen Ganglien
Cellules sympathiques interstitielles	Interstitielle sympathische Nervenzellen

Cellules sympathiques des Batraciens — *Sympathische Nervenzellen der Batrachier*

prolongement droit (efférent)	gerade Faser
» spiral (afférent?)	Spiralfaser
» à tours de spire serrés	» mit dichten Windungen
» à tours de spire lâches	» mit losen Windungen
noyaux des prolongements droit et spiral	Kerne der geraden und Spiralfaser
hile cellulaire	Hilus der Zelle
Membrane d'enveloppe nucléée	kernhaltige Hülle

Agglomérats cellulaires sympathiques (batraciens)	*Sympathische Zellkonglomerate (Batrachier)*
Cellules nerveuses (?: terminales; sous-épithéliales	Endzellen; subepitheliale Nervenzellen
Cellules nerveuses des organes des sens.	*Nervenzellen der Sinnesorgane.*

FIBRES NERVEUSES — **NERVENFASERN**

À myéline (à double contour)	markhaltige (doppeltkonturierte)
— périphériques	periphérische
Gaine de Schwann (névrilemme)	Neurilemm
Noyaux de la gaine (sous-vaginaux)	Kerne des Neurilemms (subdermale Kerne)
Couche protoplasmique périnucléaire	perinucleäre Plasmaschicht
Gaine de myéline	Markscheide (Myelinscheide)
Réticule de neurokératine	Neurokeratinnetz
Étranglements annulaires (de Ranvier)	Schnürringe (Ranvier)
Incisures de la gaine de myéline (Schmidt-Lantermann)	Marx — Einkerbungen
Entonnoirs et fibres de soutènement (Golgi)	Trichter und Stützfasern (Golgi)
Segments interannulaires	interannuläre Segm.
« uninucléés	einkernige »
« plurinucléés	mehrkernige »
Segments cylindro-coniques	zylindro-konische Segmente
Cylindraxe	Axencylinder
Fibrilles primitives du cylindraxe	Neurofibrillen (Axenfibrillen)
Gaine de *Mauthner*	*Mauthner'sche* Scheide
Renflements biconiques	bikonische Anschwellung
Disques intersegmentaires (?)	intersegmentäre Scheiben (?)
Stries de *Frommann*	*Frommann'sche* Streifen
Croix intersegmentaires (*Ranvier*)	intersegmentäre Kreuze
Fibres nerveuses centrales (sans névrilemme)	zentrale Nervenfasern (ohne Neurilemm)
Renflements cylindraxiles	Axencylinderanschwellungen
Étranglements annulaires (?)	Schnürringe (?)

Fibres nerveuses sans myéline (grises, de Remak)	*Marklose Nervenfasern (graue, Remak'sche)*
Cylindraxe	Axencylinder
Fibrilles primitives	Axenfibrillen
Noyaux des fibres grises	Kerne der grauen Nervenfasern
Névrilemme (?)	Neurilemm (?)
Gaine périneurale	perineurale Scheide
Fibrilles nerveuses terminales	nervöse Endfibrillen
Cylindre-axes nus	nackte Axencylinder

Tissu interstitiel et enveloppant des nerfs	*Interstitielles und umhüllendes Gewebe*
Nerfs périphériques	periphérische Nerven
Gaine de *Henle*	*Henle*'sche Scheide
Endonèvre	Endoneurium
Périnèvre	Perineurium
.. lamelles	.. Lamellen
.. endothelium	.. Endothelium
Épinèvre	Epineurium
Système nerveux central	centrales Nervensystem
Névroglie	Neuroglia
.. cellules névrogliques	Gliazellen
.. fibres névrogliques	Gliafasern
Cellules névrogliques primitives (embryonnaires, épendymaires)	primäre (embryonale, ependymale) Gliazellen
Cellules névrogliques définitives (secondaires)	sekundäre
Corps cellulaire	Zellleib
Noyau	Kern
Prolongements	Fortsätze
.. à long trajet	langgestreckte
.. à court trajet	kurzgestreckte
Cellules névrogliques des vertébrés infér.	Gliazellen der niederen Vertebraten
Cellules des vertébrés sup.	.. der höheren Verbraten
Cellules en araignée	Spinnenzellen
Cellules névrogliques rayonnantes (Astrocytes)	Astrocyten
Astrocytes type ramassé	kurzstrahler
.. type étalé	langstrahler
Plexus névroglique	Gliageflecht
tissu	..
Travées conjonctives prolongements de la pie-mère	bindegewebige Scheiden (Pialfortsätze)
Méninges	Hüllen des Centralnervensystems

TERMINAISONS NERVEUSES
EN GÉNÉRAL

NERVENENDIGUNGEN IM ALLGEMEINEN

Terminaisons nerveuses en général	*Nervenendigungen im Allgemeinen*
Périphériques:	Peripherische:
dans les tissus épithéliaux	in epithelialen Geweben
.. inter-épithéliales	interepitheliale
.. intra-épithéliales	intraepitheliale
.. sous-épithéliales	subepitheliale
kérato-axonales	keratoaxonale
dans le tissu musculaire	im Muskelgewebe
stries et faser	(gestreiftes und glattes)

dans les lamelles électriques	in den elektrischen Platten
dans les tissus du groupe conjonctif	in den Geweben der Bindesubstanz
Centrales:	Zentrale:
dans le système nerveux central et gan- glionnaire	im Centralnervensystem und den Gan- glien

Modes de terminaisons nerveuses périphériques

Formen der peripherischen Nervenendigungen

Plexus nerveux préterminaux:	Praeterminale Nervenplexus:
„ dans le chorion	„ im Chorion
„ dans le tissu interstitiel ou adventitiel	„ im interstitiellen oder ad- ventitiellen Bindegewebe
Réseaux (ou plexus) terminaux	Endnetze (resp. Plexus)
Terminaisons libres	freie Endigungen
Varicosités	Varicositäten
Boutons terminaux	Endknöpfe
Arborisations terminales	Endbäumchen (Endgeflechte Telolen- drien)
„ ramassée (serrée)	dichtes
„ lâche, étalée	loses
„ en buisson	buschartiges
„ en bois de cerf	geweihartiges
„ en grappe	traubenförmiges
„ en bouquet (panicule)	doldenförmiges
péricellulaire	pericelluläre
adcellulaire	adcelluläres
Taches et boutons terminaux	Endflecken – Knöpfe
plaques terminales	– Platten
calices terminaux	Endkelche
Disques et ménisques tactiles (termi- naux)	Endscheiben, Tastscheiben (*Merkel*)
Corpuscules terminaux encapsulés:	eingekapselte Nervenendkörperchen:
„ à gaine simple	mit einfacher Hülle
„ renfermant des cel- lules propres	„ specifische Zellen enthaltend
„ sans cellules pro- pres	„ ohne specifische Zellen
„ à gaine multilamellaire et bulbe central (massue centrale)	mit konzentrischlamellöser Hülle und zentralem Innenkolben
„ à bulbe central dépourvu de noyaux	mit kernlosem Innenkolben
„ à bulbe central nuclée	mit kernhaltigen Innenkolben
Corpuscules de *Grandry*	*Grandry*'sche Körperchen
„ simples	„ einfache
„ composés	„ zusammengesetzte
Gaine (capsule) périneurale	Hülle (perineurale)
Noyaux de la gaine	Kerne der Hülle

Cellules dites tactiles	Tastzellen
Disque tactil	Tastscheibe
Appareil nerveux terminal	Endnervenapparat
Fibre nerveuse afférente	zutretende Nervenfaser
Bulbes terminaux (de *Krause*)	Endkolben
» oblonga	längliche
» globuleux	abgerundete
Gaine nucléée	kernhaltige Hülle
Bulbe central	Innenkolben
Cylindre-axe	Axencylinder
(fibre terminale)	(Terminalfaser)
Cellules du bulbe (?)	Kolbenzellen (?)
Corpuscules de *Wagner-Meissner*	*Wagner-Meissner'*sche Körperchen
» simples	einfache
» lobés	zusammengesetzte
Gaine nucléée	kernhaltige Hülle
Substance endo-capsulaire	endokapsuläre Substanz
Noyaux du bulbe	Kolbenkerne
Cellules du bulbe (?)	Kolbenzellen (?)
Fibres nerveuses afférentes	zutretende Nervenfäserin
Fibres cylindraxiles spirales	Spiralwindungen des Axencylinders
Ramifications	Verzweigungen
Corpuscules de *Herbst*	*Herbst'*sche Körperchen
Gaine à lamelles concentriques	Konzentrisch lamelläre Hülle
Lamelles	Lamellen
Revêtement endothélial	Endothel
Bulbe central	Innenkolben
Noyaux du bulbe central	Kerne des Innenkolbens
Cylindre-axe (fibre axile)	Axencylinder (axile Faser)
portion intracapsulaire de la fibre afférente	intrakapsulärer Teil der zutretenden Faser
portion extracapsulaire	extrakapsulärer Teil
Corpuscules de *Vater-Pacini*	*Vater-Pacini'*sche Körperchen
Gaine à lamelles concentriques	konzentrisch lamelläre Hülle
Lamelles	Lamellen
Revêtement endothélial	Endothel
Bulbe central	Innenkolben
Cylindre-axe (fibre axile)	Axencylinder (axile Faser)
Panneaux terminaux	Endzweige
Boutons terminaux	Endknöpfe
Portion intracapsulaire de la fibre afférente	intrakapsulärer Teil der zutretenden Faser
Portion extracapsulaire	extrakapsulärer Teil
Vaisseaux de la gaine	Hüllengefässe

Terminaisons nerveuses centrales	*Zentrale Nervenendigungen*
Arborisation libre	freies Teledendrion
péricellulaire	pericelluläre

(panier péricellulaire)	(Endkorb)
glomérule	Endknäuel
réseau nerveux (Gerlach)	Nervennetz

HISTOGENÈSE DES ÉLÉMENTS NERVEUX — HISTOGENESE DER NERVÖSEN BESTANDTEILE

Centres nerveux — *Zentralnervensystem*

Épithélium des lames médullaires	Epithel der Medullarplatten
Neuroblastes (centraux)	Neuroblasten
Prolongement axogène	axogener Fortsatz
Massue d'accroissement	Wachstumskeule
Prolongements dendriogènes	dendriogene Fortsätze
Fibres cylindraxiles nues	nackte Axencylinder
Cellules myéloformatrices	myelinbildende Zellen (?)
» mésenchymateuses (?)	mesenchymatöse (?) Zellen
Chaînes de neuroblastes périphériques	periphärische Neuroblastenketten
Spongioblastes (gliablastes)	Spongioblasten (Gliablasten)

Ganglions cérébro-spinaux — *Cerebrospinale Ganglien*

Crête ganglionnaire	Ganglienleiste
Neuroblastes ganglionnaires	Ganglien-Neuroblasten
Prolongements axogènes	axogene Fortsätze
» centripète	centripetaler »
» centrifuges	centrifugaler »
Fusion des prolongements nerveux	Verschmelzung der Nervenfortsätze
Bourgeons sympathiques secondaires	Sekundäre sympathische Auswüchse

TISSU MUSCULAIRE. MUSKELGEWEBE

LISSE — GLATTES

Cellule musculaire lisse (Myocyte)	glatte Muskelzelle (Myocyt)
Zone moyenne (à noyau)	Mittelzone (Kernzone)
Extrémités	Zahnausläufer
Contour denticulé	Zackenkontour
Fibrilles musculaires	Myofibrillen
Sarcoplasma	
Noyau en bâtonnet	stäbchenförmiger Kern
Nucléole	Kernkörperchen
Charpente nucléaire	Kerngerüst
Centrosome	
Ponticules intercellulaires	Zellbrücken
Substance cimentaire	Kittsubstanz
Tissu muscul. lisse interstitiel	interstitielles gl. Muskelgewebe
Travées muscul. lisses	gl. Muskelbälkchen
Couche myoépithéliale	myo-epitheliale Schicht
Muscles lisses cutanés	glatte Hautmuskeln
Tuniques musc. lisses	gl. Muskelhäute
musculaire muqueuse	Muscularis mucosae

Tuniques musculo-élastiques	elastische Muskelbänte
Dartos	Tunica Dartos
Tissu conjonctif enveloppant (Périmy-sium)	Umhüllendes Bindegewebe
Cloisons conjonctives	bindegewebige Septa »
Nerfs et terminaisons nerveuses	Nerven-Nervenendigungen
Plexus adventitiel	adventitieller Plexus
» fondamental	Grundplexus
» myentérique	Plexus myentericus (Auerbach)
» périmusculaire	perimuskulärer
» intra musculaire (endomysaire)	intra muskulärer
Fibres terminales	Endfasern
Varicosités	Varikositäten
Taches motrices (?)	motorische Endflecken
Ganglions des plexus nerveux	Ganglien der Nervengeflechte
Cellules nerveuses sympathiques	sympathische Nervenzellen
Vaisseaux sanguins	Blutgefässe
» des travées conjonctives	Septagefässe
réseaux capillaires	Kapillarnetze
» branches longitudinales	Längsäste
» » transversales	quere Längsäste
» » obliques	schiefe »
Vaisseaux perforants	durchtretende Gefässe

CELLULES MUSCULAIRES STRIÉES, MYOCYTES STRIÉS, CELLULES MYO-CAR-DIAQUES — HERZMUSKELZELLEN, GESTREIFTE MYOCYTEN

Variétés : fusiforme	Arten : spindelförmige
» fusiforme ramifiée	spindelförmig-verzweigte
» segment musculaire	Muskelsegment
Stries transversales	Querstreifen
» longitudinales	Längsstreifen
Sarcoplasma périnucléaire	perinucleäres Sarcoplasma
Myofibrilles	Myofibrillen
Colonnes myo-fibrillaires	Muskelsäulchen
Disque sombre	dunkele Scheibe
» clair	helle »
Noyaux des cellules ou segments musculaires	Kerne der Muskelzellen u. -segmente
Disques cimentaires	Kittlinien
Substance cimentaire	Kittsubstanz
Filaments unissants (?)	Verbindungsfäden
Cellules des fibres de *Purkinje*	Zellen der *Purkinje*'schen Fasern
regno striée	gestreifte Regno
» myofibrillaire	» myofibrilläre
» moyenne	» mittlere
» périnucléaire	» perinucleäre
Granulations endoplasmiques	endoplasmatische Granula

Noyaux	Kerne
Fibres myocardiques plexiformes	Myokardfasern (netzförmige)

FIBRE MUSCULAIRE STRIÉE — GESTREIFTE MUSKELFASER

Sarcolemme	Sarkolemma
Noyaux myocytaires	Muskelkerne
» pariétaux	parietale
» profonds	tiefe
Stries transversales	Querstreifen
» longitudinales	Längsstreifen
» longitudinales granuleuses	granulierte Längsstreifen
Sarcoplasma	Sarcoplasma
Granulations réfringentes	lichtbrechende Körnchen
Fibrilles musculaires primitives (Myofibrilles)	primitive Muskelfibrillen (Myofibrillen)
Casiers musculaires	Muskelkästchen
Disque sombre (anisotrope)	dunkle Scheibe (anisotrope)
Disque clair (isotrope)	helle Scheibe (isotrope)
Lame médiane	Mittelband
» terminale	Randscheibe
Disque accessoire	Nebenscheibe
Strie intermédiaire	Zwischenband
Colonnes myofibrillaires	myofibrilläre Säulchen (Muskelsäulchen)
Champs de Cohnheim	*Cohnheim'sche* Felder
Disques de Bowman	
Fibres musculaires à contour distinct et à colonnes fibrillaires rapprochées	Scharfkonturierte Muskelfasern mit dichtständigen Säulchen
à contour indistinct et colonnes éloignées	blasskonturierte mit lockeren Säulchen
Fibres musculaires ramifiées	verästelte Muskelfasern
Faisceaux musculaires (primaires, secondaires, tertiaires...)	Muskelbündel (primäre, sekundäre, tertiäre...)
Périmysium externe	
Cloisons interfasciculaires	Bündelsepta
Périmysium interne (Endomysium)	(Endomysium)
Ciment musculo-tendineux	Muskel-Sehnenkitt
Muscles rouges	rote Muskeln
» blancs	weisse »

Terminaison nerveuses — *Nervenendigungen*

» motrices	motorische
» sensitives	sensible
Nerfs des travées conjonctives	Septa Nerven
Fibres nerveuses terminales à gaine périneurale	Endnervenfasern mit perineuraler Scheide
Plaque motrice terminale	motorische Endplatte

Arborisation nerveuse terminale	nervöse Endverzweigung (hypolemmale)
serrée	dichte
lâche	lose
Coussinet noyau	kernhaltiger Polster
Faisceaux neuro-musculaires	neuro-muskuläre Stämmchen
Arborisations nerveuses subtendineuses	nervöse Sehnenendbäumchen

HISTOGENÈSE   HISTOGENESE

Cellule myoépithéliale	myoepitheliale Zelle
Myoblaste	Myoblastzelle
Myoblaste strié	gestreifte Myoblastzelle
Exoplasma strié	gestr. Exoplasma
Axoplasma	Axoplasma
Granulations sarcoplasmiques (sarco-microsomes)	Sarkomikrosomen
granulations vitellines	Dotterkörnchen
Lignée nucléaire	Kernreihe
Cellules interstitielles	interstitielle Zellen
Myoblastes secondaires (Sarcoplastes de *Marzo-Panth*)	sekundäre Myoblasten
Chaînes de myoblastes	myoblasten Ketten

SANG   BLUT

Éléments figurés	geformte Elemente
Plasma sanguin	Blutplasma
Sérum	Blutserum
Caillot	Blutgerinnsel

GLOBULES ROUGES   ROTE [FARBIGE] BLUTZELLEN

avec hématies	
érythrocytes	Erythrocyten
anucléées	„ kernlose
discoïdales	discoidale
Couche corticale plasmique	Rindenschicht
Stroma globulaire	Zellstroma
Pigment sanguin	Blutpigment
Hémoglobine	Hämoglobin
Excavation centrale	zentrale Delle
Bourrelet marginal	Randwulst
Formes altérées :	veränderte Formen
crénelées	eingekerbte
épineuses	stechapfelartige
Micro-érythrocytes	Mikro-Erythrocyten
érythrocytes anucléés ovalaires	ovale kernlose Erythrocyten
Empilement des érythrocytes	Einzellenrollen
Globules rouges embryonnaires	embryonale Erythrocyten

nucléés (elliptiques)	kernhaltige (elliptische)
Renflement central	centrale Anschwellung
Noyau	Kern
Réticule nucléaire	Korngerüst
Erythrocytes nucléés globuleux	kernhaltige kugelige Erythrocyten

GLOBULES BLANCS — FARBLOSE BLUTKÖRPERCHEN

Leucocytes	Leukocyten
Lymphocytes	Lymphocyten
Corps cellulaire contractile	Kontraktiler Zelleib
Mouvements amiboïdes	amöboide Bewegungen
Granulations protoplasmiques:	Granula:
fines	feine
épaisses-réfringentes	dicke-lichtbrechende
acidophiles	acidophile
(éosinophiles)	(eosinophile)
basophiles	basophile
neutrophiles	neutrophile
Centrosoma	
Lymphocytes mononucléés	mehrkernige
à petit noyau, chromophile	
à gros noyau pâle	
plurinucléés	mehrkernige
à noyaux polymorphes	mit polymorphen Kernen
Microlymphocytes	Micro- und
Macrolymphocytes	Makrolymphocyten

LYMPHE LYMPHE

Lymphocytes	Lymphocyten
Plasma lymphatique	Lymphplasma
Sérum	serum
Caillot	gerinnsel
Chyle	Chylus
Plaquettes sanguines (de *Bizzozero*)	Blutplättchen
Syn. Thrombocytes	Thrombocyten
discoïdes et anuclées	discoïdale und (kernlose)
ovalaires oblongs et nucléés	länglich-ovale und kernhaltige
altérés (anguleux)	veränderte (eckige)
Amas thrombocytaires (amas granulaires de *Hayem*)	Thrombocyten-Häufchen
Granulations	Körnchen
Vacuoles	Vacuolen
Filaments de fibrine	Fibrinfäden
Cristaux d'hémoglobine	Hämoglobinkrystalle
Cristaux de Teichmann	Häminkrystalle

Cristaux d'hématoïdine	Hämatoïdinkrystalle
Ilots sanguins	Blutinseln
Erythroblastes incolores	farblose Erythroblasten
„ colorés	farbige „
Leucoblastes (?)	Leukoblasten (?)
Organes hématopoétiques	blutbildende Organe
Vaisseaux sanguins	Blutgefässe
Vaisseaux des cloisons	Septa-Gefässe
Réseaux capillaires	Kapillarnetze
Mailles quadrangulaires	rechtwinkelige Maschen
Sinuosités	Schlingen
Dilatations ampullaires	Erweiterungen
Vaisseaux lymphatiques	Lymphgefässe

TISSU CONJONCTIF. BINDEGEWEBE

Quelques catégories cellulaires générales:	Einige allgemeine Zell-Kategorien:
Cellules plastiques:	plastische Zellen:
Inoblastes	Inoblasten
Ostéoblastes	Osteoblasten
Odontoblastes	Odontoblasten
Cellules chondrogènes	Chondrogene Zellen
Chromatophores	Chromatophoren
Cellules de la nutrition	Nutritialzellen
Cellules résorbantes	resorbierende Zellen
„ Ostéoclastes	Osteoklasten
„ Sarcolytes	Sarkolyten
„ Lymphocytes phagocytaires	phagocytäre Lymphocyten
Cellules géantes formatrices	formative Riesenzellen

VARIÉTÉS CELLULAIRES CONJONCTIVES — BINDEGEWEBSZELLARTEN

Cellules du tissu conjonctif fœtal	Zellen des fœtalen Bindegew
„ „ gélatineux	„ des Gallertgewebes
„ „ réticulé	„ des retikulären Bindegewebes
Cellules ramifiées du tissu conjonctif adulte:	verzweigte Bindegewebszellen
Cellules à prolongements filiformes	mit fadenförmigen Ausläufern
Cellules pigmentaires:	Pigmentzellen:
„ étoilées	sternförmige
„ digitées	palmatae
„ autres (fusiformes)	spindelförmige
„ aplaties	abgeplattete
„ libres	freie
„ anastomosées	anastomosierende
Cellules conjonctives lamelleuses (plates)	lamellose Bindegewebszellen-platte
fusiformes	Spindelzellen

rubanées (tendineuses)	bandförmige (Sehnenzellen)
à crêtes	mit Rippen ausgestattete Zellen
irisantes	Irisierende (Glanzzellen)
chromophiles	chromophile
ramassées	abgerundete
fusiformes	spindelförmige
à prolongements	verzweigte
Cellules plasmatiques	Plasmazellen
Cellules dites d'engrais (granulo-plasmatiques)	Mastzellen (granulo-plasmatische)
Cellules adipogènes	fettbildende Zellen
„ globuleuses	runde
„ irrégulières	unregelmässige
cellules adipeuses	Fettzellen
„ séro-adipeuses	seröse Fettzellen
„ adipeuses à noyau central	Fettzellen mit mittelständigem Kern
Lymphocytes	Lymphocyten
Myélocytes	Markzellen
Cellules géantes	Riesenzellen
(Mégacaryocytes)	(Megakaryocyten)
„ à noyau unique	mit einzigem Kern
„ à noyau polymorphe	mit polymorphem Kern
„ à noyaux multiples	mit mehreren Kernen
Endothélium conjonctif	bindegewebiges Endothel

Substance fondamentale	*Grundsubstanz*
Fibres conjonctives	Bindegewebsfasern
Fibrilles conjonctives	„ fibrillen
Fibres annulaires	Ringfasern
„ spirales	Spiralfasern (umspinnende Fasern)
Fibres élastiques	elastische Fasern
Réseaux „	„ Netze
membranes „	„ Häute
grains	„ Körner
Substance amorphe	amorphe Substanz

Catégories de tissus conjonctifs	*Bindegewebskategorien*
Tissu conjonctif embryonnaire	embryonales Bindegewebe
„ gélatineux (muqueux)	Gallertgewebe
„ réticulé	retikuläres
„ adipeux	Fettgewebe
„ fibreux	faseriges Bindegewebe

Tissu conjonctif gélatineux (muqueux)	*Gallertgewebe (Schleimgewebe)*
Tissu transitoire	transitorisches
„ permanent	permanentes
Cellules ramifiées (anastomotiques)	verzweigte (anastomosierende) Zellen
Cellules globuleuses	runde Zellen
Substance amorphe intercellulaire	amorphe Zwischensubstanz

Français	Deutsch
Tissu conjonctif réticulé	*Retikuläres Bindegewebe*
Tissu proprement dit	eigentliches
„ myélo-réticulé	myelo-retikuläres
„ lymphadénoïde (?)	lymphadenoides (?)
Tissu adipeux	*Fettgewebe*
Panicule adipeux (sous-cutané)	Panniculus adiposus
Ilots adipeux	Fettzellen-Haufen
Cloisons conjonctives	bindegewebige Septa
Trame conjonctive intercellulaire	zwischenzelliges Gerüst
Réseau capillaire sanguin intercellulaire	zwischenzelliges Gefässnetz
Tissu adipeux interstitiel	interstitielles Fettgewebe
Tissu adip. périvasculaire	gefässangehendes Fettgewebe
T. adip. adviscéral	adviszerales Fettgewebe
T. adip. blanc	weisses Fettgewebe
T. adip. gris (granulo-adipeux)	graues Fettgewebe
Tissus conjonctifs à trame fibreuse	*Faserige Bindegewebsarten*
Tissu conjonctif lâche (interstitiel)	lockeres Bindegewebe (interstitielles)
„ trabéculaire	balkenförmiges
Tissu des membranes séreuses	Gewebe der serösen Häute
„ du grand épiploon	„ des grossen Netzes
Tissu membraneux de l'arachnoïde	Gewebe der Arachnoidea
Tissu conjonctif à lamelles concentriques	konzentrisch-lamelläres Gewebe
Membranes vasculaires	Gefässhäute
„ „ pigmentées	pigmentierte Gefässhäute
„ „ villeuses et papillaires	zottige, papilläre Häute
Membranes synoviales	Synovialhäute
Gaines tendineuses	Sehnenscheiden
Enveloppes parenchymateuses (viscérales)	Parenchymhüllen (viscerale Hüllen)
Membranes fibreuses	fibröse Häute
„ ostéogènes	osteogene „
„ chondrogènes	chondrogene „
Tissu tendineux	Sehnengewebe
Ligaments fibreux	fibröse Bänder
Ligaments élastiques	elastische Bänder
Tissu caverneux	Gitterbalkengewebe (?)
Vascularisation	*Gefässverteilung*
Tissu conjonctif vascularisé	gefässhaltiges Bindegewebe
„ „ non vascularisé	gefässloses
Vaisseaux autochtones	autochthone Bindegewebsgefässe

Vaisseaux traversants	durchtretende
Plexus vasculaires	Gefässgeflechte
Réseaux admirables	Wundernetze
Réseaux papillaires	Gefässnetze der Papillen

Vaisseaux lymphatiques	*Lymphgefässe*
Plexus lymphatiques	Lymphgefässgeflechte
Réseaux lymphatiques capillaires	lymphatische Kapillarnetze
Sinus et fentes lymphatiques	Lymphsinus, Lymphspalten
Fentes péricellulaires	pericelluläre Spalträume
Système canaliculé anastomotique	anastomosierende Saftkanälchen

Innervation. Terminaisons nerveuses	*Nerven. Nervenendigungen*
Troncs nerveux	Nervenstämme
Plexus nerveux	Nervengeflechte
Anses nerveuses	Nervenschlingen
Cellules nerveuses interstitielles	interstitielle Nervenzellen
Terminaisons nerveuses péricellulaires	pericelluläre Nervenendigungen
Arborisations terminales	Endbäumchen
Pelotons nerveux encapsulés	eingekapselte Nervenknäuel
Corpuscules nerveux	Nervenkörperchen

TENDONS	SEHNEN
Tendons cylindriques	zylindrische
„ membraneux	platte, häutige
Fibres tendineuses primitives	Sehnenfasern
Cellules tendineuses séries	Sehnenzellenreien
Faisceaux tendineux primaires	primäre Sehnenbündel
„ „ secondaires	sekundäre „
„ „ tertiaires	tertiäre „
„ „ quaternaires	
Cloisons conjonctives interstitielles	Sehnensepta
Enveloppe péritendineuse	Peritenonium
Revêtement endothélial	Endothelüberzug
Extrémité fibro-cartilagineuse	faserknorpelige Endportion
Faisceaux tendineux	Sehnenspindel
Vaisseaux sanguins	Blutgefässe
„ lymphatiques	Lymphgefässe
Tendons à couche enveloppante chondroïde (oiseaux)	Sehnen mit chondroider Überschicht (Vögel)
Tendons osseux	verknöcherte Sehnen
Nodules sésamoïdes tendineux (Batraciens)	sesamoide Sehnenknötchen (Batrachier)
Gaines tendineuses	Sehnenscheiden

MEMBRANES SÉREUSES	SERÖSE HÄUTE
Feuillet parietal	parietales Blatt
„ viscéral	viscerales „
Couche sous-séreuse	subseröse Schicht

Membrane fondamentale	Grundmembran
Revêtement endothélial (épithélial)	Endothel- (Epithel-) Ueberzug
Stomates (pores)	Stomata (Poren)
Fossettes (amphibiens)	Grübchen
Cellules des stomates	Stomazellen
„ des fossettes	Grübchenzellen
Rosaces endothéliales	Endothel-Rosetten
Ilots adipogènes	fettbildende Zellinseln
Vaisseaux sanguins	Blutgefässe
„ lymphatiques	Lymphgefässe
Terminaisons nerveuses sensitives	sensitive Nervenendigungen

MEMBRANES SYNOVIALES	SYNOVIALHÄUTE
(v. connexions du squelette)	(s. Verbindungen der Knochen)
Endocarde et tunique vasculaire interne	*Endocardium und Intima*
(v. système vasculaire)	(s. Gefässsystem)
MEMBRANES MUQUEUSES (MEMBR. CONJONCT. COMPOSÉES, HÉTÉROGÈNES)	SCHLEIMHÄUTE (ZUSAMMENGESETZTE, HETEROGENE MEMBRANEN)

Chorion (tunique propre)	Tunica propria
Revêtement épithélial	Epithelüberzug
Couche sous-muqueuse	Submucosa
Musculaire muqueuse	Muscularis mucosae
Membr. muq. sans papilles	Schleimhäute ohne Papillen
„ „ à papilles	„ mit Papillen
Papilles simples	einfache Papillen
Papilles composées	zusammengesetzte Papillen
Papilles libres	freie Papillen
„ cachées	überdeckte Papillen
Villosités	Zotten
Muqueuses dermoïdes	dermoide Schleimhäute
„ lymphadénoïdes	lymphadenoide Schleimhäute
Cryptes des membr. muq.	Krypten der Schleimhäute
Glandes de la tunique propre	Drüsen der Tunica propria
„ de la sous-muqueuse	„ der Submucosa
Réseaux capillaires des papilles ou villosités	Kapillarnetze der Papillen res. Zotten
Réseaux vascul. de la tunique propre	Gefässe der Tunica propria
Vaisseaux de la sous-muqueuse	Tunica der Submucosa
Vaisseaux de la couche glandulaire	Gefässe der Drüsenschicht
„ des follicules lymphadénoï	„ der lymphadenoiden Follikels
„ des	
Vaisseaux lymphatiques	Lymphgefässe
superficiels	oberflächliche
profonds	tiefe

Fentes lymphatiques	Lymphspalten
Plexus nerveux	Nervengeflechte
Cellules nerveuses interstitielles	interstitielle Nervenzellen
Terminaisons nerveuses	Nervenendigungen
„ dans le chorion	„ in der Tunica propria
„ dans l'épithélium	„ im Epithel

TÉGUMENT EXTERNE   HAUTDECKE

(v. Peau)   (s. Haut)

TISSU CARTILAGINEUX. KNORPELGEWEBE

Cellules :	*Zellen :*
cellules cartilagineuses (chondrocytes)	Knorpelzellen (Chondrocyten)
Capsules cartilagineuses	Knorpelkapseln
Chondrocytes ramifiés	verzweigte Chondrocyten
Substance fondamentale :	Grundsubstanz :
„ hyaline	hyaline
„ fibreuse	faserige
„ élastique	elastische

CARTILAGES HYALINS   HYALINE KNORPEL

à périchondre	mit Perichondrium
sans périchondre	ohne Perichondrium
(articulaire)	(Gelenkknorpel)
fœtal	fœtaler
transitoire	transitorischer
permanent	permanenter
calcifié	verkalkter
ossifiant	verknöchender
squelettaire	Skeletknorpel
„ viscéral	viscerale Skeletknorpel
Cartilage à capsules soudées	Knorpel mit verschmolzenen Kapseln
„ à capsules séparées	„ mit getrennten Kapseln
Territoires chondrocytaires	Chondrocytenterritorien
Files chondrocytaires	Chondrocytenreihen
Capsule commune (capsule-mère)	Gemeinschaftliche Knorpelkapsel (Mutterkapsel)
Capsules secondaires (filles)	sekundäre Kapseln (Tochterkapseln)
Fibres de la substance fondamentale hyaline	Fasern der hyalinen Grundsubstanz
Faisceaux conjonctifs perforants	durchbohrende Faserbündel
Vaisseaux perforants	durchbohrende Gefässe
Couche conjonctive périvasculaire	perivasculäre Bindegewebsschicht

FIBRO-CARTILAGES   FASERKNORPEL

de recouvrement	Belegfaserknorpel
interosseux	interossärer „
interarticulaire	interartikulärer „

d'insertion	
des tendons	Schnenfaserknorpel
des ligaments	Band

CARTILAGE ÉLASTIQUE (RÉTICULÉ)	**ELASTICHER KNORPEL (NETZKNORPEL)**
Cutané	Haut-Netzknorpel
Viscéral	visceraler Netzknorpel
Périchondre	Perichondrium
Couche externe	äussere Schicht
„ interne	innere „
Fibres élastiques du périchondre	elastische Fasern des Perichondriums

CARTILAGES MIXTES.	**GEMISCHTER KNORPEL.**
TRANSFORMATIONS PHYSIOLOGIQUES	**PHYSIOLOGISCHE**
DU CARTILAGE	**KNOCHELUMBILDUNGEN**
Calcification	Verkalkung
Points de calcification	Verkalkungs-punkte
Ossification	Verknöcherung
Points d'ossification	Verknöcherungs-punkte
Ramollissement	Erweichung
Transformation pseudo-fibreuse	pseudofibröse Veränderung (Zerklüf-tung)
Dégénérescence graisseuse (des cellu-les)	Fettige Entartung (der Zellen)

TISSU CHONDROÏDE À CELLULES RAMIFIÉES	**CHONDROIDES GEWEBE MIT VESZWEIGTES ZELLEN**
Substance fondamentale hyaline	hyaline Grundsubstanz
Cellules ramifiées	verzweigte Zellen
Fentes et canalicules péricellulaires	pericellulare Spalträume und Kanälchen

OSSIFICATION	**VERKNÖCHERUNG**
Enchondrale,	Enchondrale
néoplastique	neoplastische
directe	direkte
sous-périostique	subperiostale (periostaidrale)
intra-membraneuse	intramembranöse
fibreuse directe	direkte Verknöcherung des Bindegewe-bes
Ossification tendineuse	(Schnenverknöcherung)
Os enchondraux	enchondrale Knochen
Os conjonctifs	bindegewebige
métaplasiques	metaplastische
autoplastiques	autoplastische

Ossification des os longs	*Verknöcherung der langen Knochen*
Ossification enchondrale	enchondrale
centrodiaphysaire	zentrodiaphysäre
télodiaphysaire	telodiaphysäre

épiphysaire	épiphysäre
Cartilage de conjugaison	Knorpelfuge
Foyer de calcification	Verkalkungsherd
Capsules agrandies	vergrösserte Kapseln
Amas chondrocytaires	Chondrocytenhaufen
Files de chondrocytes	Chondrocytensäulen
Résorption de la subst. fondam. cartilag.	Resorption der knorpeligen Grundsubstanz
Fonte des capsules cartilag.	Auflösung der Kapseln
Espaces médullaires cartilagineux	Knorpelmarkräume
Travées cartilagineuses fondamentales	knorpelige Grundsubstanzbalken
Moelle cartilagineuse	Knorpelmark
Vaisseaux de la moelle cartilagineuse	Gefässe des Knorpelmarkes
Couche des ostéoblastes	Osteoblastenschicht
Lamelles osseuses premières	erste Knochenlamellen
Travées osseuses enchondrales	enchondrale Knochenbalken
Couche osseuse récurrante	Knochenbelegschicht
Ilots cartilagineux festonnés	ausgebuchtete Knorpelreste
Ostéoclastes	Osteoklasten (v. *Kœlliker*)
Fossettes de *Howship*	Gröbchen

Ossification sous périostale	*Sub-periostale Verknöcherung*
Couche fibreuse du périoste	Faserschicht des Periost
Couche ostéogène	osteogene Schicht
Fibres arciformes (du périoste)	bogenförmige Periostfasern
Rainure d'implantation	Ansatzrinne
Moelle sous-périostée	subperiostales Mark
Vaisseaux de la couche ostéogène du périoste	Gefässe der osteogenen Periostschicht
Travées osseuses sous-périostiques	subperiostale Knochenbalken
Couche des ostéoblastes	Osteoblastenschicht
Fibres constitutives	Konstitutionsfasern
fibres perforantes	durchtretende Fasern

Accroissement osseux	Knochenwachstum
» » par apposition	durch Apposition
» » interstitiel	interstitielles
Résorption modelante	modellirende Resorption

Ossification intra-membraneuse	*Intra-membranöse Verknöcherung*
Membrane ostéogène	Osteogene Membran
Couche fibreuse externe	äussere Faserschicht
» » interne	innere »
» » moyenne riche en cellules	mittlere zellreiche Schicht
Myélocytes de la couche moyenne	Markzellen der mittleren Schicht
Vaisseaux sanguins	Gefässe
Travées fibreuses calcifiées	verkalktes Fasergerüst
Couche des ostéoblastes	Osteoblastenschicht
Fibres constitutives	Konstitutionsfasern

Os spongieux intra-membraneux	Spongiöse intra-membranöse Knochensubstanz
Espaces médullaires	Markräume
Cellules géantes	Riesenzellen

TISSU OSSEUX. KNOCHENGEWEBE

Substance fondamentale	*Grundsubstanz*
Lamelles osseuses	Knochenlamellen
„ périphériques	äussere Grundlamellen
„ concentriques	konzentrische Lam.
» intermédiaires	Schalt- „ (interstitielle)
„ périmédullaires	innere Grundlamellen Marklamellen
Lamelles lisses (homogènes)	glatte Lamellen
„ striées	gestreifte »
Fibres de la substance fondamentale	Fasern der Grundsubstanz
„ conjonctives	Bindegewebsfasern
„ calcifiées	verkalkte
„ non calcifiées	unverkalkte
„ élastiques	elastische
Fibres de *Sharpey*	Fasern
Corpuscules osseux	Knochenkörperchen (höhlen)
Canalicules osseux	Knochenkanälchen
„ ondulés	gewundene
„ recourbés	geknickte
„ récurrents	rückläufige
Canaux vasculaires (de *Havers*)	Gefässkanäle
Canaux perforants (de *Volkmann*)	perforirende

Cellules osseuses	*Knochenzellen*
Os longs	lange Knochen
Diaphyse	Diaphyse
Epiphyses	Epiphysen
Os courts	kurze Knochen
Os plats	platte „
Table externe	tabula externa
Table interne	„ interna
Diploé	Diploe
Substance compacte	Subst. compacta
„ spongieuse	„ spongiosa
Canal médullaire	Markkanal
espaces médullaires (aréoles)	Markräume
Os dermiques	Haut Knochen
„ viscéraux	viscerale „
Périoste	Periost
Couche externe	äussere Schicht
„ interne	innere „
(v. Ossification)	(s. Verknöcherung)
Bourrelets fibro-cellulaires sous-périostiques (poissons)	subperiostale faserige Zellwülste

Moelle osseuse	*Knochenmark*
rouge	rothes
jaune	gelbes
gélatineuse	Gallertmark
Myélocytes	Myelocyten
» à petit noyau	kleinkernige
» à gros noyau	grosskernige
Cellules géantes (Myéloplaxes, *Robin*)	Riesenzellen
Ostéoblastes (*Gegenbaur*)	Osteoblasten
Lymphocytes	Lymphocyten
Cellules éosinophiles	eosinophile Zellen
Cellules adipeuses	Fettzellen
Globules rouges nucléés (*Neumann*)	kernhaltige Erythrocyten
Cellules de la trame de soutènement	Gerüstzellen
Réticule	Reticulum

Vaisseaux sanguins	*Blutgefässe*
Vaisseaux périostiques	periostale Gefässe
Vaisseaux de la substance compacte	Gefässe der Subst. compacta
Vaisseaux des canaux de *Havers*	Gefässe der *Havers*'schen Kanäle
Artères nourricières	Arteriae nutriciae
Vaisseaux de la moelle osseuse	Gefässe des Knochenmarkes
Vaisseaux lymphatiques du périoste	periostale Lymphgefässe
Fentes lymphatiques périvasculaires de l'os compact	perivasculäre Lymphspalten der Compacta
Fentes lymphatiques de la moelle osseuse	Lymphspalten des Knochenmarkes
Nerfs du périoste	Periostnerven
Nerfs des trous nourriciers	Nerven der Ernährungslöcher (Foramina nutritia)
Corpuscules nerveux terminaux	terminale Nervenkörperchen

TISSU OSTÉO-CARTILAGINEUX (TISSU OSSEUX MIXTE, KNOCHEN-KNORPELIGES GEWEBE (GEMISCHTES KNOCHENGEWEBE

CONNEXIONS DU SQUELETTE, KNOCHENVERBINDUNGEN

Sutures (Synarthroses)	Naht
Couche fibreuse interosseuse	faserige Zwischenschicht (Nahtband)
Syndesmoses	Bandverbindung
Ligaments fibreux	fibröse Bänder
» interosseux	
» périarticulaires	peri articulaire
Ligaments élastiques	elastische Bänder
Synchondroses	Knorpelhaft
cartilagineuse	
fibro-cartilagineuse	Faserknorpelhaft
(amphiarthroses, symphyses)	

Disques intervertébraux	Randscheiben
Cartilage hyalin d'encroûtement	hyaliner Belegknorpel
Fibro-cartilage	Faserknorpel
Couche externe (à fibres croisées)	äussere Schicht (mit gekreuzten Fasern)
Couche interne	innere Schicht
Noyau muqueux (gélatineux)	nucleus pulposus (Gallertkern)
Diarthroses	Gelenkverbindung
Cartilage articulaire	Gelenkknorpel
Capsule articulaire	Gelenkkapsel
Couche fibreuse	Stratum fibrosum
Membrane synoviale	Stratum synoviale (Synovialhaut)
Couche intermédiaire (sous-synoviale)	Stratum intermedium (sub-synoviale)
Plis synoviaux	Synovialfalten
„ adipeux	Plicae adiposae
„ vasculaires	„ vasculosae
Villosités synoviales (franges)	Synovialzotten
Revêtement cellulaire plat	innere platte Zellschicht
Vaisseaux sanguins de la synoviale	Synovial-Blutgefässe
„ lymphatiques	„ Lymphgefässe
Vaisseaux profonds	tiefe Gefässe
„ superficiels	oberflächliche Gefässe
Nerfs	Nerven
Terminaisons nerveuses	Nervenendigungen

Corps vertébral de la queue des amphi-   *Wirbelkörper des Salamanders*
biens urodèles (salamandre)   *(Schwanzgegend)*

Anneau osseux	Knochenring
Anneau chondroïde	Chondroider Ring
Couche striée externe (radiaire)	äussere radiär gestreifte Schicht
Couche principale	Hauptschicht
Substance intercellulaire hyaline	hyaline Zwischen-Substanz
Cellules cartilagineuses	Knorpelzellen
Membrane limitante hyaline (gaine de la corde)	hyaline Grenz-membran
Couche épithéloïde externe (épithélium de la corde)	äussere epitheloide Schicht (Chorda-Epithel)
Couche vésiculaire centrale (cellules de la corde)	blasige Zentralschicht (Chorda-Zellen)
Corde dorsale (embryons d'Amphibiens)	Chorda
grandes cellules vésiculaires	grosser blasige Zellen
Cellules plates sous-vaginales	platte subvaginale Zellschicht
épithélium de la corde dorsale	Chorda-Epithel
Gaine de la corde	Chordascheide

Corps vertébral (amphicoele) des poissons   *Wirbelkörper der Knochenfische*
osseux

Anneau osseux bicorne	bikonischer Knochenring
Noyau or (fixation osseux) central	zentraler Knorpelkern

Tissu fibro-capsulaire propre (chorde dorsale)	faserkapseliges Gewebe (chorda)
zone centrale	zentrale Zone
zone moyenne	mittlere Zone
zone externe	äussere Zone
Substance intercellulaire fibroïde	gallertfaserige Zwischensubstanz
Cellules hyalines	hyaline Zellen
noyau excentrique	exzentrischer Kern
couche protoplasmique étoilée	sternförmige Plasmaschicht

TISSU OSSEUX DU CÉMENT DENTAIRE, ZEMENTKNOCHEN

Dentine (Ivoire)	*Zahnbein*
non vasculaire	gefässloses
Vaso-dentine	Vaso-Dentin
Ostéo-Dentine	Osteo-Dentin

TISSU LYMPHADÉNOÏDE, SYSTÈME LYMPHADÉNOÏDE, LYMPHADÉNOÏDES GEWEBE, LYMPHADÉNOÏDES SYSTEM

Réticule lymphadénoïde	lymphadénoïdes Reticulum
Fibrilles de la trame de soutènement	Gerüstfibrillen
Cellules ,, ,, ,, ,, ,, ,,	Gerüstzellen
Fibres en treillis	Gitterfasern
Globules lymphoïdes	lymphoïde Zellen[*]
(épithélium lymphadénoïde?)	lymphadénoïdes Epithel?)
Lymphocytes à noyaux irréguliers	Lymphocyten mit unregelmässigen Kernen
Cellules à gros noyau	grosskernige Zellen
Cellules globuleuses pigmentées	runde pigmentirte Zellen
Tissu lymphadénoïde diffus	diffuses lymphadénoïdes Gewebe
Follicules lymphadénoïdes	lymphadénoïde Knötchen
,, solitaires	solitäre
,, agminés	gehäufte
,, sousépithéliaux	sub-epitheliale
,, cryptobordants	Kryptenumschliessende
,, intra-glandulaires	intraglanduläre
,, parenchymateux	parenchymatöse
,, interstitiels	interstitielle
Nodules secondaires	Sekundärknötchen
,, germinatifs	Keimknötchen
Cordons lymphadénoïdes	lymphadénoïde Stränge
Vaisseaux folliculaires	Follikelgefässe
Branches circulaires (tangentielles)	zirculäre Aeste (tangentielle)
Branches radiaires	radiäre Aeste
Anses capillaires profondes	tiefe Kapillarschlingen
Sinus périfolliculaires	perifollikuläres Lymphsinus
Sinus médullaires	Marksinus

Cryptes lymphadénoïdes	*Lymphadenoïde Krypten*
simples	einfache
composées	zusammengesetzte
Diverticule épithélial primaire	primäre Epitheleinstülpung
Diverticules épithéliaux secondaires	sekundäre Epitheleinstülpungen
Coque lymphadénoïde	lymphadenoïde Belegschicht
Gaine conjonctive	bindegewebige Hülle
Parenchymes lymphadénoïdes	*lymphadenoïde Organe*

SYSTÈME VASCULAIRE SANGUIN. BLUTGEFÄSSSYSTEM

CŒUR	HERZ
Péricarde	Pericardium
feuillet pariétal	parietales Blatt
feuillet viscéral. Syn. épicarde, exocarde	viscerales Blatt (Epicardium, Exocardium)
endothélium	Endothel
Couche sous-séreuse	Subserosa
Panicule adipeux sous-séreux	subseröses Fettgewebe
Myocarde	Myocardium
Fibres de *Purkinje*	*Purkinje'sche Fasern*
Muscles papillaires	Musculi papillares
Muscles pectinés	Musculi pectinati
Endocarde	Endocardium
couche externe	äussere Lage
couche intermédiaire	Zwischenschicht
couche interne (lamelleuse) (hyaline)	innere Lage (lamellöse) Schicht
endothélium	Endothel
Anneaux fibreux auriculo-ventriculaires	Annuli fibrosi
Valvules auriculo-ventriculaires	Atrioventrikular-Klappen
Couche endocardique pariétale	parietale Endokardlage
Couche fasciculée plexiforme	flechtförmige Faserschicht
Couche intermédiaire	Zwischenschicht
Couche endocardique ostiale	ostiale Endokardlage
Cordages tendineux	Chordae tendineae
Valvules sigmoïdes	Semilunarklappen
Couche endartérielle pariétale	parietale Intimalage
Couche fasciculée plexiforme	flechtförmige Faserschicht
Couche cellulo fibrillaire	zellig-fibrilläre Schicht
Couche intermédiaire	Zwischenschicht
Couche endocardique ostiale	ostiale Endokardlage
Nodule d'*Arantius*	Nodulus Arantii
Cloison interauriculaire	Scheidewand der Vorhöfe
„ interventriculaire	„ der Kammern
Vaisseaux sanguins	Blutgefässe
sous-péricardiques (sous-séreux)	subseröse „
myocardiques	Myocardgefässe
endocardiques	Endokard „

Couche subcardique non vascularisée	gefässlose Endokardschicht
Vaisseaux lymphatiques	Lymphgefässe
sous-péricardiques (sous-séreux)	subseröse
myocardiques (?)	Myokard-Lymphgefässe (?)
Fentes lymphatiques périvasculaires du myocarde	perivaskuläre Lymphspalten des Myokards
endocardiques	Endokard-Lymphgefässe

Nerfs	*Nerven*
Plexus cardiaque	Plexus cardiacus
Ganglion de *Remak*	*Remak*'sches Ganglion
" de *Ludwig*	*Ludwig*'sches "
" de *Bidder*	*Bidder*'sches "
Plexus sous-péricardique (sous-séreux)	subseröser Plexus
Plexus myocardique interstitiel (fondamental)	interstitieller Myokardplexus (Grundplexus)
Plexus myocardique intermédiaire	intermediärer Plexus
Plexus myocardique terminal	terminaler Myokardplexus
Plexus sous-endocardique	subendokardialer Plexus
endocardique	Endokardplexus
sous-endothélial	subendothelialer Endokardplexus
Terminaisons nerveuses	Nervenendigungen
motrices	motorische
sensitives	sensible
Arborisations terminales myocytaires	motorische Telodendrien
Terminaisons sensitives	sensible Nervenendigungen
" sous-péricardiques	subseröse "
" myocardiques	myokardiale "
" endocardiques	endokardiale "
Histogénèse	*Histogenese*
Endothélium endocardique	Endokardendothel
Endothélium péricardique	Perikardendothel
Couche myocardique embryonnaire	embryonal-Myokardschicht
zone externe	äussere Lage
zone interne	innere Lage
Myoblastes cardiaques ramifiés	verzweigte Myoblasten
Syncytium myocardique	Myokardsyncytium
Myofibrilles	Myofibrillen
Couche myofibrillaire pariétale	myofibrilläre Wandschicht
Sarcoplasme	Sarcoplasma
Zone nucléaire centrale	zentrale Kernzone

ARTÈRES	ARTERIEN
Type élastique	elastischer Typus
" musculaire	muskulöser "
" intermédiaire (mixte)	Uebergangstypus (gemischter)
Tuniques:	Gefässhäute:
externe (adventice)	Adventitia
moyenne	Media

interne (endartère)	Intima
Endothélium	Endothel
Membranes élastiques fenêtrées	gefensterte elastische Häute
Lame élastique interne	innere elastische Haut (Elastica interna)
Réseaux élastiques	elastische Netze
Couche musculaire annulaire	Ringmuskelschicht
Faisceaux muscul. longitudinaux	Längsmuskelbündel
Artères hélicines	Rankenarterien
„ pénicillées	Pinselarterien
„ terminales	terminale Arterien
Artérioles	Arteriolen
Artérioles précapillaires	präkapilläre Arteriolen
Réseaux admirables	Wundernetze
„ glomérulés	Gefässknäuel

VAISSEAUX CAPILLAIRES   KAPILLAREN (HAARGEFÄSSE)

Capillaires artériels	arterielle Kapillaren
„ veineux	venöse „
Tube endothélial capillaire	Endothelrohr
Stomates	Stomata (Poren)
Adventice des capillaires	Adventitia der Kapillaren (Perithelium)
Réseaux capillaires	Kapillarnetze
„ à mailles allongées	„ mit länglichen Maschen
„ „ quadrangulaires	„ mit viereckigen „
„ „ polygonales	„ mit polygonalen „
„ „ arrondies	„ mit rundlichen „
„ „ radiaires	„ mit radiären „
„ „ tourbillonnées	„ mit wirbeligen „
Diverticules capillaires	Kapillardivertikel

VEINES   VENEN

Type musculaire	muskulöser Typus
„ sans éléments musculaires	muskelloser „
Tuniques:	Gefässhäute:
externe (adventice)	Adventitia
moyenne	Media
interne	Intima
Endothélium	Endothel
Lamelles élastiques	elastische Lamellen
Réseaux élastiques	elastische Netze
Couche musculaire annulaire	Ringmuskelschicht
Faisceaux musculaires longitudinaux	Längsmuskelbündel
„ externes (adventitiels)	äussere (adventitielle)
„ internes	innere
Valvules veineuses	Venenklappen
Veinules	kleinste Venen
Veines tourbillonnaires	Venae vorticosae

Sinus veineux (de la dure-mère)	Venensinus der Dura
Sinus sanguins des poils tactiles	Blutsinus der Fühlhaare
Sinus sanguins du placenta	Blutsinus der Placenta

TISSU ÉRECTILE	SCHWELLGEWEBE

Sinus sanguins	Blutsinus
Endothélium	Endothel
Travées	Septa
Cellules musculaires lisses	glatte Muskelzellen
Fibres élastiques	elastische Fasern
Tunique albuginée	Albuginea
Vaisseaux afférents des sinus sanguins	zuführende Gefässe
Vaisseaux efférents	abführende „
Nerfs des vaisseaux sanguins	Nerven der Blutgefässe
Plexus adventitiel (fondamental)	adventitieller Plexus (Grundplexus)
„ intermédiaire (supramusculaire) admusculaire	intermediärer „
„ intramusculaire	intramuskulöser „
„ terminal (pénicellulaire)	Endplexus (perizellulärer)
Taches motrices (?)	motorische Flecken (?)
Terminaisons nerveuses sensitives dans l'adventice	sensible Nervenendigungen in der Tunica adventitia
Fibrilles terminales	Endfibrillen
Buissons, bouquets terminaux	Endbüschel, Endknoten
Corpuscules de *Vater-Pacini*	*Vater-Pacini*'sche Körperchen
Terminaisons sensitives	sensible Nervenendigungen
dans la tunique moyenne	in der Muscularis
dans la tunique interne (plexus sous-endothélial)	in der Intima (subendothelialer Plexus)
Vasa vasorum	
Pointes d'accroissement	spitze Gefässsprossen
„ nuclées	kernhaltige „
„ anuclées	kernlose „
Cordons vasculaires pleins	solide Gefässstränge
Canalisation	Aushöhlung
Cellules vaso-formatives (?)	vasoformative Zellen

SYSTÈME VASCULAIRE LYMPHATIQUE. LYMPHGEFÄSSSYSTEM

Vaisseaux lymphatiques	*Lymphgefässe*
Tunique externe (adventice)	Adventitia
„ moyenne	Media
„ interne	Intima
Endothélium	Endothel
Valvules	Klappen
Capillaires lymphatiques	Lymphkapillaren
Endothélium sinueux	ausgeschnittenes Endothel
Gaines lymphatiques périvasculaires	perivaskuläre Lymphscheiden
Fentes lymphatiques périvasculaires	perivaskuläre Lymphspalten

Sinus lymphatiques cloisonnés	Lymphsinus
Fentes lymphatiques péricellulaires	perizelluläre Lymphspalten
Système lymphatique canaliculé	Saftkanälchensystem
Nerfs (v. Vaisseaux sanguins)	Nerven (s. Blutgefässe)
Vasa vasorum des lymphatiques	—
Pointes d'accroissement	spitze Gefässprossen

Ganglions lymphatiques   Lymphknoten

Gaine (capsule)	Hülle (Kapsel)
Travées corticales	Rindensepta
„ médullaires	Marksepta
Substance corticale	Rindensubstanz
„ médullaire	Marksubstanz
Follicules corticaux (lymphadénoïdes)	Rindenknötchen (lymphadenoide)
Nodules secondaires (germinatifs)	sekundärknötchen (Keimknötchen)
Sinus périfolliculaires	Rindensinus
Cordons médullaires	Markstränge
Sinus médullaires	Marksinus
Réticule des sinus lymphatiques (Trabécules)	Reticulum (Bälkchen) der Lymphsinus
Vaisseaux lymphatiques afférents	zuführende Lymphgefässe
„ „ efférents	abführende „
Hile	Hilus
Pigment des ganglions lymphatiques	Pigment der Lymphknoten
Vaisseaux sanguins	Blutgefässe
„ superficiels (capsulaires)	oberflächliche (Kapselgefässe)
„ profonds	tiefe
„ du hile	Hilusgefässe
„ des travées conjonctives	Septagefässe
Réseaux capillaires des follicules	Kapillarnetze der Rindenknötchen
„ des cordons médullaires	„ der Markstränge
Nerfs	Nerven
Plexus nerveux périvasculaires	perivaskuläre Nervenplexus
Nerfs des travées	Septanerven
Nerfs des cordons médullaires (?)	Nerven der Markstränge

Cœurs lymphatiques   Lymphherzen

Couche musculaire	Muskelschicht
Intima	Intima
Endothélium	Endothel

PARENCHYMES LYMPHADÉNOÏDES   LYMPHADENOIDE ORGANE

I. Intravasculaires   I. Intravasculär

Ganglions lymphatiques   Lymphknoten

(v. système vasculaire)	(s. Gefässystem)

Rate	*Milz*
Gaine (capsule)	Hülle (Kapsel)
Travées	Milzsepta
Follicules spléniques	Milzfollikel
Cordons spléniques	Milzstränge
Pulpe splénique	Milzpulpa
Cellules folliculaires	Follikelzellen
Cellules des cordons spléniques	Milzstrangzellen
Cellules de la pulpe splénique	Pulpazellen
Cellules de la trame de soutènement	Gerüstzellen
Lymphocytes éosinophiles	eosinophile Lymphocyten
„ plurinucléés	mehrkernige „
Cellules géantes	Riesenzellen
Cellules pigmentées	pigmentierte Zellen
Granulations pigmentaires	Pigmentkörnchen
Globules rouges nuclées	Kernhaltige Blutzellen
Cellules à hématocytes	hematocytenhaltige Zellen
Trame de soutènement	Stützgerüst
Fibres ou treillis	Gitterfasern
Vaisseaux sanguins	Blutgefässe
Vaisseaux superficiels (capsulaires)	oberflächliche Gefässe
„ profonds	tiefe „
„ du hile	Hilusgefässe
„ des travées spléniques	Septagefässe
Artères pénicillées	Penicillgefässe
Réseaux capillaires des follicules	Follikelkapillarnetze
Vaisseaux de la pulpe	Pulpagefässe
Gousses artérielles	Hülsenarterien (Schweigger-Seidel)
Capillaires artériels	arterielle Kapillaren
Voies vasculaires de la pulpe	Gefässbahnen der Pulpa
Capillaires veineux	venöse Kapillaren
Cellules vasendymaires fusiformes	vasendymäre Spindelzellen
Veines de la pulpe	Pulpavenen
Fibres élastiques transversales des vei-nes	elastische Querfasern der Venen
Vaisseaux lymphatiques	Lymphgefässe
Lymphatiques superficiels	oberflächliche Lymphgefässe
„ profonds	tiefe „
„ du hile	Hilus-Lymphgefässe
„ des travées (?)	Septa „ (?)
Voies lymphatiques de la pulpe (?)	Lymphwege der Pulpa (?)
Nerfs	Nerven
Plexus splénique	Plexus lienalis
Nerfs vasculaires	Nerven der Penicilli
Terminaisons motrices vasculaires	motorische Gefässnervenendigungen
Nerfs des travées spléniques	Septanerven
„ de la pulpe splénique (?) (v. Kölliker)	Pulpanerven (?)

II. Organes lymphoïdes para-épithéliaux	II. Lymphadenoide paraepitheliale Organe
Thymus	*Thymus*
Lobules thymiques	Thymusläppchen
Tissu interlobulaire	Läppchensepta
Cordon central (?)	Zentralstrang (?)
Substance corticale	Rindensubstanz
Substance médullaire	Marksubstanz
Travées de la subst. corticale	Rindensepta
Cellules thymiques	Thymuszellen
„ de la substance corticale	„ der Rindensubstanz
„ de la subst. médullaire	„ der Marksubstanz
Corpuscules de *Hassal*	*Hassal*'sche Körperchen
cellules pariétales	Randzellen
cellules centrales	Zentralzellen
Cellules de la trame de soutènement	Gerüstzellen
Trame de soutènement	Gerüst
Cellules thymiques pigmentées (*lézard*)	pigmentierte Thymuszellen (*Eidechse*)
Cellules thymiques à structure gra-	Thymuszellen mit konzentrische fibril-
nulo-fibrillaire concentrique (*ger-*	lärer Plasmastruktur (*Frosch, Ei-*
mandie, lézard)	*dechse*)
Vaisseaux sanguins	Gefässe
Vaisseaux interlobulaires	interlobuläre Gefässe
„ parenchymateux	parenchymatöse „
Vaisseaux de la substance médullaire	Gefässe der Marksubstanz
Réseaux capillaires de la substance corticale	Kapillarnetze der Rindensubstanz
Veines interlobulaires (périphériques)	interlobuläre Venen (periphärische Läppchenvenen)
Veines profondes (médullaires)	Markvenen
Vaisseaux lymphatiques	Lymphgefässe
Troncs efférents	abführende Lymphstämme
Vaisseaux lymphatiques interlobulaires	interlobuläre Lymphgefässe
Lymphatiques périlobulaires	perilobuläre Lymphräume
Nerfs	Nerven
Nerfs vasculaires	Gefässnerven
Nerfs des travées interlobulaires	Septanerven
Amygdales. Follicules lymphadénoïdes agminés	*Tonsillen. Gehäufte lymphadenoide Follikel*
s. Appareil digestif	s. Verdauungs-Apparat

SYSTÈME TÉGUMENTAIRE. INTEGUMENTUM

PEAU (MAMMIFÈRES)	HAUT (SÄUGETHIERE)
Derme, chorion	*Cutis, Corium, Lederhaut*
Couche fondamentale	Grundschicht

Couche papillaire	Papillarschicht (Stratum papillare)
Crêtes dermiques	Hautleisten
Papilles	Papillen
Papilles vasculaires	Gefäss-Papillen
— à corpuscules nerveux	Nervenkörperchen-Papillen
Vallécules	Zwischengratforchen
Bourgeons épithéliaux interpapillaires	interpapilläre Epithelzapfen
Lame basale (?)	Basalmembran (?)
Muscles lisses cutanés	glatte Hautmuskeln
Os dermiques	Hautknochen
— *Hypoderme*	— *Unterhaut*
Pannicule adipeux sous-cutané	Panniculus adiposus
Bois adipeux	Fettzellenhaufen
Cloisons limitantes	Grenzscheiden
Derme et hypoderme embryonnaire	embryonale Cutis und Subcutis
Stade gélatineux	Gallertstadium
Cellules conjonctives plastiques (Ino-blastes)	plastische Bindegewebszellen (Inoblas-ten)
Cellules globuleuses	runde Zellen
Substance fondamentale gélatineuse	gallertartige Grundsubstanz
Ilots de cellules adipogènes	Fettbildende Zellherde
Stade fibreux	fasergewebiges Stadium
— *Épiderme*	— *Epidermis, Oberhaut*
— Plan muqueux (germinatif)	— Schleimschicht, Keimschicht (Stratum germinativum, Stratum mucosum)
Couche de cellules prismatiques (basales)	prismatische Zellschicht (Basalschicht)
Couche de cellules polyédriques (cellules crénelées)	polyedrische Zellschicht (Stilzellen)
Fentes intercellulaires	Interzellulargänge
Ponts plasmatiques	Plasmabrücken
Couche de cellules granuleuses (stratum granuleux)	Stratum granulosum (platte Körnerzellenschicht)
Granulations kératohyalines (d'éléidine)	keratohyaline Granula
— Plan corné	— Hornschicht
Stratum lucidum (couche hyaline)	Stratum lucidum (homogene Hornschicht)
Couche cornée stratifiée	Stratum corneum (lamellöse Hornschicht)
Crêtes des cellules racornies	Leisten der Hornzellen
Pigment épidermique	Oberhautpigment
Corpuscules de *Langerhans*	*Langerhan'sche* Körperchen
Vaisseaux sanguins	Gefässe
Vaisseaux dermiques profonds	tiefe Cutisgefässe
Rameaux ascendants	aufsteigende Aeste
Réseau sous-papillaire	subpapillares Gefässnetz
Vaisseaux des papilles	Papillengefässe
Vaisseaux de l'hypoderme	Unterhautgefässe
— du pannicule adipeux	Gef. des Panniculus adiposus

Vaisseaux lymphatiques	Lymphgefässe
„ profonds	tiefe „
„ superficiels	oberflächliche „
„ des papilles (?)	der Papillen (?)
Nerfs	Nerven
„ de l'hypoderme	Unterhautnerven
„ du derme	Cutisnerven
Nerfs papillaires ascendants	aufsteigende Papillen-Nerven
Plexus papillaires	papilläre Nervengeflechte
Branches sous-épidermiques horizontales	subepidermale Horizontalzweige
Corpuscules de *Vater-Pacini*	*Vater-Pacini'sche* Körperchen
„ de *Meissner*	*Meissner'sche* Körperchen
Pelotons nerveux encapsulés	eingekapselte Nervenknäuel
Anses pelotonnées	geknäuelte Nervenschlingen
Ménisques tactiles *(de Merkel)*	Tastscheiben
Organe de *Eimer*	*Eimer'sches* Organ
Plexus intra-épithéliaux	intraepitheliale Nervenplexus
Terminaisons intra-épithéliales libres	freie intraepitheliale Nervenendigungen
Boutons terminaux	Endknöpfe

PEAU (REPTILES) HAUT (REPTILIEN)

— *Derme*	— *Cutis*
Lamelle dermique marginale	dermale Grenzschicht
Couche vasculo-pigmentaire superficielle	oberflächliche Pigment- und Gefäss-schicht
Couche fasciculée	flechtförmige Faserschicht
Couche compacte (lame-Paste)	kompakte Schicht
— *Hypoderme*	— *Unterhautgewebe*
Couche vasculo-pigmentaire profonde	tiefe Gefäss- und Pigmentlage
Plaques osseuses cutanées	Hautknochen
„ superficielles	—oberflächliche
„ profondes	— tiefe
— *Epiderme*	— *Epidermis*
Plan squameux	Schuppenlage
„ cuticule	kuticula
„ couche squameuse de tame	abhäldbare Schuppenlage
„ couche adhérente	adhärente Schuppenlage
Plan profond sous-squameux	subsquameale Lage
Couche de cellules plates	platte Zellschicht
„ de cellules polyédriques	polyedrische „
„ de cellules prismatiques	prismatische „
Pigment épidermique	Epidermis-Pigment
Cellules pigmentaires ramifiées	verzweigte Pigment-Zellen
Poches squamifères	Schuppentaschen
plan du toit	Dachlage
plan du lit squameux	Schuppenbett
plis de la poche squamifère	Falten des Schuppenbettes

PEAU (AMPHIBIENS)	HAUT (AMPHIBIEN)
— *Derme*	— *Cutis*
Lamelle dermique limitante	dermale Grenzschicht
Couche vasculo-pigmentaire superficielle	oberflächliche Pigment- und Gefäss-schicht
Couche glandulaire	Drüsenschicht
Couche lamellaire compacte	kompakte lamelläre Schicht
Cloisons verticales	vertikale Septa
Sacs lymphatiques sous-cutanés	subdermale Lymphsäcke
— *Hypoderme*	— *Hypodermis*
— *Épiderme*	— *Epidermis*
Plan hyalin (corné)	hyaline Lage (Hornschicht)
Plan muqueux	Schleimschicht
couches des cellules aplaties	platte Zellschicht
couche des cellules polyédriques	polyedrische „
ponts intercellulaires	Interzellularbrücken
fentes intercellulaires	Interzellulargänge
couche des cellules basales	Basalzellenschicht
Cellules pigmentaires ramifiées (chromatophores)	verzweigte Pigmentzellen (Chromatophoren)
Pigment épidermique	Epidermispigment
Bourrelets épidermiques	epidermoidale Warzen

PEAU (POISSONS OSSEUX)	HAUT (KNOCHENFISCHE)
— *Derme*	— *Cutis*
Plan d'écailles	Schuppenlage
Couche dermique superficielle	oberflächliche Cutisschicht
Cellules pigmentaires superficielles	oberflächliche Pigmentzellen
Loges squamales	Schuppensäckchen
Lames dermiques intermédiaires	intermediäre Cutis-lamellen
couche lâche périsquamale	
couche lamellaire (compacte) profonde	tiefe kompakte Lamellenschicht
cloisons verticales	vertikale Septa
couche pigmentaire profonde	tiefe Pigmentschicht
— *Hypoderme*	— *Unterhautgewebe*
— *Épiderme*	— *Epidermis*
Plan de cellules pavimenteuses	Pflasterzellenlage
de cellules cylindriques(-polymorphes)	zylindrisch-polymorphe Zelllage
Couche des cellules basales	Basalzellenschicht
Cellules muqueuses. Syn. de *Leydig*, caliciformes	Schleimzellen, *Leydig*'sche Zellen, Becherzellen
Cellules pigmentaires	Pigmentzellen
— *Épiderme (torpille)*	— *Epidermis (Torpedo)*
Couche de cellules à cuticule	Zellschicht mit Kutikularsaum

Plan épidermique principal	Hauptzelllage
Cellules muqueuses	Schleimzellen
Couche de cellules basales	Basalzellenschicht

PEAU (LAMPROIE)	HAUT (PETROMYZON)
— *Derme*	— *Cutis*
Lame dermique limitante	dermale Grenzschicht
Couche pigmentée superficielle	oberflächliche Pigmentlage
Couche lamellaire compacte	kompakte Lamellenschicht
Couche pigmentaire profonde	tiefe Pigmentschicht
— *Hypoderme*	— *Subcutis*
Plan des cellules adipeuses	Fettzellenlage
Cellules pigmentaires ramifiées	verzweigte Pigmentzellen
— *Épiderme*	— *Epidermis*
Cellules en massue	Kolbenzellen
sessiles	sessile
pédonculées	gestielte
gaine	Scheide
massue centrale	Innenkolben
canalicules collatéraux	kollaterale Kanälchen
renflement terminal	Endanschwellung
noyaux gemmés	Doppelkerne
Cellules granuleuses	Körnerzellen
à pédicule simple	einfachgestielte
à pédicule géminé	doppeltgestielte
cuticule	Kutikula
hyaloplasma	Hyaloplasma
granuloplasma	Granuloplasma
réseau fibrillaire terminal	Endfadenapparat
prolongements intracellulaires	intrazelluläre Fortsätze
noyau	Kern
nucléole	Nucleolus

GLANDES CUTANÉES	HAUTDRÜSEN
Glandes sébacées	*Talgdrüsen*
Type glandulaire sacculaire-aggloméré	Drüsentypus: säckchenförmig-gehäufter
Glandes indépendantes	selbständige Drüsen
— annexées aux follicules pileux	haarbalgständige „
— agminées	gehäufte „
— composées	zusammengesetzte „
Glandes sébo-cutanées proprement dites	eigentliche Haut-Fettdrüsen
glandes de la caroncule lacrymale	Drüsen der Caruncula lacrymalis
Glandes préputiales	Vorhautdrüsen
— des petites lèvres	Drüsen der Kleinschamlippen
Glandes sébacées en grappe de Meibomius	Meibom'sche Drüsen

Membrane propre	Membrana propria
Epithélium sécrétoire	excernierendes Epithel
„ pariétal	wandständige Epithelschicht
„ sébacé à noyau central	Fettepithel mit mittelständigen Kern
„ centro-acineux	zentroacinöses Epithel
Sébum	Sebum
Epithélium des voies excrétoires	Epithel der Ausführgänge
Glandes sébacées-annexes	Adnexe Fettdrüsen

Glandes sudoripares — *Schweissdrüsen*

Type glandulaire: tubuleux glomérulé	Drüsentypus: Knäuelförmig-tubulöser

Glandes cérumineuses — *Ohrschmalzdrüsen*

Glomérule sécrétoire:	Drüsenknäuel:
couche adventitielle	Adventitialschicht
membrane propre	Membrana propria
cellules myo-épithéliales	myo-epitheliale Zellen
epithélium sécrétoire	sezernierendes Epithel
granulations pigmentaires	Pigmentkörnchen
cuticule interne	innerer Epithelsaum
Conduit excréteur	Ausführgang
couche adventitielle	Adventitialschicht
membrane propre	Membrana propria
épithélium	Epithel
portion intra-épidermique du conduit excréteur	intraepidermales Ausführgangsteil
pore excréteur	Schweisspore
Glandes sudoripares à embouchure libre	Schweissdrüsen mit freier Mündung
„ débouchant dans un follicule pileux	„ mit Haarbalgmündung
Glandes de *Moll*	*Moll*'sche Drüsen

Glandes lactigènes — *Milchdrüsen*

Glande mammaire	Milchdrüse
Type glandulaire: eury-tubuleux-acineux composé	Drüsentypus: zusammengesetzter weitröhrig acinöser
Glandes lactigènes multiples	multiple Milchdrüsen
Lobes glandulaires	Drüsenlappen
Lobules	Drüsenläppchen
Tissu interstitiel	interstitielles Binde-gewebe
vésicules adipeuses	Fettzellen
Tubes acineux	acinöse Schläuche
Epithélium sécrétoire prismatique	prismatisches Drüsenepithel
„ „ cubique	kubisches „
Granulations graisseuses	Fettkörnchen
Conduits alvéolaires	Alveolargänge
Canaux excréteurs intra-lobulaires	intralobuläre Ausführgänge
„ „ interlobulaires	interlobuläre „

Conduits galactophores	Ductus lactiferi
Sinus	sinus lactiferi
Globules du colostrum	Colostrumkörperchen
Globules du lait	Milchkügelchen
Glandes de *Montgomery*	*Montgomery*'sche Drüsen
Glandules sébacées annexes	adnexe Fettdrüschen
Mamelon	Brustwarze
Aréole	Warzenhof
Muscles lisses cutanés	glatte Hautmuskeln
Vaisseaux sanguins	Blutgefässe
„ interlobulaires	interlobuläre
„ interalvéolaires	interalveoläre
„ réseau capillaire péri-alvéolaire	perialveoläres Kapillarnetz
„ des conduits excréteurs	Gefässe der Ausführgänge
Cercle veineux de Haller	Sinus venosus Halleri
Vaisseaux lymphatiques	Lymphgefässe
Fentes lymphatiques inter-alvéolaires (?)	interalveoläre Lymphspalten
Lymphatiques interlobulaires	interlobuläre Lymphgefässe
„ des conduits excréteurs	Lymphgefässe der Ausführgänge
Réseau lymphatique de l'aréole	Warzenhof-Lymphgefässnetz
Nerfs	Nerven
Plexus interlobulaire	interlobulärer Nervenplexus
„ interalvéolaire	interalveolärer „
„ épidermal	epidermaler „
rameaux perforants	Rami perforantes
plexus hypodermal	hypodermaler Plexus
arborisations terminales adcellulaires	adzelluläre Telodendrien

Glande uropygienne (du croupion) — *Gland. uropygica (Bürzeldrüse)*

Type glandulaire: Tubuleux-acineux à confluents glandulaires	Drüsentypus: schlaftubulöser mit Sammelgängen
Corps glandulaire	Drüsenkörper
Mamelon glandulaire	Drüsenwarze
Tubes glandulaires	Drüsenschläuche
Travées conjonctives inter-tubulaires	bindegewebige Septa
Fond glandulaire	Drüsenfundus
Corps glandulaire	Drüsenkörper
Embouchures dans les confluents glandulaires	Mündungen in die Sammelgänge
Confluents sous-mamillaires	submammilare Sammelgänge
Constrictions glandulaires	Drüsenkonstrictionen
Confluents mamillaires (externes)	mammillar Sammelgänge
Canalicules excréteurs	Ausführkanälchen
Tissu interstinel du mamelon	interstitielles Warzengewebe
Corpuscules de *Herbst*	*Herbst*'sche Nervenkörperchen
Revêtement cutané du mamelon	Hautdecke der Warze

Glandes fémorales sous-cutanées du lézard	*Subkutane Schenkeldrüsen der Eidechse*
Type glandulaire: sacculaire à conduit glandulaire commun	Drüsentypus: säckchenförmig, gemeinschaftlicher Drüsengang
Sacculus glandulaires	Drüsensäckchen
Travées inter-sacculaires	bindegewebige Septa
Conduit glandulaire commun	gemeinschaftlicher Drüsengang
Crypte excrétoire	exkretorische Krypte
Epithélium des sacrules glandulaires	Epithel der Drüsensäckchen
» couche épithéliale pariétale	wandständige Epithelschicht
» couche principale	Hauptschicht
Enveloppe glandulaire	Drüsenhülle
Epithélium du conduit glandulaire commun	Epithel des gemeinschaftlichen Drüsenganges
zone de cellules à noyau ratatiné	Zellzone mit geschrumpften Kernen
zone de cellules granulo-hyalines	körnig-hyaline Zellzone
zone de globes hyalins	hyaline Schollenzone
Paroi du conduit glandulaire commun	Wandung des gemeinschaftlichen Drüsenganges
couche dermique	dermale Lage
couche épidermique	epidermale Lage
Glandes cutanées des amphibiens	*Hautdrüsen der Amphibien*
Type glandulaire: vésiculaire simple	Drüsentypus: einfach-acinöser
Glandes superficielles (petites) (dites muqueuses)	oberflächliche (kleine) Schleimdrüsen
» profondes (gl. granuleuses)	tiefe Körnerdrüsen
Vésicule glandulaire	Drüsenacinus
couche adventitielle	Adventitialschicht
membrane propre	Membrana propria
cellules myo-épithéliales	myoepitheliale Zellen
épithélium du fond vésiculaire	Fundusepithel
épithélium de la région apicale	Epithel der apikalen Region
conduit intra-épidermique	intraepidermaler Gang
Glandes cutanées parotidiennes	*Parotiden*
Glandes latérales (salamandre) (glandes venimeuses)	*Seitendrüsen (Salamandra macula) (Giftdrüsen)*
Glandes cutanées du pouce (grenouille)	*Daumendrüsen (Frosch)*
Type glandulaire: sacculaire simple à diverticules secondaires	Drüsentypus: einfachsäckchen förmiger mit sekundären Ausstülpungen
Sacs glandulaires	Drüsensäckchen
Cloisons interglandulaires	Zwischendrüsensepta
Membrane propre	Membrana propria

Cloisons intraglandulaires	Innensepta
Diverticules épithéliaux secondaires	sekundäre Epitheldivertikel
Épithélium glandulaire	Drüsenepithel
portion granuleuse	Körniger Teil
granulations protoplasmiques	Granula
portion hyaline	hyaliner Teil
couche de noyaux pariétaux	wandständige Kernschicht
Épithélium de la région glandulaire apicale	Epithel der apikalen Drüsenregion
Conduit intra-épidermique	intraepidermaler Ausführgang

Glandes paracutanées — *Paracutane Drüsen*

(v. conjonctive, cloaque, prépuce) — (v. Conjunctiva, Kloake, Vorhaut)

ONGLES — NÄGEL

Lame onguéale	Nagelplatte
Stries inguéales	Nagelstreifen
Racine onguéale	Nagelwurzel
Lunule	Lunula
Bords latéraux	Seitenränder
Bord libre	Nagelrand
Écailles onguéales	Nagelschüppchen
Cellules onguéales	Nagelzellen
Matrice de l'ongle	Matrix
Loge onguéale	Nageltasche
Lit de l'ongle	Nagelbett
Sillons latéraux	Nagelfalz
Bourrelets latéraux	Nagelwall
Lame recouvrante de la racine	Wurzeldecke
Éponychium	Eponychium
Épidermicule de l'ongle	Hornstreifen
Plan épithélial supérieur de la racine	Oberwurzelepithellage
couche germinative	stratum germinativum
couche granuleuse	stratum granulosum
couche cornée	stratum corneum
Plan épithélial de la matrice	Matrixepithellage
Plan épithélial du lit de l'ongle	Nagelbettepithellage
couche germinative	strat. germinativum
granulations kératohyalines (ony- chogènes)	keratohyaline Granula
couche cornée	strat. corneum
Crêtes dermiques du lit onguéal	Nagelbettleisten
Vaisseaux sanguins du lit onguéal	Blutgefässe des Nagelbettes
Anses vasculaires des crêtes dermiques	gefässschlingen der Nagelbettleisten
Vaisseaux lymphatiques du lit onguéal (Tomsa)	Lymphgefässe des Nagelbettes
Nerfs du lit onguéal	Nerven des Nagelbettes
Histogénèse	*Histogenese*

Stade du bourrelet onguéal	Stadium des Nagelwalles
Rainure onguéale	Nagelrinne
Lame épidermique rétro-onguéale	retroungueale Epidermisplatte
couche prismatique	prismatische Zelllage
couche moyenne	mittlere Zelllage
couche supérieure	obere Zelllage
Bourrelet onguéal	Nagelwall
couche prismatique	prismatische Zelllage
couche de cellules polyédriques	polyedrische Zelllage
couche de grandes cellules kératinisées	Lage von grossen Hornzellen
couche épidermique superficielle	oberflächliche Epidermislage
Sillon préonguéal	Vornagelfurche
Stade de la lame onguéale	Stadium der Nagelplatte
Eponychium (couche épidermique sus-onguéale)	Eponychium (supraungueale Epidermislage)
Lame onguéale	Nagelplatte
zone radiculaire	Wurzelzone
zone moyenne	Mittelzone
sillon intermédiaire	Zwischenrinne
zone antérieure	Vorderzone
Bourrelet épidermique préonguéal	vorderer Epidermiswall
Epithélium de la région de la racine (matrice)	Epithel der Wurzelzone (Matrixepithel)
plan sus-onguéal	supraungueale Lage
plan sous-onguéal	infraungueale Lage
Epithélium du lit onguéal	Epithel des Nagelbettes
Crêtes épithéliales du lit	Epithelleisten des Nagelbettes

POILS   **HAARE**

Follicule pileux	Haarbalg
région papillaire	Papillarzone
" radiculaire	Wurzelzone
" du collet folliculaire	Halszone
" infundibulaire terminal	Endtrichter
Papille	Papille
collet	Hals
plaque sous-papillaire	Subpapillare Platte
Tunique folliculaire	Balgfaserhaut
couche externe	äussere Lage
couche interne	innere Lage
Membrane vitrée	Glashaut
Gaines épithéliales radiculaires	epitheliale Wurzelscheiden
G. ép. externe (folliculaire)	äussere Balgepithel
couche prismatique	prismatische Zellschicht
plan de cellules polyédriques et plates	polyedrisch platte Zelllage
G. ép. interne (radiculaire)	innere Wurzelepithelscheide

couche de *Henle* — *Henle'sche* Schicht
couche de *Huxley* — *Huxley'sche* „
Granulations kérato-hyalines — keratohyaline Granula
Cuticule interne de la gaine — Oberhäutchen der Wurzelscheide

Poil — *Haar*

Bulbe — Haar-Zwiebel
Racine — Wurzel
Tige (flèche) — Schaft
Cuticule du poil (épidermicule) — Haarcuticula (Oberhäutchen)
Cellules de la matrice — Matrixzellen
Substance corticale — Rindensubstanz
Substance médullaire — Marksubstanz
Fibres pileuses corticales — Rindenfasern (des Haares)
Granulations pigmentaires — Pigmentkörper
Stries pigmentaires — Pigmentstreifen
Cellules pigmentaires du bulbe — Pigmentzellen des Bulbus
Noyaux de la substance corticale — Kerne der Rindensubstanz
Fissures à air — Luftspalten
Cellules médullaires — Markzellen
Granulations kérato-hyalines — keratohyaline Granula
Glande sébacée — Haarbalgdrüse
Muscle arrecteur du poil — Arrector pili
Cils palpébraux — Lidrandcilien
Vibrisses — Nasenhaare (vibrissae)
Poils sans substance médullaire — marklose Haare
Vaisseaux sanguins — Gefässe
Vaisseaux du follicule pileux — Gefässe des Haarbalges
„   de la couche externe — „ der äusseren Lage
„   de la couche interne — „ der inneren Lage
Vaisseaux de la papille — Gefässe der Haarpapille
Vaisseaux lymphatiques du follicule pileux — Lymphgefässe des Haarbalges

Nerfs — *Nerven*

Anneau nerveux (Collier nerveux) — Nervenring
Fibres épilemmales — epilemmale Fasern
„   perforantes — durchbohrende „
„   hypolemmales — hypolemmale „
Arborisation terminale — Telodendron
Boutons terminaux — Endknöpfe
Plaques terminales — Endplatten
Disques tactiles — Tastscheiben

Histogénèse — *Histogenese*

Germe pileux — Haarkeim (Haarknospe)
Bourgeon pileux — Haarzapfen
Couche périféale prismatique — prismatische Wandschicht
Renflement terminal — Endanschwellung

Région bulbaire du germe	Zwiebelregion des Haarkeimes
Invagination bulbaire	Bulbus-Einstülpung
Germe de la papille	Papillenanlage
Papille	Papille
Couche dermique folliculaire	dermale Balgschicht
Renflement sébo-glandulaire	Balgdrüsenanlagen
Région sus-glandulaire du germe pileux	Supraglanduläre Haarkeimregion
Cône intérieur	Innenkegel
Gaine du cône intérieur	Scheide des Innenkegels
Epithélium de la matrice du poil	Matrixepithel
Gaine épithéliale externe (folliculaire)	äussere Epithelscheide (Balgepithel)
Bourgeons sébacés secondaires	sekundäre Balgdrüsenknospen
Eminence myo-épithéliale (?)	myo-epitheliale Knospe (?)
Eruption des poils	Durchbruch der Haare
Poils du duvet, Lanugo	Wollhaare, Lanugo
Vernix caseosa	Vernix caseosa
Chute des poils	Haarwechsel
Poils à bulbe plein	Kolbenhaare
Touffe pileuse	zerfasertes Haarende
Poils de remplacement	Ersatzhaare

Mammifères

Säugetiere

Poils à canal médullaire cloisonné	Haare mit gefensterten Markkanal
Soies	Borstenhaare
Poils à sinus vasculaires	Sinushaare
Follicule	Balg
Tunique fibreuse	Faserhaut
Tunique caverneuse	kavernöse Scheide
plan externe (à sinus sanguins), externe sanguine supérieure	äussere Lage (Blutsinuslage), oberer Blutraum
plan interne (compact, à vaisseaux fins)	innere Lage (kompakte, mit feinem Gefässnetzen)
Bourrelet du plan interne de la tun. caverneuse	Wulst der inneren Lage
Couche lâche intermédiaire	lockere Zwischenschicht
Tunique vitrée	Glashaut
Gaine épithéliale folliculaire	Balgepithelscheide
Gaine épithéliale radiculaire	Wurzelepithelscheide
Cuticule du poil	Haaroberhäutchen
Couche corticale du poil	Rindenschicht
Canal médullaire	Markkanal
Substance médullaire	Marksubstanz
Réseau vasculaire de la moelle pileuse	Gefässnetz des Haarmarkes
Glande sébacée	Talgdrüse
Tunique fibreuse engainante	äussere Faserhaut

Piquants (Hérisson)	*Stacheln (Igel)*
Follicule	Stachelbalg
Tunique folliculaire	Balgfaserhaut
Membrane vitrée	Glashaut
Gaine épithéliale folliculaire	epitheliale Balgscheide
Gaine épithéliale radiculaire	epitheliale Wurzelscheide
Piquant	Stachel
bulbe	Zwiebel (Bulbus)
encoche sus-bulbaire	suprabulbäre Einkerbung
collet	Hals
racine	Wurzel
tige	Stachelschaft
pointe	Stachelspitze
stries longitudinales	Längstreifen
cuticule	Oberhäutchen
substance corticale	Rinde
pigment de la subst. corticale	Pigment
Travées cortico-médullaires externes	äusseres Balkensystem der Marksubstanz
Travées centrales	zentrale Balken
Compartiments médullaires externes	äussere Markfelder
Compartiments méd. internes	innere Markfelder
Espace médullaire de la racine et du bulbe	Markraum der Wurzel und des Bulbus
Cellules de la substance médullaire	Markzellen
Stries médullaires convexes	gewölbte Markstreifen
Papille	Balgpapille
Région bulbaire du follicule	Zwiebelregion des Balges (Balggrund)
Épithélium du fond folliculaire	Balggrundepithel
„ papillaire	Papillenepithel
(Épithélium de la matrice)	(Matrixepithel)
Couche bulbaire sus-épithéliale	supraepitheliale Zwiebelschicht
Muscle folliculaire (arrecteur)	Balgmuskel (Arrector)
„ faisceaux descendants	absteigende Bündel
„ faisceaux latéraux	laterale „
„ faisceaux ascendants	aufsteigende „
Utricules sébacées folliculaires	Balgfettsäckchen

PLUMES	FEDERN
Follicule et racine de la plume	*Federbalg und Federwurzel*
Tunique folliculaire	Balgscheide
Lame vitrée	Glashaut
Gaine épithéliale folliculaire	epitheliale Balgepithelscheide
Gaine épithéliale radiculaire	Wurzelepithelscheide
Tuyau de la racine	Spule
Papille folliculaire	Balgpapille

Collet de la papille	Hals
Ombilic inférieur	Umbilicus inferior
Trame papillaire fondamentale	Grundsubstanz der Papille
Couche papillaire marginale	Randschicht
Épithélium papillaire	Papillenepithel
Lamelles épithéliales péripapillaires	peripapilläre Epithellamellen
Lamelles cornées du canal médullaire (Lamelles choronnantes)	Horndamellen des Markkanals (Markhornscheiden)
Muscles folliculaires	Balgmuskeln
faisceaux de la base	Basalbündel
faisceaux latéraux	Seitenbündel

Plume propr. dite — *Eigentliche Feder*

Hampe	Scapus (Kiel)
Tuyau de la racine	Spule
Strie médullaire cornée (âme de la plume)	Markhornstreifen (Federseele)
Tige	Schaft (Rachis)
Ombilic supérieur	oberer Nabel
Face convexe de la tige (antérieure, supérieure)	konvexe Fläche (vordere, obere)
Face concave (postérieure, inférieure)	konkave Fläche (hintere, untere)
sillon longitudinal	Längsfurche
Substance corticale (de la tige)	Rindenschicht
médullaire	Markschicht
Vexillum	Fahne
Barbes	Federn (Rami)
Barbules	Federchen (Radii)
Crochets	Näcken (Hamuli)

Follicule plumigène — *Federkeim*

Tuniques folliculaires	Balgscheiden
Tunique fibreuse	Faserhaut
plan externe	äussere Lage
interne	innere Lage
Membrane vitrée	Glashaut
Gaine épithéliale folliculaire	epitheliale Balgscheide
couche cylindrique	Zylinderzellschicht
couche polyédrique aplatie	polyedrisch platte Zelllage
Gaine épithéliale radiculaire (gaine de la plume)	epitheliale Wurzelscheide (Federscheide)
plan externe (corné)	äussere Lage (Hornschicht)
plan interne	innere Lage'
Papille folliculaire	Balgpapille
collet	Hals
prolongements latéraux basilaires	seitliche Basalfortsätze
sommet	Spitze

Matrice épithéliale plumigère	Matrixepithel des Federkeimes
renflement bulbaire	Bulbus
épithélium papillaire	Papillenepithel
„ latéral	Seitenepithel
„ apical	apikales „
Crêtes épithéliales	Epitheleisten
(Rayons épithéliaux)	(Epithelstrahlen)
„ primaires	primäre
„ secondaires	sekundäre
Cellules axiles (médullaires)	axile Zellen (Markzellen)
Cellules pariétales (corticales)	Wandzellen (Rindenzellen)
Prolongements papillaires intermédiaires	intermediäre Papillenfortsätze
Gaine cornée commune des crêtes épithéliales	gemeinschaftliche Hornscheide der Epitheleisten
Cellules pigmentaires marginales de la papille	Randpigmentzellen der Papille
Cellules pigmentaires des crêtes épithéliales	Pigmentzellen der Epitheleisten
Région génératrice de la hampe	kielbildende Region
couche épithél. germinative (prismatique)	Keimschicht
couche alvéolaire	Alveolarschicht
couche cornée	Hornschicht

ORGANES DES SENS

I. Intra-épithéliaux

ORGANE DE LA GUSTATION	GESCHMACKSORGAN
Gobelets gustatifs	Schmeckbecher
Syn. Bourgeons gustatifs	Geschmacksknospen
Corpuscules du goût	
Bourgeons épithéliaux	Epithelknospen
Bourgeons terminaux	Endknospen
Bulbes gustatifs	Geschmackskolben
Base	Basalende
Sommet	Spitze
Faces latérales	Seitenflächen
Pore gustatif	Porus
„ externe	äusserer
„ interne	innerer
Couronne ciliée	Härchenkranz
Cellules pariétales. Syn. recouvrantes	Wandzellen. Deckzellen
extérieures	äussere
de soutenement externes	äussere Stützzellen
Extrémité profonde	tiefes Zellende
„ périphérique	Oberflächliches „
Noyau	Kern

Cellules centrales	zentrale Zellen
Cell. gustatives	Geschmackszellen
— sensorielles	Sinneszellen
— neuro-épithéliales	Neuroepithelzellen
Cellules en bâtonnet	Stäbchenzellen
Cellules en pointe	Stiftchenzellen
Cellules fusiformes	Spindelzellen
Prolongement périphérique de la cellule gustative, cil gustatif	äusserer Fortsatz
Prolongement profond (basal)	tiefer (basaler)
Zone nucléée	Kernzone
Cellules de soutènement internes	innere Stützzellen
Cellules basales	Basalzellen
Plexus nerveux sous-basal	subgemmaler Plexus
Fibres périgemmales	perigemmale Fasern
— intragemmales	intragemmale
— intergemmales	intergemmale

Disque gustatif (grenouille)	*Geschmacksscheibe (Frosch)*
Région du bord	Seitenrandregion
Région principale	Hauptregion
Zone épithéliale périphérique (nucléée, striée)	peripherische Epithelzone (kernlosa, gestreifte)
zone profonde (nucléée)	tiefe Zone (kernhaltige)
strie intermédiaire	Zwischenstreifen
zone fibrillaire (cupule nerveuse)	fibrilläre Zone (Nervenschale)
chorion sous-épithélial	subepitheliales Chorion
zone claire du chorion	helle Choriumzone
zone vasculo-nerveuse	Gefäss Nervenzone
Cellules épithéliales cylindriques	Zylinderzellen
région striée	gestreifte Zone
région nucléée	Kernzone
prolongement profond	tiefer Fortsatz
Cellules à bâtonnet (neuro-épithéliales)	Stäbchenzellen (neuroepitheliale)
Cellules fusiformes	spindelförmige Zellen
Cellules à noyau basilaire	Zellen mit basalem Kern
Cellules de soutènement	Stützzellen
Cellules fourchues	Gabelzellen
Cellules à ailes	Flügelzellen
Nerfs papillaires	Papillarnerven
Plexus sous-basal	Basalplexus
Plexus sous-gemmal cupuliforme (Poissons)	Schalenförmiger Nervenplexus (Fische)
Plexus sous-épithélial	sub-epithelialer Plexus
Plexus intra-épithélial	intraepithelialer Plexus
Terminaisons libres	freie Nervenendigungen
Réseaux péricellulaires	perizelluläre Netze
Terminaisons nerveuses de continuité	Nervenendigungen per continuitatem

Plaques terminales	Endplatten
Manteau nerveux (?)	nervöse Mantelschicht
Cellules ganglionnaires sous-épithéliales	subepitheliale Ganglienzellen

ORGANE DE L'OLFACTION — GERUCHSORGAN

Epithélium de la muqueuse olfactive	Epithel der Riechschleimhaut
Bordure ciliée	Ciliensaum
Plateau cuticulaire	Kutikularsaum
Zone sans noyaux	kernlose Zone
Zone à noyaux superposés	mehrzeilige Kernzone
Cellules olfactives	Riechzellen
prolongement périphérique	peripherischer Fortsatz
cil olfactif	Riechcilie
prolongement profond (nerveux?)	tiefer Fortsatz (Nervenfortsatz)
zone nucléaire	Kernzone
noyau	Kern
nucléole	Nucleolus
Cellules de soutenement	Stützzellen
prolongement cylindrique cannelé	gefurchter Zylinderfortsatz
prolongement festonné	ausgeschnittener Fortsatz
Cellules basales	Basalzellen
Tunique propre de la muqueuse olfactive	Tunica propria der Riechschleimhaut
couche sous-épithéliale	subepitheliale Schicht
plan glandulaire	Drüsenlage
Glandes de *Bowman*	*Bowman*'sche Drüsen
Culs de sac glandulaires	Drüsensäckchen
membrane propre	Membrana propria
épithélium sécrétoire	Drüsenepithel
conduit excréteur intra-épithélial	intraepithelialer Ausführgang
épithélium du conduit	Ausführgangsepithel
Travées interglandulaires	Zwischendrüsensepta
Plan nerveo-vasculaire profond	tiefe Nerven- und Gefässlage
Faisceaux nerveux olfactifs	Riechnervenbündel
Fibrilles olfactives	Riechfibrillen
Arborisations intra-épithéliales libres	intraepitheliale Endedendrien

Fossette olfactive de la grenouille — *Riechgrübchen des Frosches*

Muqueuse olfactive	Riechschleimhaut
Cellules olfactives	Riechzellen
Cils olfactifs	Riechcilien
Cellules de soutenement intermédiaires	Stützzellen (Zwischenzellen)
partie cylindrique	zylindrischer Zellteil
partie nucléée	Kernzone
nucléole	Nucleolus
prolongement festonné (profond)	ausgeschnittener Fortsatz

Cellules basales	Basalzellen
Tunique propre (chorion)	Tunica propria
couche sous-épithéliale	subepitheliale Lage
plan profond	tiefe Lage
Glandes de *Bowman*	*Bowman*'sche Drüsen
sacs glandulaires	Drüsensäckchen
membrane propre	Membrana propria
épithélium à grosses granulations	grobkörniges Epithel
extrémité cellulaire profonde	tiefes Zellende
onglet	Hacken
noyau basilaire	Basalkern
nucléole	Nucleolus
conduit excréteur intra-épithélial	intraepithelialer Ausführgang
Cellules pigmentaires de la tunique propre	Pigmentzellen der Tunica propria
Faisceaux nerveux olfactifs	Riechnervenbündel
sous-épithéliaux	
profonds	
Vaisseaux sanguins	Blutgefässe
superficiels (plan sous-épithélial)	subepitheliale Lage
profonds	tiefe Gefässlage

<table>
<tr><td align="center">II. Organes des sens tégumentaires</td><td align="center">II. Integument-Sinnesorgane</td></tr>
<tr><td align="center">CANAUX LATÉRAUX (POISSONS)</td><td align="center">SEITENKANÄLE (FISCHE)</td></tr>
</table>

Enveloppe conjonctive	Bindegewebshülle
Couche cellulaire plate limitante	platte Zellgrenzschicht
Fente cloisonnée péricanaliculaire	Spaltraum und Balkengewebe
Membrane basale	Basalmembran
Épithélium de revêtement	Deckepithel
couche externe à noyaux plats	äussere plattkernige Schicht
de cellules cubiques	kubische Zellschicht
plateau cuticulaire	Kutikularsaum
Éminences neuro-épithéliales	Neuroepitheliale Hügel
Disque épithélial	Epithelscheibe
excavation centrale	centrale Einsenkung
bordure ciliée	Cilienzone
plateau cuticulaire	Kutikularsaum
cellules cylindriques évasées	Kolbenzellen
cellules intermédiaires	Zwischenzellen
cellules basales	Basalzellen
recouvrantes latérales	seitliche Belegzellen
Couche vasculo-nerveuse sous-épithéliale	subepitheliale Gefäss- und Nervenschicht

<table>
<tr><td align="center">III. Organes des sens composés</td><td align="center">III. Zusammengesetzte Sinnesorgane</td></tr>
<tr><td align="center">APPAREIL DE L'AUDITION</td><td align="center">GEHÖRAPPARAT</td></tr>
<tr><td align="center">*Oreille interne (Mammifères)*</td><td align="center">*Inneres Ohr (Säugetiere)*</td></tr>
</table>

Labyrinthe osseux	knöchernes Labyrinth
membraneux	häutiges

Périlymphe	Perilymphe
Endolymphe	Endolymphe

Canaux semicirculaires	*Bogengänge*
Canaux osseux	knöcherne Gänge
périoste	Periost
espace cavitaire (lymphatique)	Lymphraum
tissu trabéculaire cloisonnant	Balkengewebe
tissu rétiforme	netzförmiges Gewebe
Canaux membraneux	häutige Bogengänge
extrémité ampullaire	Ampullenende
« non ampullaire	ampullenfreies Ende
tunique propre	Tunica propria
couche basale	Basalschicht
épithélium de revêtement	Deckepithel
Ampoules	Ampullen
postérieure	hintere
antérieure	vordere
externe	äussere
Crêtes acoustiques	Cristae acusticae (Hörleisten)
Vestibule osseux	knöcherner Vorhof
Vestibule membraneux	häutiger
Utricule	Utriculus (elliptisches Säckchen)
Saccule	Sacculus (rundes Säckchen)
Conduit utriculo-sacculaire	Ductus utriculo-saccularis
Conduit endolymphatique	Ductus endolymphaticus
Canalis reuniens	—
Taches acoustiques	Maculae acusticae (Hörflecken)
Otolithes	Otolithen
Otoconie	Otoconia (Gehörsand)
Épithélium des crêtes et taches acoustiques	Epithel der Cristae u. Maculae
Disque neuro-épithélial	Epithelwall
Couche de cils	Cilienschicht
Plateau cuticulaire	Kutikularsaum
Couche sans noyaux	kernfreie Epithelschicht
Couche de noyaux superposés	Kernanlage
Cellules ciliées	Haarzellen
Cellules intermédiaires (intercalaires) (de soutènement)	Zwischenzellen (Stützzellen)
Cellules à noyau basal	basalkernige Zellen
Épithélium marginal	Grenzepithel
Intumescence de la tunique propre (crêtes et taches acoustiques)	Verdickung der Tunica propria (Cristae u. Maculae)
couche basale (sous-épithéliale)	Basalschicht
couche fibrillaire hyaline	hyaline Faserschicht
couche fasciculée	grobfaserige Schicht
Vaisseaux superficiels (sous-épithéliaux)	oberflächliche Gefässige

Vaisseaux profonds	tiefe Gefässlage
Nerfs des taches et crêtes acoustiques	Nervenäste Maculae u. Cristae
Plexus nerveux de la tunique propre	Nervenlage der Tunica propria
Fibres perforantes	durchtretende Nervenfasern
Plexus intraépithélial	intraepithelialer Plexus
Fibrilles terminales	Endfibrillen
Calices nerveux (?)	Endkelche (Nervenkelche) (?)
Terminaisons en chandelier	leuchterförmige Nervenendigungen

Limaçon osseux

Knöcherne Schnecke

Membraneux	Häutige
Axe osseux a. columelle	Modiolus
Crible de la base	Cribrum basale
Rampe vestibulaire	Scala vestibuli
„ tympanique	„ tympani
Canal cochléaire	Ductus cochlearis (Schneckengang)
Lame spirale osseuse	Lamina spiralis ossea
bord adhérent	adhärenter Rand
lèvre de la lame spir.	Labium laminae spiralis
couche osseuse vestibulaire	vestibuläre Knochenlage
couche osseuse tympanique	tympanale
canal nerveux	Nervenkanal
travées osseuses rhizonantes	Knochensepta
espaces périnerveux	perinervöse Spalträume
pertuis nerveux	Foramina nervina
Bandelette sillonnée	Lamina sulcata s. Limbus spiralis
lèvre vestibulaire	Labium vestibulare (Limbus)
crête spirale	Crista spiralis
dents auditives (de Huschke)	Hörzähne
sillon spiral (interne)	Sulcus spiralis (internus)
prolongement basilaire de la bande-	Basalfortsatz der Lam. sulc.
lette	
zone perforée	Habenula perforata
couche principale de la band. sil.	Hauptschicht der Lam. sulc. (grobfa-
fasciculée	serige Schicht)
couche fibro-hyaline	hyaline Faserschicht
vaisseaux de la couche principale	Gefässe der Hauptschicht
couche cellulaire prismatique du limbe	prismatische Zellschicht des Labium
de la lèvre vestibulaire	vestibulare
cuticule	Kutikula
Epithélium du sillon spiral	Epithel des Sulcus spiralis
Membrane de Corti	Membrana tectoria
bord adhérent	adhärenter Rand
partie principale	Hauptteil
bord libre	freier Rand
renflement terminal	Endanschwellung
stries de la membrane	Streifen
Membrane basilaire	Membrana basilaris

zone lisse	zona laevis (tecta)
zone pectinée	zona pectinata
couche limitante sous-épithéliale	subepitheliale Grenzschicht
couche des fibres radiaires	Radiärfaserschicht
Lame neuro-épithéliale du canal cochléaire	*Neuroepithel-platte* des Ductus cochlearis
Épithélium limitant interne	inneres Grenzepithel
Cellules ciliées internes	innere Haarzellen
bâtonnets auditifs	Haarstäbchen
plateau cuticulaire	Kutikularsaum
extrémité cellulaire périphérique	peripherisches Zellende
région nucléaire	Kernzone
extrémité cellulaire profonde	tiefes Zellende
Cellules intermédiaires (intercalaires) (de soutènement)	Zwischenzellen (Stützzellen)
Arc de Corti	*Corti'scher Bogen*
Tunnel	Tunnel
Pilier interne	innere Pfeilerzelle
Pilier externe	aussere Pfeilerzelle
extrémité céphalique (tête)	Kopfteil (Kopf)
pilier	Pfeiler
base (pied)	Basal (s. Fuss) platte
partie hyaline de la base	hyaliner Teil
partie granuleuse	granulierter „
région nucléaire	Kernzone
articulation des piliers	Pfeilergelenk
facette concave du pilier interne	konkave Gelenkfläche
facette convexe du pilier externe	konvexe gelenkfläche
plateau céphalique du pilier interne	innere Kopfplatte
prolongement phalangien du pilier externe	Phalangenfortsatz
espace de *Nuel*	*Nuel'scher Raum*
Cellules ciliées externes	*äussere Haarzellen*
bâtonnets auditifs	Hörstäbchen
plateau cuticulaire	Kutikularsaum
extrémité cellulaire périphérique	peripherisches Zellende
corps hyalin (de *Hensen*)	hyaliner Körper
région nucléaire	Kernzone
prolongement profond	tiefer Fortsatz
éminence nerveuse interne	innerer Nervenhügel
strie granuleuse	Körnerstreifen
Cellules de *Deiters*	*Deiters'sche Zellen*
région basilaire	Basalteil
Noyau gemmé	Kern
Col	Halsteil
prolongement filiforme	Endenfortsatz
strie de *Retzius*	*Retzius'scher Streifen*
stries limitantes	Grenzstreifen
cône basal des stries limitantes	Basalkegel der Grenzstreifen

Membrane réticulée	Membrana reticularis
Phalanges	Phalangen
de la 1re rangée	erster Reihe
de la 2e	zweiter
de la 3e	dritter
cadre terminal	Schlussrahmen
Épithélium limitant externe	äusseres Grenzepithel
Cellules de *Hensen*	*Hensen*'sche Zellen
cellules de *Claudius*	*Claudius*'sche
Revêtement cellulaire de la face tympa-	tympanale Zellbelegschicht der Membr.
nique de la membrane basilaire	basilaris
Vaisseau spiral	vas spirale
Ligament spiral	Ligamentum spirale
plan profond	tiefe Lage
plan superficiel	oberflächliche
bord d'insertion	Insertionsrand
Bandelette vasculaire	Stria vascularis
couche épithéliale	
couche cellulo-vasculaire	
plateau cuticulaire	Kutikularsaum
lame épithéliale	Epithelplatte
couche lacunaire (vésiculaire)	Stratum lacunosum (vesiculare)
vaisseaux capillaires intra-épithé-	intraepitheliale Kapillargefässe
liaux	
vaisseaux de la couche lacunaire	Gefässe des Stratum lacunosum des
	Epitheli
pigment de l'épithélium de la bande-	Pigment der Stria vascularis
lette vasculaire	
Promontoire	Promontorium
épithélium du promont.	Epithel
Sillon spiral externe	Sulcus spiralis externus
Membrane de *Reissner* (Membrane vés-	*Reissner*'sche Membran (Membrana ves-
tibulaire)	tibularis)
couche fondamentale	Grundschicht
revêtement cellulaire vestibulaire	vestibuläre Zellbelegschicht
revêtement cochléaire	cochleäre
Vaisseaux des rampes vestibulaire et	Gefässe der Scalae vestib. und tymp.
tympanique	
Vaisseaux de la lame spirale osseuse	Gefässe der Lam. spir. ossea
Vaisseaux périostique de la lame spir.	Gefässe des Periostes
osseuse	
Vaisseaux de la bandelette sillonnée	gefässe der Lamina sulcata
Vaisseau spiral	Vas spirale
Vaisseaux du ligament spiral	Gefässe des Ligam. spir.
Vaisseaux de la bandelette vasculaire	Gefässe der Stria vascularis
sous épithéliaux	subepitheliale
intra-épithéliaux	intraepitheliale
Vas prominens	

Canaux semi-circulaires membraneux (oiseaux)	*Häutige Bogengänge (Vögel)*
Tunique adventice vasculaire	adventicielle Gefässschicht
tunique propre chondroïde	chondroïde Tunica propria
épithélium de revêtement	Deckepithel
Espace cavitaire cloisonné	äusserer Lymphraum
tissu rétiforme	Netzgewebe
périoste interne	inneres Periost
Crêtes acoustiques	Cristae acusticae
région de la base	Basalregion
du col	Halsregion
bourrelets latéraux	Seitenwülste
éminence médiane	Mittelwulst
région du toit	Dachregion
Intumescence de la tunique propre	Anschwellung der Tunica propria
Lame épithéliale de la crête	Epithelplatte des Hörhügels
épithélium cilié de l'éminence médiane	Haarepithel des Mittelwulstes
épithélium cilié du col	der Halsregion
épithélium des bourrelets latéraux	Epithel der Seitenwülste
cellules en bouteille (en cruche)	flaschenförmige (krugförmige) Zellen
cellules cylindro-coniques	konisch-cylindrische Zellen
épithélium de la base de la crête	Epithel der Basalregion der Crista
épithélium du toit	Dachepithel

LIMAÇON	*Schnecke*
Rampe vestibulaire	Scala vestibularis
Rampe tympanique	Scala tympani
Paroi osseuse	knöcherne Wand
Périoste interne	inneres Periost
Fente cavitaire cloisonnée	Lymphraum
Tissu rétiforme	Netzgewebe
Bandelette vasculo-épithéliale de la rampe vestibulaire	Gefäss-Epithelpolster der Scala tympani
Couche conjonctive externe à noyaux aplatis	äussere plattförmige Schicht
Plan épithélial	Epithellage
Flots épithéliaux	Epithelinseln
Cellules épithéliales vésiculaires	blasige Epithelzellen
Cellules granuleuses fuseolaes	lichtbrechende Körnerzellen
vaisseaux sous-épithéliaux	Subepitheliale Gefässe
vaisseaux intra-épithéliaux	intraepitheliale Gefässe
Lame chondroïde externe	äusserer Knorpelrahmen
Côte pariétal	wandständige Scale
Lexne de la l. chaud ext.	Lаmina

Lame chondroïde interne	innerer Knorpelrahmen
côté pariétal	wandständige Seite
face vestibulaire	vestibuläre Fläche
face tympanique	tympanale
promontoire	Promontorium
sillon interne	Sulcus internus
région perforée	Zona perforata
lèvre de la l. chond. int.	Labium des inn. Knorpelrahmens
canal nerveux	Nervenkanal
loge du ganglion cochléaire	Ganglionkanal
Lame basilaire	Membrana basilaris
Epithélium du promontoire et du sillon interne	Epithel des Promontoriums und des Sulcus internus
Lame neuro-épithéliale de la membrane basilaire	Neuroepitheliale Platte der Memb. basilaris
Revêtement vestibulaire de la lame chondr. externe	Vestibulare Epithelschicht des äuss. Knorpelrahmens
Membrana tectoria	
Renflement terminal du limaçon	Endanschwellung der Schnecke
Tache nerveuse terminale	Macula terminalis
Arc chondroïde	Knorpelbogen
Région de la lame neuro-épithéliale basilaire	Ableitung der basilaren Neuroepithel-platte
Tunnel sous basilaire	subbasilarer Tunnel
Région de la tache nerveuse terminale	Abteilung der Macula terminalis
Faisceaux nerveux de la tache terminale	Nervenbündel der Macula
Lame neuro-épithéliale de la tache	neuroepitheliale Platte der Macula
Epithélium bordant externe	äusseres Grenzepithel
Epithélium bordant interne	inneres
couche des otolithes	Otolithenschicht

Labyrinthe membraneux (Amphibiens)	*Häutiges Labyrinth (Amphibien)*
Canaux semi-circulaires	Bogengänge
Epithélium de revêtement	Deckepithel
Tunique propre chondroïde	Chondroide Tunica propria
substance fondamentale hyaline	hyaline Grundsubstanz
cellules ramifiées	verzweigte Zellen
fentes péricellulaires	perizelluläre Spalträume
Couche adventice vasculaire	adventielle
Cellules pigmentaires	gefässchicht Pigmentzellen
Espace cavitaire cloisonné	äusserer Lymphraum
Tissu réiforme	Netzgewebe
Crêtes acoustiques	Cristae acusticae
région basale	Basalregion
collicule	Hügel
excavation cupuliforme	schalenförmige Einsenkung (cupula)
rigole latérale	Seitenrinne

Lame neuro-épithéliale	Neuroepitheliale Platte
cellules ciliées périphériques	oberflächliche Haarzellen
cellules ciliées profondes (grêles)	tiefe Haarzellen
cellules filiformes (de soutènement)	Fadenzellen (Stützzellen)
Épithélium de la rigole latérale	Epithel der Seitenrinne
Utricule	Utriculus
segment post-endolymphatique (postérieur)	hintere Abteilung
segment pré-endolymphatique (antérieur)	vordere ,,
conduit endolymphatique	Ductus endolymphaticus
Excroissances de l'utricule:	Ausbuchtungen des Utriculus
—Postérieure (à parois épaisses) basilaire	hintere (dickwandige) Pars basilaris
tache nerveuse	Macula
—Latérale-interne	Laterale-innere (Pars neglecta)
,, région postérieure	hintere Abteilung
,, région moyenne (sulciforme)	mittlere (rinnenförmige)
,, région antérieure	vordere
tache nerveuse	Macula
—Inféro-postérieure (dite lagena)	Untere-hintere (sogenannte Lagena)
tache nerveuse	Macula
—Inféro-antérieure (sacculiforme)	Untero-vordere (Sacculus)
tache nerveuse	Macula
Tache nerveuse du fond de l'utricule	Macula des Fundus utriculi
Taches nerveuses à 2 plans de noyaux	Maculae mit 2 Kernreihen
,, à plusieurs (3 à 5) plans de noyaux	,, mit mehrzeiliger Kernzone
Pigment des taches nerveuses	Pigment der Nervenflecken
Otolithes	Otolithen
Épithélium strié du labyrinthe membraneux (cellules à bâtonnets basaux)	Stäbchenepithel des häutigen Labyrinthes
Nerfs:	Nerven:
Division postérieure du n. acoustique:	hintere Abteilung des N. acusticus:
,, branche ampullaire postérieure	Zweig für die hintere Ampulle
,, de l'excroissance basilaire	für die Pars basilaris
,, de l'excroissance latérale-interne	für die Pars neglecta
,, de l'excroissance inféro-postérieure	für die Lagena
Division antérieure du n. acoust.	Vordere Abteilung des N. acusticus
,, branche de l'excroissance sacculaire	für den Sacculus
,, de la tache du fond de l'utricule	für die Boden-Macula des Utriculus
,, ampullaire antérieure	für die vordere Ampulle
,, ampullaire externe	für die äussere Ampulle
Coupole gélatineuse (poissons)	gelatinöse Kappe (Velum gelatinosum)
Cellules granuleuses en cruche (poissons)	krugförmige Körnerzellen

Oreille moyenne. Syn. Caisse du tympan | *Mittleres Ohr. Paukenhöhle*

Tunique muqueuse	Schleimhaut
tunique propre (chorion)	Tunica propria
épithélium de revêtement	Deckepithel
„ „ à cils vibratiles	Flimmerepithel
„ „ non cilié	flimmerloses
Osselets	Gehörknöchelchen
Marteau	Hammer
Manche	Manubrium
Enclume	Amboss
Apophyse lenticulaire	Processus lenticularis
Étrier	Steigbügel
„ base	Basis
Muscles des osselets	Muskeln der Gehörknöchelchen
Articulation du marteau avec l'enclume	Hammer-Amboss-Gelenk
„ de l'enclume avec l'étrier	Amboss-Steigbügel-Gelenk
Ligaments des osselets	Bänder der Gehörknöcheln
Trompe d'Eustache	Tuba Eustachii (Ohrtrompete)
portion osseuse	knöchernen Teil
„ fibreuse	fibröser
„ cartilagineuse	knorpeliger
Cartilage élastique	elastischer Knorpel
Cartilage hyalin	hyaliner
Muqueuse	Schleimhaut
tunique propre (chorion)	Tunica propria
Glandes tubaires	Drüsen der Tuber
infiltrations lymphadénoïdes	lymphadenoïde Herde
épithélium à cils vibratiles	Flimmerepithel

Oreille externe | *Äusseres Ohr.*

Pavillon	Ohrmuschel
Revêtement cutané	Hautdecke
de l'hélix	der Helix
de l'anthélix	der Anthelix
de la fossette naviculaire	
du tragus	des Tragus
de l'antitragus	des Antitragus
de la conque	der Concha
du lobule de l'oreille	des Ohrläppchens
Follicules pileux	Haarbälge
Poils follets	Wollhaare
Glandes sébacées	Balgdrüsen
Glandes sudoripares	Schweissdrüsen
Cartilage de soutènement	Stützknorpel
Cartilage élastique	elastischer Knorpel

Ilots cartilagineux ramollis	erweichte Knorpelherde
Ilots cartilagineux hyalins	hyaline Knorpelherde
Périchondre	Perichondrium
Conduit auditif externe	äusserer Gehörgang
portion cartilagineuse	knorpeliger Teil
portion osseuse	knöcherner Teil
Lame cartilagineuse élastique	elastische Knorpelplatte
Périchondre	Perichondrium
Couche sous-cutanée	Unterhautgewebe
Revêtement cutané	Hautschicht
— Région externe	— äussere Region
folicules pileux	Haarbälge
Glandes sébacées	Talgdrüsen
" à conduit évasé	" mit erweiterten Ausführgänge
Glandes cérumineuses	Ohrschmalzdrüsen
Cérumen	Ohrschmalz
— Région interne	— innere Region
Membrane du tympan	Membrana tympani
Couche propre	Grundmembran
Syn. Lame fibreuse	Faserhaut
fibres radiaires	radiäre Fasern
fibres circulaires	kreisförmige Fasern
anneau tympanique (fibro-cartilagineux)	Annulus fibrocartilagineus
région du manche du marteau	Region des Hammerhandgriffs
revêtement épidermique	epidermale Deckschicht
revêtement épithélial interne	inneres Deckepithel

APPAREIL DE LA VISION — SEHAPPARAT

Globe oculaire (œil) sclérotique — *Augapfel. Sclera (Sclerotica)*

Couche adventitielle externe	äussere Adventitialschicht
Tunique fibreuse	Faserhaut
" région limitante antérieure	vordere Grenzzone
" région d'insertions tendineuses	Sehnenansatzregion
" principale	Hauptregion
Cellules pigmentaires de la tunique fibreuse	Pigmentzellen der Fibrosa
Vaisseaux de la couche adventice	Gefässe der Adventitia
Vaisseaux de la tunique fibreuse	Gefässe der Fibrosa
Vaisseaux de la région limitante antérieure	Gefässe der vorderen Grenzzone
Sclérotique (vertébrés)	Sclera (Wirbeltiere)
Plaques cartilagineuses	Scleraknorpel
Cartilage pigmenté hyalin	hyaliner Pigmentknorpel
Plaques osseuses	Scleraknochen
" antérieures	vorderer Knochenring
" postérieures	hinterer "

Espaces médullaires	Markräume
Lamelles périmédullaires	perimedulläre Lamellen
Lamelles fondamentales	Grundlamellen
Médullocelles	Markzellen
Cellules adipeuses	Fettzellen
Cellules géantes	Riesenzellen

Cornée — *Hornhaut (Cornea)*

Épithélium antérieur	vorderes Deckepithel
Membrane basale ou limitante antérieure (de *Bowman*)	vordere Basal- (s. grenz-) Membran
Tunique propre	Tunica propria
lamelles de la t. propre	Lamellen
cellules "	Zellen der Propria
espaces péricellulaires	perizelluläre Spalträume
canalicules	Kanälchen
Membrane basale ou limitante postérieure (de *Demours*, de *Descemet*)	Vordere Basal- (s. grenz-) Membran
Épithélium (endothélium) postérieur	hinteres Deckepithel (Endothel)
Nerfs de la cornée	Nerven der Hornhaut
plexus fondamental	Grundplexus
" sous-basal	Basalplexus
rameaux perforants	
plexus sous-épithélial	subepithelialer Plexus
" intra-épithélial	intraepithelialer
fibrilles terminales	Endfibrillen
renflements terminaux	Endanschwellungen

Choroïde — *Chorioidea (Gefässhaut)*

Région principale ?	Hauptzone
Membrane suprachoroïdienne	M. suprachorioidea
Cellules pigmentaires de la Lamina fusca	Pigmentzellen der L. fusca
Couche des gros vaisseaux	äussere Gefässlage
Couche chorio-capillaire	Lamina chorio-capillaris
Membrane vitrée de *Bruch*	Glashaut
Cellules de la choroïde	Zellen der Chorioidea
Pigment choroïdien	Pigment
Cellules musculaires lisses (*H. Müller*)	platte Muskelzellen
Vaisseaux de la couche externe	Gefässe der Aussenschicht
Vaisseaux tourbillonnés	Vasa vorticosa
Capillaires tourbillonnés	Wirbelkapillaren
Tapis (Mammifères)	Tapetum (Sanguiera)
fibreux	fibrosum
celluleux	cellulosum
Région antérieure Corps ciliaire	Vordere Zone, Corpus ciliare
Plan externe ou musculaire	äussere s. Muskellage

Plan interne. Procès ciliaires	innere Lage. Processus ciliaris
Muscle tenseur de la choroïde (de *Brücke*)	Tensor chorioideae *Brücke*'scher Muskel
Muscle de *Müller*	*Müller*'scher Muskel
Tissu conjonctif interstitiel	interstitielles Bindegewebe
Cellules pigmentaires	Pigmentzellen
Procès ciliaires	Processus ciliares
Plis	Falten
Trame conjonctive (de soutènement)	Stützgewebe
Vaisseaux sanguins	Blutgefässe
Portion ciliaire de la rétine (v. rétine)	Pars ciliaris retinae

Peigne (Oiseaux)	*Pecten (Vögel)*
Plis	Falten
Trame de soutènement	Stützgewebe
Pigment	Pigment
Revêtement cellulaire	Deckzellschicht
Muscle de *Crampton*	*Crampton*'scher Muskel

Bourrelet falciforme (Perches)	*Processus falciformis (Barsch)*
Couche fibro-vasculaire	Gefässfaserschicht
Plan pigmentaire	Pigmentlage
Plan de cellules en colonne	Säulenzellenlage

Iris	*Regenbogenhaut*
Endothélium antérieur (revêtement cellulaire plat antérieur)	vorderes Endothel (vordere Plattzellschicht)
Couche limitante antérieure (?)	vordere Grenzschicht (?)
Plan fibro-pigmentaire antérieur	vordere Pigment-Faserlage
Plan vasculo-pigmentaire moyen (principal)	mittlere Gefäss- und Pigmentlage
Plan fibro-musculaire	Muskellage
fibres circulaires. Sphincter pupillaire	Musculus Sphincter
fibres radiaires. Dilatateur de la pupille	M. dilatator pupillae
Couche limitante postérieure	hintere Grenzschicht
Épithélium pigmenté postérieur	hintere Pigment-Epithelschicht
Cellules conjonctives pigmentaires de l'iris	Pigmentzellen der Iris
globuleuses, ovoïdes	abgerundete, ovoide
étirées, fusiformes	gestreckte, spindelförmige
ramifiées	verzweigt
Angle cornéo-irien	Iriswinkel

Ligament pectiné	Ligamentum iridis pectinatum
tissu trabéculaire cornéo-iridien	Irido-cornéales Balkengewebe
Bourrelet cellulaire post-cornéen (*Poissons*)	postcornealer Zellwulst (*Fische*)

Rétine   *Netzhaut, Retina*

I. Région visuelle	Regio optica
Couches :	Schichten :
Plan pigmentaire	Pigmentlage
Plan des cellules visuelles (neuro-épithélial)	Sehzellenlage (neuro-epithélial)
Couche des bâtonnets et des cônes (couche de *Jacob*)	Stäbchen- und Zapfenschicht
Membrane limitante externe	äussere Grenzmembran (Limitans externa)
Couche des grains externes	äussere Körnerschicht
Plan nerveux (cérébral)	nervöse Lage (Gehirnlage)
Couche spongieuse externe	äussere Spongiosa
Syn. moléculaire externe	Molekularschicht
plexiforme	äussere
réticulaire	retikuläre
intermédiaire	Zwischenkörnerschicht
sous-épithéliale	subepitheliale
Plexus basal (*Ranvier*)	Basalplexus
Couche des grains internes	innere Körnerschicht
Couche spongieuse interne	innere Spongiosa
Syn. „ réticulaire	„ retikulare
„ moléculaire	„ Molekularschicht
Couche des cellules ganglionnaires	Ganglienzellenschicht
Couche des fibres optiques	Optikusfasernschicht
Membrane limitante interne	Limitans interna
Épithélium pigmenté de la rétine	Pigmentepithel
zone nucléée	Kernzone
zone pigmentée	Pigmentzone
lambeaux cellulaires	Zellfetzen
granulations pigmentaires baciliformes	stäbchenförmige Pigmentkörnchen
gouttelettes colorées	farbige Kügelchen
Cellules visuelles	Sehzellen
Cell. vis. à bâtonnet	Sehstäbchenzellen
a) Région exo-limitante	Exolimitantieller Teil
Bâtonnet	Stäbchen
— Segment externe	— Aussenglied
striation longitudinale	Längsstreifung
striation transversale	Querstreifung
Altérations postmortales	postmortale Veränderungen
incurvation	Krümmung
division en disques	Scheibenzerklüftung

— Segment interne	Innenglied
Corps ellipsoïde	Stäbchen-Ellipsoid
Syn. corps lenticulaire	Corpus lentiforme
b) Région endo-limitante	Endolimitantieller Teil
portion intermédiaire	Zwischenstück
noyau du bâtonnet	Stäbchenkern
stries chromatiques	Chromatinstäbe
prolongement profond	tiefer Fortsatz
renflement terminal	Endanschwellung
Cellules visuelles à cône	Zapfenzellen
a) Région exo-limitante	Exolimitantieller Teil
Cône	Zapfen
— Segment externe	Aussenglied
striation longitudinale	Längstreifung
striation transversale	Querstreifung
Altérations postmortales	postmortale Veränderungen
incurvation	Krümmung
gonflement	Quellung
segmentation en disque	Scheibzerklüftung
— Segment interne	Innenglied
Ellipsoïde	Zapfenellipsoid
Syn. Corps lenticulaire	Linsenkörper
intercalaire	
b) Région endo-limitante	Endolimitantieller Teil
portion intermédiaire	Zwischenstück
noyau du cône	Zapfenkern
prolongement profond	tiefer Fortsatz
plateau basal	Fussplatte
Cellules visuelles (Oiseaux)	Sehzellen (Vögel)
Cellules à bâtonnet	Stäbchenzellen
Segment interne	Innenglied
Ellipsoïde cylindrique	Zylinder-Ellipsoid
Corpuscule baciliforme	Stäbchenförmiges Körperchen
Strie médiane	Mittelstreifen
Cellules visuelles à cône (Oiseaux)	Zapfenzellen (Vögel)
Variété baciliforme	stäbchenähnliche Varietät
Segment interne cylindrique	Zylindrisches Innenglied
Ellipsoïde cylindrique	Zylindrisches Ellipsoid
Gouttelettes huileuses colorées	Farbige Oelkugel
Cônes doubles (hétéromorphes)	Doppelzapfen (heteromorphe)
— Cône grêle	— Schlanker Zapfen
gouttelette colorée	farbige Oelkugel
corps ellipsoïde	Zapfenellipsoid
— Cône épais	dicker Zapfen
corps ellipsoïde	Ellipsoid
corps hyalin ergoïde (accessoire)	accessorischer hyaliner Körper
Cellules visuelles à cône (Reptiles)	Zapfenzellen (Reptilien)
Cônes simples	Einfache Zapfen
corps ellipsoïde granuleux	körniges Ellipsoid

gouttelette huileuse colorée	farbige Oelkugel
Cônes doubles (hétéromorphes)	Doppelzapfen (heteromorphe)
cône à gouttelette colorée	Zapfen mit Oelkugel
corps ellipsoïde granuleux	körniges Ellipsoid
cône sans gouttelette colorée	Zapfen ohne Oelkugel
amas de granules pigmentés (ellipsoïde?)	Pigmentkörschenhaufen
corps hyalin profond (accessoire)	accessorischer hyaliner Körper
noyaux géminés	Doppelkerne
Cellules visuelles à cône (*Batraciens*)	Zapfenzellen (*Batrachier*)
Cônes simples	einfache Zapfen
Gouttelette huileuse non colorée	farblose Oelkugel
Cônes doubles (hétéromorphes)	Doppelzapfen
Cône long ellipsoïde	langer Zapfen Ellipsoid
Gouttelette huileuse	Oelkugel
Cône épais ellipsoïde	dicker Zapfen Ellipsoid
Cellules visuelles (*Poissons*)	Sehzellen (*Fische*)
Cellules à bâtonnet	Stäbchenzellen
Segment externe	Aussenglied
renflement sous-bacillaire (corps ellipsoïde?)	subbacillare Anschwellung (Ellipsoid?)
segment fibrillaire	Stäbchenfaden
noyau	Stäbchenkern
prolongement fibrillaire profond (interne)	tiefer (innerer) Fibrillenfortsatz
Cellules à cône	Zapfenzellen
Segment externe bacilliforme	stäbchenförmiges Aussenglied
Segment interne	Innenglied
— région exolimitante (ou colonne)	—exolimitanhelle Abteilung (scioleudermige)
portion hyaline (corps ellipsoïde?)	hyaliner Teil (Ellipsoid)
portion granuleuse	körniger Teil
région endolimitante	— endolimitanielle Abteilung
portion intermédiaire	Zwischenstück
noyau	Zapfenkern
prolongement profond (interne)	innerer (tiefer) Fortsatz
pied	Fussplatte
fibrilles basales	Basalfibrillen
Cellules jumelées à cône	Doppelzapfenzellen (Zwilling —)
homomorphes	homomorphe
Massues de *Landolt*	*Landolt*'sche Kolben
Couche spongieuse externe	aeussere Spongiosa
Cellules horizontales	Horizontalzellen
petites	kleine
grandes	grosse
Cellules nerveuses étoilées	sternförmige Nervenzellen
Cellules à prolongements descendants	Zellen mit absteigenden Fortsätzen]
Cellules concentriques (*Schifferdecker*)	konzentrische Zellen
Couche des grains internes	innere Körnerschicht

Cellules bipolaires	bipolare Zellen
prolongement externe	äusserer Fortsatz
arborisation terminale externe (adépithéliale)	äusseres Telodendrion
prolongement interne	innerer Fortsatz
arborisation terminale interne (adganglionnaire)	inneres Telodendrion
région nucléée	Kernzone
Cellules amacrines (dites spongioblastes)	amakrine Zellen (sogenann. Spongioblasten)
étagées	schichtbildende
diffuses	diffuse
Couche spongieuse interne	innere Spongiosa
prolongement des cellules bipolaires	Fortsätze der bipolaren Zellen
prolongements des cellules amacrines	Fortsätze der Amakrinen
prolongements des cellules ganglionnaires	Fortsätze der Ganglienzellen
Cellules ganglionnaires	Ganglienzellen
corps	Zellleib
noyau	Kern
nucléole	Nucleolus
prolongements dendritiques	Dendriten
prolongement nerveux	Nervenfortsatz
Fibres optiques centripètes	zentripetale Opticus Fasern
" " centrifuges	zentrifugale
Trame de soutènement de la rétine	Stützsubstanz der Retina
fibres de *Müller*	*Müller'sche* Fasern
cône terminal interne	innerer Endkegel
fibre	Faser
ramifications collatérales	collaterale Fortsätze
segment des couches des fibres et cellules ganglionnaires	Teil der Nerven und Ganglien Zellschicht
Segment de la spongieuse interne	Teil der inneren Spongiosa
segment de la couche des grains internes (région nucléée)	Teil der inneren Körnerschicht (Kernzone)
Segment de la spongieuse externe	Teil der äusseren Spongiosa
Segment de la couche des grains externes	Teil der äusseren Körnerschicht
Fibres en panier	Faserkörbe
Tache jaune de la rétine	Macula lutea
couche des fibres de *Henle*	*Henle'sche* Faserschicht
pigment	Pigment
Fossette centrale	Fovea centralis
couche neuro-épithéliale	Neuroepithelschicht
cônes modifiés	modifizierte Zapfen
membrane limitante externe	Limitans externa
couche des grains externes	äussere Körnerschicht
couche spongieuse externe	äussere Spongiosa
membrane limitante interne	Limitans interna

Région de l'Ora serrata	Region der Ora serrata
II. Portion ciliaire de la rétine	Pars ciliaris retinae
Couche d'épithélium pigmenté	Pigmentepithellage
Couche des cellules cylindriques	Zylinderzelllage
Portion irienne de la rétine	Pars iridica retinae
(Épithélium pigmenté de l'iris)	(Pigmentepithel der Iris)
Papille du nerf optique	Sehnervpapille
Lame criblée	Lamina cribrosa
Artère centrale de la rétine	Arteria centralis
Veine centrale	Vena centralis
Vaisseaux du plan nerveux (cérébral) de la rétine	Gefässe der nervösen (cerebralen) Lage der Retina
plan interne	innere Lage
plan externe (profond)	äussere Lage (tiefe)
Réseaux capillaires rétiniens	Kapillarnetze
à mailles plus lâches	weitmaschiges Netz
à mailles serrées (réseau profond)	feinmaschiges (tiefes)
Arbuscules vasculaires	Gefässbäumchen
Arcades capillaires	bogenförmige Kapillarschlingen
Nerf optique	Sehnerv
gaine durale	Duralscheide
gaine arachnoïdienne	Arachnoidealscheide
gaine piemérienne	Pialscheide
Espace sous-dural	Subduraler Raum
Espace sous-arachnoïdien	Subarachnoidealer ..
Espace lymphatique *Tenonien*	*Tenon*'scher Lymphraum
Espace lymphatique suprachoroïdien	Suprachoroidealer Lymphraum
Canal de *Schlemm*	*Schlemm*'scher Kanal
Espaces de *Fontana*	*Fontana*'sche Räume
Espace de *Petit*	*Petit*'scher Raum

Cristallin	*Linse (Lens)*
Capsule	Kapsel
région antérieure	vordere Region
région postérieure	hintere ..
Épithélium du cristallin	Linsenepithel
antérieur	vorderes
de la zone équatoriale	der Aequatorialzone
Fibres cristalliniennes	Linsenfasern
larges	breite
étroites	schmale
de la couche corticale du cristallin	der Kortikalschicht
du noyau du cristallin	des Linsenkernes
denticules marginaux	Randzähnchen
fibres multinuclées (Reptiles, Amphibiens)	mehrkernige Fasern (Reptilien, Amphibien)
fibres anuclées	kernlose Fasern
Étoiles du cristallin	Linsensterne
antérieure	vorderer Stern

postérieure	hinterer
Tunique vasculaire du cristallin	Tunica vasculosa lentis
Membrane pupillo-capsulaire	Membrana capsulo-pupillaris
Zonule de *Zinn*	Zonula Zinnii (ciliaris)

Corps vitré — *Glaskörper (Corpus vitreum)*

Substance amorphe (humeur vitrée)	amorphe Substanz (Humor vitreus)
Cellules du corps vitré	Glaskörperzellen
globuleuses (lymphatiques)	runde (Lymphkörperchen)
fixes	fixe Zellen
Membrane hyaloïde	Glashaut (Hyaloidea)
Artère hyaloïde	Arteria hyaloidea
Canal de *Cloquet*	Canalis hyaloideus

ANNEXES DE L'ŒIL — ADNEXAE DES SEHAPPARATES

Paupières — *Augenlider*

Plan cutané	Hautlage
follicules pileux	Haarfollikel
poils follets	Wollhaare
glandes sébacées	Balgdrüsen
glandes sudoripares	Schweissdrüsen
Plan fibro-musculaire	Muskellage
Muscle de *Riolan*	Musculus Riolani
Muscles lisses de la paupière	glatte Augenlidmuskeln
Muscle de *Müller*	*Müller*'scher Muskel
Plan fibro-glandulaire propre	Tarsus- und Drüsenlage
Lame tarse	Tarsus,
Glandes de *Meibomius*	*Meibom*'sche Drüsen
Vésicules glandulaires	Drüsenbläschen
Épithélium glandulaire sébacé	Fettdrüsenepithel
Conduit excréteur	Drüsengang
Épithélium du conduit excréteur	Epithel des Ausführganges
Plan de la muqueuse conjonctive	Bindehautlage (Conjunctiva palpebralis)
Tunique propre (chorion)	Propria
Infiltrations lymphadénoïdes	Lymphdrüsenode Herde
Revêtement épithélial	Conjunctiva-Epithel
Épithélium stratifié mixte	Uebergangs Epithel (gemischtes)
Cellules caliciformes	Becherzellen
Cryptes épithéliaux (glandes de *Henle*)	Epithelkrypten (*Henle*'sche Drüsen)
Épithélium cylindrique stratifié	Geschichtetes Zylinderepithel
Glandes affluentes de la conjonctive	akzessäre Conjunctiva-Drüsen (Fornix
(cul de sac de la conjonctive)	drüsen)
Région du bord palpébral	Lidkante
Cils	Cilien (Lidwimperhaare)
Glandes sébacées des cils	Balgdrüsen der Cilien
Glandes de *Moll*	*Moll*'sche Drüsen
Revêtement épidermique	Lidrandepidermis
Cil secondaire	Pilus secundarius

Caroncule lacrymale	Caruncula lacrimalis
follicules pileux	Haarbälge
glandes sébacées	Talgdrüsen
Terminaisons nerveuses de la conjonctive	Nervendigungen der Conjunctiva
Bulbes terminaux (de *Krause*)	Endkolben
Terminaisons intra-épithéliales	Intraepitheliale

Troisième paupière (Mammifères)   *Drittes Augenlid (Säugetiere)*

Cartilage de la 3e paup.	Knorpel des 3. Augenlides
Couche périchondriale	perichondriale Schicht
Trame conjonctive fondamentale	bindegewebige Grundschicht
Membrane muqueuse	Schleimhaut
de la face extérieure	der äusseren Fläche
de la face intérieure (oculaire)	der inneren Fläche (bulbäre)
Chorion (tunique propre)	Tunica propria
infiltrations lymphadénoïdes	lymphadenoide Herde
follicules lymphatiques clos	solitäre Lymphfollikel
follicules lymphatiques agminés	gehäufte Lymphfollikel
Revêtement épithélial	Deckepithel
de la face extérieure	der äusseren Fläche
intérieure	der inneren
Epithélium pavimenteux stratifié	geschichtetes Plattenepithel
Epithélium stratifié mixte	gemischtes Epithel
Epithélium cylindrique stratifié	geschichtetes Zylinderepithel
Interstices épithéliaux	Epithellücken
Cryptes muqueuses intra-épithéliales	intraepitheliale Schleimkrypten
Epithélium pigmenté	Pigmentepithel
Cellules pigmentaires ramifiées sous-et intra-épithéliales	Subepitheliale und intraepitheliale Pigment Zellen
Racinettes pigmentaires	Pigmentwürzelchen

Glandes de la 3e paupière (Mammifères)   *Drüsen des 3. Augenlides (Säugetiere)*

Couche glandulaire rétro-cartilagineuse	retrochondrale Drüsenschicht
Couche glandulaire de la région basale	Drüsenschicht der Basalregion
des régions marginales supérieure et inférieure de la lame cartilagineuse	der oberen und unteren Randregion der Knorpelplatte
Lobules glandulaires	Drüsenläppchen
Travées conjonctives interlobulaires	bindegewebige Septa
Cellules adipeuses interstitielles	interstitielle Fettzellen
et Glandes homomorphes	et. Homomorphe Drüsen
Alvéoles glandulaires	Drüsenalveolen
Conduits excréteurs perforants	durchbohrende Ausführgänge
terminaux	Endgänge
Embouchures	Mündungen
Follicules lymphadénoïdes adjacents	adnexe lymphadenoide Follikel

b) Hétéromorphes (hétérogènes)	b) Heteromorphe (heterogene)
Lobules sténo-alvéolaires	engalveoläre Läppchen
Lobules eurytubulaires	weitraumige acinöse Schläuche

Glande lacrimale	*Thränendrüse*
Enveloppe commune	Gemeinschaftliche Hülle
Lobes	Lappen
Travées interlobaires	interlobäre Septa
Lobules	Läppchen
Travées interlobulaires	interlobuläre Septa
Îlots de cellules adipeuses	Fettzellen-Inseln
Travées interalvéolaires	interalveoläre Septa
Alvéoles glandulaires	Drüsenalveolen
„ à lumen étroit	mit engem Lumen
„ à lumen plus large	mit weiterem Lumen
„ à cellules gonflées	mit aufgeblasenen Zellen
„ à cellules prismatiques	mit prismatischen Zellen
Granulations sécrétoires	Sekretgranula
Canalicules intercalaires	Schaltröhrchen
Canaux excréteurs intralobulaires	intralobuläre Gänge
„ interlobulaires	interlobuläre
„ terminaux	Endausführgänge
Infiltrations lymphadénoïdes	Lymphadenoide Herde
Conduits lacrymaux	Thränenröhrchen
tunique muqueuse	Schleimhaut (Tunica propria)
revêtement épithélial	Deckepithel
Conduit nasal	Thränennasengang
Couche périostique	periostale Lage
Tunique muqueuse	Schleimhaut (Tunica propria)
Infiltrations lymphadénoïdes	lymphadenoide Herde
Epithélium de revêtement	Deckepithel
Diverticules glandulaires	Drüsenkrypten

Autres glandes de la cavité orbitaire	*Andere Drüsen der Augenhöhle*
Mammifères	*(Säugetiere)*
1. Glandes s'ouvrant dans la région extérieure de la cavité orbitaire	1. Drüsen mit exorbitärer Mündung
Glande sous orbitaire	*Glandula infra orbitalis*
a) Variété sténo-alvéolaire, type séreux	a) Engalveoläre Art, seröser Typus
Alvéoles glandulaires	Drüsenalveolen
Epithélium glandulaire (pyramidal-tronqué)	Drüsenepithel (abgestuzt pyramidenförmig)
zone cellulaire externe	äussere Zellzone
zone cellulaire interne	innere Zellzone
Conduits intra-lobulaires (à épithélium cubique)	intra-lobuläre Gänge (mit kubischem Epithel)
Conduits interlobulaires (à épithélium cylindrique)	interlobuläre Gänge (mit zylindrischem Epithel)

Glande sous-orbitaire accessoire (lapin)	Gl. infra-orbitalis accessoria (Kaninchen)
b) Variété hétéromorphe	b) Heteromorphe Art
Glande sous-orbitaire du rat blanc	Gl. infra-orbitalis der weissen Ratte
— Lobules sténo-alvéolaires	— Engalvéolare Läppchen
Épithélium glandulaire mégacellulaire	grosszelliges Drüsenepithel
Noyaux géants	Riesenkerne
Noyaux polymorphes	polymorphe Kerne
Cellules multinucléées	mehrkernige Zellen
Cinèses	Kinesen
— Lobules curv-tubulaires	— Weitröhrige Läppchen
Épithélium prismatique sébacé	prismatisches Fettepithel
Conduits exo-parenchymateux	Exo-parenchymatöse Ausführgänge
Conduit terminal	Terminalgang
Embouchure commune avec le conduit de la glande orbitaire externe	gemeinschaftliche Mündung mit dem Ausführgange der gl. orbitalis externa

Glande orbitaire externe (adparotidienne) — *Glandula orbitalis externa (adparotica) (Nebenohrspeicheldrüse)*

Type glandulaire: sténo-alvéolaire composé	Drüsentypus: zusammengesetzer eng alveolarer
Épithélium mégacellulaire	grosszelliges Drüsenepithel
Noyaux géants	Riesenkerne
Noyaux polymorphes	polymorphe Kerne
Cinèses	Kinesen
Canalicules excréteurs intercalaires	Schaltröhrchen
Canaux excréteurs	Ausführgänge
— interlobulaires	interlobulär
— exo-parenchymateux	exo-parenchymatöse
Conduit terminal	Endgang
embouchure commune avec le conduit de la glande sous-orbitaire	gemeinschaftlich Mündung mit dem Endgange der Gl. infra-orbitalis

II. Glandes s'ouvrant dans la région interne de la cavité orbitaire — II. Drüsen mit eno-orbitärer Mündung

Glande de Harder — *Harder'sche Drüse*

a) Variété homomorphe curvi-tubulaire	a) Weitröhrige homomorphe Art
Tubes glandulaires acineux	acinöse Drüsenschläuche
Épithélium glandulaire prismatique	prismatischer Drüsenepithel
à gouttelettes graisseuses (rat blanc) (épithélium glandul. sébacé)	mit Fetttröpfel (weisse Ratte) (fettiges Drüsenepithel)
à granulations hyalines (cobaye)	mit hyalinen Granulis (Meerschweinchen)
Concrétions pigmentaires glandulaires (rat)	Drüsenpigmentkonkremente
Conduits alvéolaires	Alveolargänge

Conduits excréteurs interlobulaires	interlobuläre Ausführgänge
Conduit terminal	Endgang
Infiltrations lymphadénoïdes (colizge)	lymphadenoide Herde (Meerschweichen)
b) Variété hétéromorphe	b) Heteromorphe Art
Glande de *Harder* du *hérisson*	*Harder'sche* Drüse des *Igels*
Parties eurytubulaires acineuses	Weitröhrig-acinöse Teile
Epithélium prismatique sébacé	prismatisches Fettdrüsenepithel
Ilots disséminés sténo-alvéolaires (sé- reux)	zerstreute engalveoläre Inselchen (se- rös)
Tissu interstitiel adipeux	Fettzwischengewebe
Conduits alvéolaires	Alveolärgänge
Conduits interlobulaires	Interlobulärgänge
Conduits lobaires	Lobärgänge
Conduit terminal	Endgang
Embouchure	Mündung
Infiltrations lymphadénoïdes (folliculos)	Lymphadenoide Herde (Follikel)
Glande de *Harder* du *Porc*	*Harder'sche* Drüse des *Schweins*
Lobules glandulaires compacts à con- duits rayonnés	kompakte Drüsenläppchen mit radiären Ausführgängen
Parties sténo-alvéolaires	Engalveoläre Drüsenteile
Ilots eurytubuleux à épithélium sébacé	Weitröhrige Drüsenteile mit fettigem Epithel
Conduits intra-lobulaires rayonnés	radiäre intralobuläre Ausführgänge
Conduits exo-parenchymateux	Exoparenchymatöse Gänge
Conduit terminal	Endgang
Embouchure	Mündung
Glande de *Harder* du *lapin*	*Harder'sche* Drüse des *Kaninchens*
a) Partie rose (plus grande)	Rosapartie (Pars rubicunda major)
Tubes glandulaires acineux	acinöse Drüsenschläuche
Epithélium prismatique	prismatisches Drüsenepithel
structure protoplasmique aréolaire irrégulière	unregelmässig alveoläre Zellleib-struktur
granulations hyalines	hyaline Granula
molécules graisseux	Fettkörnchen
b) Partie blanche	weisser Teil (Pars albescens minor)
Tubes glandulaires acineux	acinöse Drüsenschläuche
Epithélium cylindrique	Zylinderepithel
Structure protoplasmique aréolaire fine	feine alveoläre Zellleibstruktur
Noyaux pariétaux opposé-basales	wandständige Kerne
Conduit excréteur terminal. Glandule accessoire	Endgang. Accessorisches Drüschen
type alvéolaire séreux	seröser Alveolartypus
Embouchure du conduit excré. termi- nal	Mündung des Endganges
Glande de *Harder* du *canard*	*Harder'sche* Drüse (*Ente*)
Type glandulaire tubuleux aginge composé à radiants centro-lobu- laires	Drüsentypus: gehault-tubulöser zu- sammengeastelter, mit lobulären Sekundärästen

Lobules glandulaires	Drüsenläppchen
Tubes glandulaires primaires	primäre Drüsenröhren
Membrane propre	Membrana propria
Épithélium cylindrique à noyau basal (apposéocrade)	Zylinderepithel mit basal ständigen Kern
Tubes glandulaires secondaires	sekundäre Drüsenröhren
Confluents ramifiés contro-lobulaires	verzweigte tubuläre Sammelgänge
Glandes de Harder (grenouille)	Harder'sche Drüse (Frosch)
Type glandulaire: tubulo-saccaire, aciné subcomposé	Drüsentypus: röhrigsäckchenförmiger, gehäufter
Canaux glandulaires	Drüsenschläuche
Saccules glandulaires	Drüsensäckchen
Épithélium cylindrique à noyau opposo-siturale	Zylinderepithel mit apposobasalem Kern
Granulations hyalines protoplasmiques	hyaline Zellenbgranula
Canaux collecteurs	Sammelgänge
Conduit collecteur terminal	Endsammelgang
Sinuosités	Ausbuchtungen
Entonnoir terminal	Endtrichter

REMARQUES EXPLICATIVES

Abréviations : Syn. — Synonyme, s. — sen, v. — vide

Granulations homogènes. Il est tout indiqué de distinguer entre les granulations faisant partie intégrante du protoplasma ou du noyau, et celles qui se forment dans l'intérieur du protoplasma et représentent des inclusions hyalines.

L'ancienne dénomination : éléments anatomiques, tout en n'ayant pas de sens très précis, peut être appliquée indifféremment soit aux cellules proprement dites, soit aux dérivés des cellules (fibres-cellules, fibres). On pourrait encore proposer comme dénomination plus générale : Unités biotoniques, c'est à dire pouvant au besoin être isolées d'une manière indépendante et sans être désorganisées : ces unités, à la fois structurales et physiologiques, se composent de parties plastiques élémentaires.

Mentionnons encore d'autres dénominations proposées pour désigner les unités anatomiques et physiologiques: Probioblastes (v. Kœlliker); Elementarorganismen (Brücke); Plastides (Haeckel).

Fibrocytes simples et composés: Cellules transformées ayant la forme d'une fibre formée soit aux dépens d'une seule, soit aux dépens d'un certain nombre de cellules.

Enveloppes cellulaires. Couche corticoplasmique: on pourrait donner ce nom à la couche protoplasmique extérieure plus dense, mais pas isolable, qu'on constate aux différentes cellules.

Capsules: cette dénomination, il faut le dire, n'a pas de sens précis : capsules cartilagineuses, capsules des viscères (rate, rein, testicule), capsule des cellules ganglionnaires, capsules articulaires ... Il semblerait indiqué de réserver ce nom aux enveloppes rigides de la cellule, telles que les capsules cartilagineuses.

Corps cellulaire, Protoplasma. Cette dernière dénomination tend à être remplacée par celle de corps cellulaire (Zelleib), vu que le protoplasma n'est pas encore une matière simple et unitaire, mais ce n'est pas une raison suffisante. On ne saurait disconvenir que le terme : corps cellulaire ne suffit pas pour caractériser cette matière propre douée de propriétés physiologiques dites vitales.

Mitoplasma : en modifiant un peu le nom proposé par *Flemming* (Mitom). Les dénominations : mitoplasma et spongioplasma (*Leydig*) ne sont pas entièrement équivalentes ; chacune d'elles invoque une conception particulière.

Citons encore un certain nombre d'autres dénominations se rapportant au protoplasma : Idioplasma (*Naegeli*), plasma germinatif (Keimplasma, *Weismann*), Archoplasma (*Boveri*), énergides (Energiden, *Sachs*), Kinoplasma, trophoplasma (*Strasburger*). Bien qu'à ces dénominations soient attachées des conceptions d'une grande portée générale, il y a à dire cependant qu'elles ne correspondent pas à des entités morphologiques constatables au microscope.

Deuto- ou paraplasma (Kupffer). Ces dénominations ont cela de commode qu'elles permettent de spécifier d'un seul mot les différentes inclusions qu'on peut constater dans le corps cellulaire.

Granulations nucléoïdes : elles ne sont pas à confondre avec les granulations dites chromophiles (de *Ehrlich*, *Altmann*, *Benda-Nissl* et d'autres) ; il s'agit des granulations qui fixent les matières colorantes nucléaires.

Cristalloïdes : il s'agit des inclusions signalées plus récemment par *Reinke*, *Plato*, *v. Lenhossék* et *v. Bardeleben* dans les cellules interstitielles du testicule.

Canalicules trophiques ; Trophospongien : particularités de structure signalées par *Holmgren* dans diverses espèces cellulaires. Il est permis de se demander s'il s'agit dans tous les cas d'une formation identique ?

Filaments ergastoplastiques : Ces filaments signalés par *Garnier* dans les cellules glandulaires (Des filaments basaux des cellules glandulaires, *Bibliog. anat.* 1897) se distinguent en effet des fibrilles protoplasmiques ordinaires. L'auteur pense avec *Bouin* que ces filaments sont « l'expression morphologique d'un processus d'élaboration chimique ». Des structures fibrillaires de ce genre ont été signalées déjà auparavant par *E. Solger* dans la sous-maxillaire d'homme (Anatom. Anzeiger, IX, 1894).

Des centrosomes multiples ont été décrits par *A. Heidenhain* dans certaines cellules géantes. L'ensemble de ces centrosomes forme un « Mikrocentrum » ou « Centralkörper Gruppe ». (Arch. f. mikr. Anat. 43, 1894).

Hyalome polaire : on pourrait désigner ainsi l'espace clair entourant les centrosomes ; la dénomination : Astrocoele invoque l'idée d'une cavité dont l'existence n'est pas établie.

Croissant (ou anneau) périnucléaire : on constate des formations de ce genre dans les cellules ovulaires en particulier. Parmi les travaux plus récents qui touchent à ce sujet, citons ceux de *Loyez* et de *Hollander* (Arch. d'Anatom. microscopique, 1904).

Structure aréolaire, Wabenstruktur de *Bütschli*. Il y a à distinguer entre la structure aréolaire élémentaire du protoplasma, et celle qui résulte de la présence d'inclusions dans le corps cellulaire (granulations de deutoplasma).

Situation du noyau : proximocoele et oppositocoele ; on pourrait spécifier par ces termes la situation du noyau dans les cellules glandulaires par rapport à la cavité du tube ou de l'alvéole. Exosomatique : noyau situé en dehors du corps cellulaire proprement dit, à la base d'un des prolongements, comme on peut le constater dans les cellules pigmentaires.

Chromosomes: on comprend généralement sous ce nom les segments ou anses chromatiques qu'on reconnaît dans le noyau pendant la division cinétique, et non pas les granules chromatiques beaucoup plus fins qu'on peut distinguer dans les filaments nucléaires. Il semblerait plus opportun de désigner sous ce nom plutôt les dits granules chromatiques élémentaires que les segments plus volumineux. La dénomination centrosoma s'applique également à un corpuscule très petit. On comprendrait sous le nom de caryosomes les granulations nucléaires achromatiques.

Nucléoles conglomérés: accolés de manière à former un petit groupe; cette disposition peut être constatée aux taches germinatives de l'ovule.

Nucléoles nucléomiens (Carnoy): on pourrait aussi les désigner sous le nom de chromatiques pour éviter la répétition du même mot.

Nucléoles composés: laissant reconnaître deux parties distinctes, comme les nucléoles de l'ovule de l'anodonte.

Mentionnons à ce propos qu'Auerbach a décrit des noyaux sans nucléole, anucléolaire Kerne (Organologische Studien, p. 79).

Des zones hyalines péri-nucléaire et nucléolaire ont été décrites plus récemment par Leydig (Zelle und Gewebe, pp. 21, 26). Eimer et Auerbach ont déjà fait des constatations analogues par rapport au nucléole.

Il est certain qu'une zone péri-nucléaire propre, plus claire et raréfiée, peut être reconnue dans les œufs des vertébrés inférieurs; on peut, de plus, reconnaître à cette zone (reptiles, oiseaux) une structure striée ou fibrillaire; mais l'action des réactifs pourrait avoir sa part dans la production de ces zones. On peut objecter cependant qu'on les observe aussi aux œufs ne présentant pas de rétraction de la vésicule germinative.

Division auto-nucléaire: limitée au noyau seul, pour le distinguer de la division nucléo-cellulaire comprenant à la fois le noyau et le corps cellulaire.

Scission caryo-métabolique. On pourrait comprendre sous ce nom plus explicite la fragmentation et scission indirectes d'Arnold (indirecte Segmentirung und Fragmentirung) vu que dans ce mode de division nucléaire on constate aussi des changements aux parties constituantes du noyau.

Cinèses multipolaires. Citons parmi les travaux plus récents la communication de Kromprecher renfermant un essai de classification de ces cinèses (Ergänzungsheft z. Bd. X Anat. Anzeiger 1895). Les travaux de Henneguy (Journ. de l'Anat. et de la Physiol. 1891) et de Kostanecki (Anatomische Hefte 1892) contiennent entre autres ces données relatives à ce genre de cinèses.

Noyaux chromato-partites et chromato-modelés. Au cours du développement des ovules en particulier, on peut distinguer des noyaux dans lesquels les parties chromatiques sont à l'état de division particulièrement fine et ne laissant pas reconnaître de structure déterminée, alors qu'à un stade plus avancé les parties chromatiques forment les structures nucléaires connues.

Atrophies nucléaires accompagnées de production de fentes: s'observe p. ex. dans la régression des ovules (lapine); on peut reconnaître en outre, dans l'espace périnucléaire, des fibrilles déliées rattachant le noyau rétracté au corps cellulaire.

Substance fondamentale lamellaire-caniculée: subst. fondamentale du tissu osseux et de la dentine.

Agencement des cellules. Cellules endo-lacunaires et endo-cavitaires: On pourrait se servir de ces termes pour spécifier les différences ayant trait aux rapports des cellules et de la substance fondamentale qui les entoure. Dans une série le cas, les cellules sont entourées de lacunes, irrégulières, mal délimitées ou largement confluentes, comme on le constate dans la plupart des variétés de tissu conjonctif; c'est le cas des cellules endolacunaires. Dans d'autres cas, les cellules sont entourées d'espaces nettement circonscrits non seulement par la substance fondamentale intercellulaire, mais encore par une couche capsulaire propre (cartilage hyalin), et ces espaces péricellulaires communiquent entre eux par l'intermédiaire des canalicules également bien délimités, comme on le constate dans le tissu osseux; c'est le cas des cellules endocavitaires.

Connexions des cellules. Pontoculo-plasmiques: par l'intermédiaire des pontcules protoplasmiques; péridendritiques: par l'intermédiaire d'un réticule ou réseau, tel que le neurospongium (réseau fin de Gerlach); péridendritique: par l'intermédiaire d'une arborisation péricellulaire (connexions entre cellules nerveuses); interdendritiques: par l'intermédiaire de deux arborisations terminales (exemple: connexions au niveau des glomérules olfactifs).

Tissus holocytaires non inoblastiques: formés entièrement de cellules ne donnant pas naissance aux fibres conjonctives.

Tissus inoblastiques: donnant naissance ou se formant aux dépens des fibres conjonctives.

Tissus d'origine mixte: c'est à dire se formant aux dépens d'un élément épithélial ou se rattachant à l'épithélium, et d'un élément inoblastique (tissu conjonctif). La fibre nerveuse à myéline est dans ce cas d'après l'état actuel de nos connaissances, en admettant l'origine mésenchymateuse des cellules formant la myéline, ce qui cependant n'est pas établi avec certitude. L'ébauche du poil comprend non seulement l'épithélium, mais encore la papille dermique, et l'évolution ultérieure de ces deux parties est liée l'une à l'autre; alors que, par exemple, l'os se forme aux dépens d'un tissu inoblastique seul. La place du tissu lymphadénoïde ne saurait être marquée pour le moment que provisoirement, vu les divergences considérables qui existent relativement à son développement (*Stöhr, Retterer, Beard, Ranhuseu et Prymak*, et d'autres).

Tissus archiblastiques, parablastiques et mésenchymateux (*His, Waldeyer et Hertwig*): Il est presque superflu de rappeler les divergences d'opinions qui existent par rapport à cette classification de tissus partant du point de vue embryologique, et notamment pour ce qui concerne le parablaste (*His*). Quant à la catégorie de tissus mésenchymateux (*Hertwig*) comprenant le groupe de tissus conjonctifs de *Reichert*, l'endothélium vasculaire et le sang, il reste à savoir si le mésenchyme correspond à une entité morphologique. D'après *Kollmann*, l'ébauche des tissus mésenchymateux est localisée à la région du feuillet germinatif (Keimwall) et constitue l'archiblaste (Archiblast).

Ovule, Ovulaste: cellules ovulaires encore actives dans l'intérieur de l'épithélium germinatif (Nagoski): cellules des nids ou cordons ovulaires. Ovules faisant partie des hélicines ovariques. Ovules de 1er ordre — faisant partie des follicules primordiaux; ovules de 2me ordre — comprenant les stades ayant trait à la formation de la zone pellucide et à la différenciation du vitellus.

Bâtonnets de la zone pellucide. On constate ces formations aux trous de poussées; les bâtonnets semblent partir de l'épithélium folliculaire et s'enfoncer dans la zone pellucide.

Vitellus. Couche stéréoplasmique présentant une striation radiaire; couche chondroplasmique renfermant les grosses inclusions vitellines.

Tissus geroncatives. Filaments ourcicaires pennés — garnis de fibrilles collatérales ressemblant à des pinceaux. Stellules — se composent de granulations ou courts filaments agencés en figures stellaires ou rosaces. Ces deux particularités de structure sont bien exprimées dans la vésicule germinative de la salamandre maculée. *Flemming* a décrit ces structures dans l'ovule de Siredon (Zellsubstanz, Kern u. Zelltheilung); *Carnoy* et *Lebrun* dans l'ovule de Salamandre (la Cellule, XII, 1897).

Granulations nucléoliformes: volumineuses ressemblant à des nucléoles qu'on constate dans le caryoplasma de la vésicule germinative des reptiles en particulier.

Zone méio-granuleuse centrale (vésicule germinative; amphibiens, reptiles); se composant de filaments ou d'anses nucléaires et de granulations.

Spermatozoïde. À la partie principale de la tête, il y a lieu de distinguer deux portions l'antérieure — hyaline; la postérieure — vitreuse (réfringente), très accusées p. ex. chez le chien et le lapin.

Coussinet cervical; bourrelet ou appendice protoplasmiques à la portion intermédiaire des spermatozoïdes en formation.

Le segment intermédiaire (Mittelstück, *Schweigger, Seidel*) est aussi désigné sous le nom de Verbindungsstück.

Le filament terminal de la queue porte aussi le nom de filament de *Retzius*.

Filament spiral de la queue: Spiralsaum (*Ballowitz*).

Amas vitellin; Bourrelet ectodermique: Amas de cellules plus globuleuses accolées à la couche cellulaire marginale et qu'on constate à la vésicule blastodermique du lapin (*van Beneden*).

Épithélium. Thèque des cellules caliciformes (Theca d'après *List*); couche enveloppante du calice.

Épithélium à alvéoles; dont la face profonde est creusée d'alvéoles; exemple: cellules superficielles du revêtement vésical.

Épithélium trapézoïdal; formé dont la coupe optique ressemble à un trapèze et qu'on constate à l'épithélium de transition de la conjonctive.

Épithélium festonné; dont la partie profonde est excisée et denticulée, comme on le constate aux cellules de soutènement de la région olfactive.

Épithélium dendroïde; pourvu de fins prolongements arborescents; exemple: épithélium de l'épendyme (ventricules inférieurs).

Épithélium simple à plusieurs rangées de noyaux; peut simuler un épithélium stratifié, les noyaux étant situés à des niveaux différents.

Dérivés épithéliaux hétéroplastiques; qui dérivent de l'épithélium mais évoluent d'une manière spéciale en donnant naissance à des tumeurs propres.

Mentionnons, à ce propos, la dénomination: cellules «chromaffines» donnée par *Kohn* à certaines cellules ou agglomérations cellulaires se trouvant au voisinage du système nerveux sympathique à cause de leur affinité pour le chrome; les cellules de la substance médullaire des capsules surrénales, des nodules carotidien et coccygien, appartiendraient à cette catégorie cellulaire. Encore auparavant *Stilling* décrivit ces cellules sous le nom de cellules «chromophiles»; mais cette dénomination vise également non pas l'affinité pour certaines matières colorantes (dans le sens ordinaire du mot), mais celle pour les solutions de bichromate de potassium. On peut objecter à ces dénominations qu'elles prêtent à la confusion.

Cellules épithéliales; groupe naturellement provisoire, vu que l'origine des variétés cellulaires respectives n'est pas encore suffisamment élucidée, mais la constitution et l'agencement de ces cellules les rapprochent de l'épithélium. Les cellu-

 NATHAN LOEWENTHAL

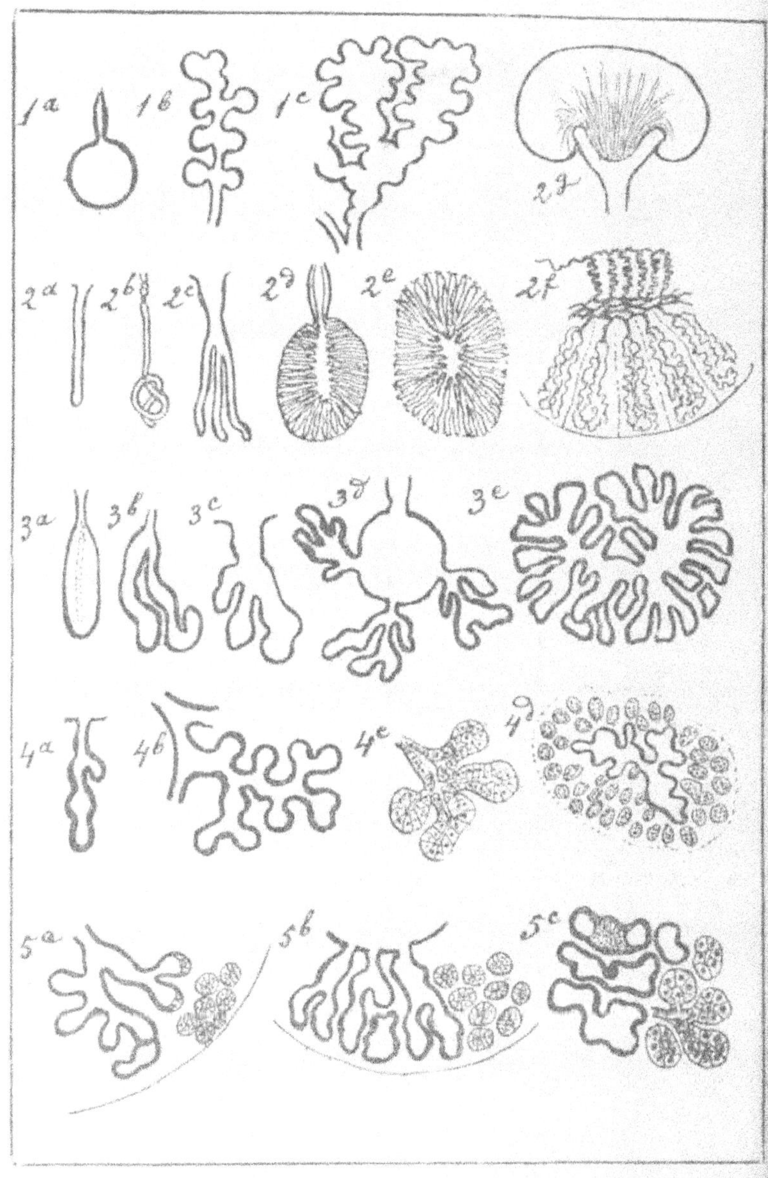

EXPLICATION DE LA PLANCHE

FIGURES SCHÉMATISÉES AYANT TRAIT AUX TYPES GLANDULAIRES

Fig. 1a — 1c Glandes acineuses.
1a Glande acineuse simple
1b " acineuse agminée en grappe simple
1c " infundibulo-acineuse, composée

Fig. 2a — 2g Glandes tubuleuses.
2a Glande tubuleuse simple
2b " " glomérulée
2c " " agminée-digitée
2d " " agminée à confluent central
2e " " agminée-composée à confluents centro-lobaires ramifiés. Un seul lobule est représenté
2f " " agminée-composée à système intermédiaire de canaux excréteurs rétiformes
2g " " agminée-composée à émonctoire commun

Fig. 3a — 3e Glandes utriculaires
3a Glande utriculaire simple
3b " divisée et enroulée
3c " agminée-pluripartite digitée
3d " agminée-composée et à conduits collecteurs
3e " agminée-composée à confluents centro-lobulaires

Fig. 4a — 4e Glandes tubulo-acineuses et tubulo-utriculaires
4a Glande tubulo-acineuse simple
4b Glande tubulo-acineuse composée eurytubulaire
4c Glande tubulo-acineuse ou utriculaire sténo-tubulaire
4d Type intermédiaire; sténo-alvéolaire à conduits intra-lobulaires dilatés.

Fig. 5a — 5c Glandes hétérogènes
5a Glande partie tubulo-acineuse eurytubulaire, partie sténo-alvéolaire ou sacculaire
5b Glande partie utriculaire, partie sténo-alvéolaire
5c Semblable au type 5a, mais à canaux larges beaucoup moins ramifiés

---

les interstitielles de l'ovaire pourraient dériver des restes épithéliaux qu'on constate dans la substance médullaire de l'ovaire (corps de *Wolff*). Pour ce qui concerne les cellules du corps jaune, elles dériveraient d'après *Sobotta* de l'épithélium folliculaire.

Glandes en général. Cryptes glandulaires : il s'agit des cryptes situés en entier ou pour une large part dans l'épaisseur du revêtement épithélial même, comme on le constate dans l'épithélium de la conjonctive.

Glandes exocrines : s'ouvrant à l'extérieur (au lieu des glandes ouvertes).

Les dénominations acinus et vésicule sont en somme équivalentes et peuvent être employées indifféremment l'une pour l'autre. Quant au mot alvéole, il a un sens bien moins précis et, pour ce qui concerne le type glandulaire, plutôt conventionnel. On l'emploie tantôt comme synonyme de la forme vésiculeuse, tantôt pour désigner la forme utriculaire. Ainsi l'on dit : alvéoles ou vésicules pulmonai res en identifiant l'alvéole avec la vésicule, on dit d'autre part aussi: alvéoles des glandes salivaires (Alveolen des auteurs allemands). Le plus souvent on ne décrit que deux types glandulaires fondamentaux: le tubuleux et l'alvéolaire ou acineux. L'étude des formes glandulaires simples démontre cependant qu'il en existe trois: le tubuleux, l'acineux (ou le vésiculeux) et l'utriculaire (c. à d. en forme de sac plus ou moins allongé).

En fait de glandes utriculaires typiques, on peut citer les glandes de l'oviducte de la grenouille et de l'orvet. Les glandes sébacées des mammifères appartiennent plutôt au type utriculaire qu'au type acineux.

Types composés de glandes: tubulo-acineux, c. à d. des vésicules greffées sur un tube; tubulo-utriculaire: des utricules greffées sur un tube; ces deux types ne sont cependant pas tout-à-fait indépendants, il n'est pas rare d'observer des formes intermédiaires. Vient en suite le type utriculo- ou infundibulo-acineux, où des vésicules sont greffées sur une utricule ou un infundibulum (pour les variétés de formes glandulaires consult. la planche schématique ci-jointe.

Glandes agminées: On pourrait nommer ainsi les glandes qui se composent d'un agrégat de glandes simples (dans le sens strict du mot) qui débouchent dans un conduit commun non subdivisé. Ces glandes ne sont plus simples vu qu'elles se composent de plusieurs unités glandulaires (tubes ou utricules); elles ne sont pas non plus composées dans le sens qu'on attribue ordinairement à ce mot, vu que le conduit n'est pas divisé et que la glande ne se compose pas de lobules.

Glandes subcomposées: à système de conduits peu ramifiés.

Glandes à confluent central. Cette catégorie glandulaire n'a pas encore été suffisamment mise en relief. Dans ce cas, une agglomération d'unités glandulaires débouchent dans un espace commun — confluent central — qui ne correspond pas encore au vrai conduit excréteur. Exemple de glandes tubuleuses non composées de ce genre: les glandes du proventricule des oiseaux (pigeon).

Glandes tubuleuses. Agminées composées à confluents centro-tubulaires ramifiés: la glande de Harder du canard.

Gl. tubuleuses à système de canaux excréteurs intermédiaires, rétiformes, exemple: le testicule de mammifères (rete testis). Cette particularité de structure devient plus facilement explicable si l'on tient compte de la constitution des glandes agminées à confluent central ramifié, et représente pour ainsi dire un stade plus différencié de ce dernier type (compar. les figures 2 — 2).

Glandes tubuleuses agminées composées à glomérules vasculaires et à émonctoire commun. Rein: cette glande aussi se laisse rattacher au type à confluent central; ce confluent est représenté par le bassinet du rein.

Glandes tubuleuses composées (véritables): foie.

 acineuses simples: Glandes cutanées des Amphibiens.
  agminées, en groupe simple: Glandes de Meibomius.
 infundibulo-acineuses) communs.
 acineuses débitrices) avance.
Glandes utriculaires simples: glandes de l'oviducte de la grenouille.
  agminées, digitées: glandes séparées.
  enroulées: glandes de l'oviducte de l'orvet.
  digito-agminées composées: glandes préputiales du rat blanc.
  agminées composées à confluents centro-lobulaires: glandes bucco-uréthrales du rat blanc.

Glandes utriculo-acineuses : glandes prostatiques (homme)

Glandes tubulo-acineuses simples. On constate des glandes de cette espèce soit simples (formées d'un seul tubulo-acinus) soit divisées dans la muqueuse utérine du hérisson.

— tubulo-enrymbulaires ; à canaux glandulaires larges ; glande de Harder, hérisson

— siège alvéolaires ou -utriculaires ; à alvéoles ou utricules à cavité étroite : glandes salivaires.

— variété intermédiaire à conduits intra-lobulaires dilatés. Un exemple de ces glandes est fourni par les glandes de la troisième paupière du chien.

Glandes hétérogènes (mixtes)

subdivision a) : Glandes de Harder et de la troisième paupière du hérisson ; glande de Harder du porc ; gl. sous-orbitaire du rat blanc

subdivision b) : Glandes bulbo-uréthrales (Méry-Cowper) du rat blanc.

Glandes séro-sébacées. Exemple : Glande de Harder du hérisson et du porc.

Glandes séro-colloïdes (?) À en juger d'après les réactions micro-chimiques il est permis de conclure à l'existence de telles glandes. La glande sous-maxillaire proprement dite du rat blanc n'est pas une glande séreuse pure, mais mixte d'après la constitution de l'épithélium, et probablement séro-colloïde.

Glandes closes atypiques. On pourrait comprendre sous ce nom la portion glandulaire de l'hypophyse (homme), vu qu'on y constate à la fois des cordons, et des îlots (follicules) pour la plupart pleins, en partie aussi pourvus de cavités.

Structure fine des glandes. Fibres en treillis, Gitterfasern signalées par v. *Kupffer* et *Oppel* dans le foie. Cellules étoilées du foie, — connues aussi sous le nom de cellules de v. *Kupffer*.

Cellules en panier : aussi cellules de *Boll-Lavdowsky*.

Cellules nerveuses interstitielles ; signalées par *Cajal* dans le pancréas, par *Karol Roff* dans les glandes salivaires.

Plexus nerveux péricellulaire. *Berkley* a signalé ce mode de terminaison dans les lobules hépatiques (Anat. Anzeiger, VIII).

La terminaison en forme de bouquets, grappes ou arborisations accolées aux cellules glandulaires a été décrite en particulier par *Arnstein* et ses élèves (gl. sudoripares, sébacées, de *Meibomius* et d'autres)

Capillaires sécrétoires. On peut objecter que cette expression évoque l'idée d'un tube à paroi propre, alors qu'il s'agit des canalicules ou rigoles dépourvus de revêtement cellulaire propre et creusés pour ainsi dire dans le corps cellulaire.

Tissu nerveux. Neurofibrilles. *Bethe* fait la distinction entre des neuro-fibrilles périphériques et centrales (Allgem. Anat. u. Physiol. des Nervensystems, 1903). Il est juste de rappeler à propos de ces formations (*Apáthy, Bethe, Cajal, Auerbach, Dcandgge* et d'autres) que la structure fibrillaire des cellules des centres nerveux a déjà été signalée par Max *Schultze* (éventails fibrillaires).

Terminaison dendritique glomérulée. Celle des grandes cellules olfactives dans les glomérules olfactifs.

Terminaison en bouquet aux prolongements protoplasmiques des grains du cervelet.

Prolongements dendritiques épineux ; garnis de ces fines excroissances généralement connues et qui se montrent à la suite de l'imprégnation par la méthode de *Golgi* ; plusieurs noms ont été donnés à ces excroissances qu'on pourrait aussi nommer pinnules.

Prolongements péri-, homo- et oppositotropes. On pourrait spécifier par ces expressions la direction des prolongements dendritiques (protoplasmiques); péritropes — partant indifféremment de toutes les parties de la périphérie cellulaire; oppositotropes — se dirigeant dans des sens opposés; homotropes — se dirigeant dans le même sens (cellules de *Purkinje*).

Parmi les divers noms donnés au prolongement nerveux, celui de neurite serait le plus recommandable s'il n'existait déjà le mot névrite ayant une tout autre signification.

Le rétrécissement intermédiaire (collet) du prolongement nerveux, au niveau de jonction du cône d'implantation et du filament cylindraxile, est très accusé par ex. aux grandes cellules pyramidales de l'écorce du cerveau.

Les prolongements nerveux : type de *Deiters* et type de *Golgi* pourraient être désignés sous les noms : prolong. nerveux axiles (vu leur continuation directe avec un cylindre axe) et prolong. nerveux arborescents (vu qu'ils se perdent dans une arborisation très fournie.

Prolongements cellulaires atypiques : pour spécifier les prolongements de quelques espèces cellulaires ne présentant pas de caractères suffisamment tranchés pour permettre de les classer en protoplasmiques et nerveux (p. ex. les prolongements des grains du cervelet).

Cellules ganglionnaires chromophiles : il s'agit des différences relatives à la colorabilité des cellules signalées par *Flesch* et ses élèves.

Des branches collatérales du prolongement nerveux des cellules ganglionnaires (cérébro-spinales) ont été signalées par *Dogiel*. Le même auteur décrit des prolongements nerveux donnant naissance à trois branches, et une espèce cellulaire dont le prolongement nerveux se ramifie à diverses reprises et se termine par des arborisations péricellulaires entourant les cellules ordinaires (pourvues d'un prolongement en T).

Cellules ganglionnaires bipolaires des poissons. A part les cellules non couvertes de myéline, il y en a d'autres qui sont entourées d'un manchon de myéline se continuant sans interruption sur les prolongements nerveux.

Des prolongements dendritiques (protoplasmiques) aux cellules ganglionnaires ont été signalés en particulier par *Fusari*, *Cannieu*, *Sclavunos* et *Spirlas*.

Cellules sympathiques de batraciens, connues aussi sous le nom de cellules de *Beale*. Les variétés de prolongement spiral à tours serrés et lâches peuvent être reconnues dans le sympathique abdominal de la grenouille.

Agglomérats sympathiques (batraciens). Ces corps représentent selon toute évidence des foyers de prolifération des cellules sympathiques; ils sont en connexion avec des faisceaux de fibres de *Remak* et sont entourés d'une gaine qui se continue sur ces faisceaux à la manière d'une gaine périneurale.

Disques intersegmentaires (du cylindre-axe). D'après *Demoor*, il y aurait au niveau des renflements bi-coniques une couche intermédiaire se comportant d'une manière spéciale par rapport au nitrate d'argent (Contrib. à l'étude de la fibre nerveuse. Institut Solvay, Bruxelles, 1891.)

La distinction entre les cellules névrogliques des vertébrés supérieurs et inférieurs a bien sa raison d'être surtout au point de vue de l'extension des prolongements cellulaires. Pour ce qui concerne les astrocytes, *Athias* pense avec *Sala* que cette forme de la cellule névroglique n'est pas du tout représentée chez les batraciens (Bibliogr. anatomique, 1897).

Terminaisons nerveuses. Texte épithéliales : dans l'épithélium de revêtement adéno-épithéliales — dans les glandes; kérato-vaginales — dans les gaines des formations cornées (poils).

Plexus nerveux préterminaux. Ceux qui précèdent les plexus terminaux.

Arborisations terminales, péricellulaire et adcellulaire: le premier mode de terminaison se rapporte au cas où les fibrilles terminales enlacent toute la périphérie cellulaire, on pourrait appeler adcellulaires celles où l'arborisation ne touche qu'à une des faces de la cellule ou à une partie de son pourtour.

Bulbes terminaux. D'après *Krause*, les bulbes de tous les corpuscules nerveux terminaux seraient pourvus de cellules nucléées; Kolbenzellen (Arch. f. mikr. Anat. XIX). Ce n'est cependant pas encore admis sans restriction. V. *Koelliker* décrit les bulbes terminaux comme étant dépourvus de noyaux et ne renfermant qu'un contenu clair (Handb. d. Gewebelehre, 6 Aufl., p. 177). Sur des préparations de corpuscules de *Pacini* examinés soit en entier soit par la méthode de coupes, il est difficile de se convaincre de l'existence des cellules ou des noyaux dans le bulbe central, alors que les noyaux sont faciles à reconnaître dans la bulbe des corpuscules de *Herbst*.

Corpuscules de *Meissner*. Le contenu endidermal (situé à l'intérieur de la gaine) de ces corpuscules est-il comparable à celui du bulbe central des corpuscules de Pacini ou même de Herbst? Le bulbe de ces derniers corpuscules paraît être clair et homogène; dans les corpuscules de Meissner, il paraît exister à l'intérieur de la gaine une substance granuleuse entourant des noyaux serrés et dirigés transversalement, et de plus, on peut reconnaître dans cette substance granuleuse des lignes plus claires semblant indiquer qu'elle est segmentée autour des noyaux.

Corpuscules de *Pacini* et de *Herbst*. La portion de la fibre afférente qui traverse les gaines de ces corpuscules pourrait être désignée sous le nom d'intra-capsulaire par opposition à la portion située en dehors des gaines (ou extra-capsulaire).

Histogénèse des éléments nerveux. On pourrait désigner sous le nom de prolongement axogène (en abrégeant le mot: axone) celui qui donne naissance au cylindre-axe, et de dendritogènes ceux qui fournissent les prolongements protoplasmiques.

La formation de la myéline est encore sujette à des controverses, de même que le rôle et l'origine des cellules dites mésenchymateuses ou de *Vignal*. Pour ce qui concerne la manière de voir généralement admise sur la formation du cylindre-axe par excroissance à partir des cellules neuroblastes (*His, Cajal*), il y a à citer les constatations plus récentes de *Bethe* qui, s'appuyant surtout sur les recherches de *Dohrn*, arrive à conclure que les cylindres-axes se forment aux dépens des cellules multiples, c'est à dire dans l'intérieur des chaînes cellulaires (Zellketten) formant la première ébauche des nerfs périphériques (Allg. Anat. u. Physiol. des Nervensystems, p. 235 u ff.)

Tissu musculaire lisse. Ponticules intercellulaires: Les images qui correspondent à ces formations ont cependant été interprétées d'une autre manière et l'existence de ces ponticules a été mise en doute. A la place des présumés ponticules il y aurait un système de fibrilles ou travées conjonctives enlaçant les cellules musculaires (compar. *J. Schaffer*, Anat. Anz. XV, *Prenant*, Arch. d'Anat. microscop. V, et d'autres). L'existence d'une substance unissante cémentaire est mise en doute. *Bohemnggui* défend l'existence des vraies ponticules protoplasmiques intercellulaires (Anat. Anz. X).

Le centrosoma des cellules musculaires lisses (ou plus exactement parlant:

diplosoma) est désigné par v. *Lenhossék* (1899) sous le nom de «Mikrocentrum» (macrocentre) dénomination admise aussi par *Heidenhain* pour les cellules géantes (v. plus haut: centrosomes multiples).

Tissu musculaire lisse. La question des taches motrices est controversée. Parmi les observations plus récentes qui touchent à ce sujet, citons la communication de Kytmanoff (méthode au bleu de méthylène) sur les terminaisons nerveuses dans le conduit thoracique et dans les vaisseaux lymphatiques du cordon séminal. L'auteur décrit des fibrilles nerveuses variqueuses qui enlacent les cellules musculaires par un renflement ressemblant aux taches motrices de Ranvier.

Sur des préparations imprégnées au chlorure d'or, de la vessie de la grenouille, on peut reconnaître également des fibrilles qui semblent s'accoler aux cellules musculaires pour s'y terminer par une extrémité renflée, mais on pourrait objecter qu'il s'agit d'imprégnations incomplètes, et que les boutons terminaux imprégnés correspondent à des varicosités au delà desquelles la fibre n'a pas été imprégnée.

Vaisseaux perforants qui traversent les tuniques musculaires, et tout en abandonnant des rameaux à ces tuniques se rendent à d'autres parties (sous-muqueuse, muqueuse de l'intestin).

Cellules musculaires striées du cœur. La variété fusiforme ramifiée peut être isolée du myocarde de la grenouille, de la salamandre ou de la tortue, et établit la transition entre la cellule fusiforme striée et le segment musculaire tel qu'on l'observe chez les mammifères.

La nomenclature ayant trait à la structure de la fibre musculaire striée est particulièrement chargée. Il y a entre autres à choisir entre les expressions: disque, bande, lame, strie et ligne, souvent appliquées à la même formation.

On pourrait désigner sous le nom de myofibrilles les fibrilles musculaires primitives. Les colonnes musculaires (Muskelsäulchen), dénomination assez vague, pourraient être appelées: colonnes myofibrillaires.

Stries longitudinales granuleuses de la fibre musculaire: stries plus épaisses et renfermant des granulations distinctes.

Lame médiane ou strie de *Hensen*. Lame terminale ou de *Merkel*. Disque accessoire ou d'*Engelmann*. Strie intermédiaire ou d'*Amici-Krause*.

Perimysium interne, on pourrait bien l'appeler endomysium, comme on dit perimètre et endomètre.

Citons quelques autres dénominations de la plaque motrice des fibres striées. Plaque terminale (*Rouget*); éminence de *Doyère*; buisson de *Kühne*.

Coussinet nucléé; cette expression conviendrait peut-être mieux que les dénominations: plaque granuleuse ou semelle granuleuse (Sohlenplatte), vu que cette couche forme, en tous cas chez les mammifères, une éminence distincte.

Faisceaux névro-musculaires. Autres noms donnés à la même formation: Fuseaux névro-musculaires, bourgeons musculaires (Muskelknospen, v. *Koelliker*), organes de *Kühne*.

Arborisations nerveuses terminales adtendineuses: Fuseaux de Golgi, fuseaux névro-tendineux.

Histogenèse de la fibre musculaire. Cellules interstitielles; il s'agit des cellules de forme irrégulière et qu'on constate soit entre les fibres musculaires en voie de développement, soit à leur surface.

Myoblastes secondaires; chaînes de myoblastes. On pourrait donner ce nom aux sarcoplastes de *Margo-Paneth* pour spécifier les cellules et les chaînes cellu-

...laires prenant part à la formation du tissu musculaire en dehors de la période embryonnaire (régénération, néoplasie musculaire). Des chaînes de myoblastes se détachant des fibres musculaires déjà formées ont été figurées aussi par *Lawdowsky* (Éléments d'anatomie microscopique, en russe). D'autre part, les sarcoplastes ont été aussi interprétés comme des sarcolytes entrant en jeu dans la dégénérescence musculaire (*Sig. Mayer*).

Sang. Globules rouges. Couche cortico-plasmique: on pourrait appeler ainsi la couche marginale plus dense mais non isolable de ces globules.

Érythrocytes nucléés globuleux. On constate dans des préparations de la moelle osseuse de la grenouille des globules rouges plus petits que les globules elliptiques ordinaires, à contour arrondi ou oval-arrondi, et à noyau également moins allongé que celui des hématies ordinaires; ce noyau est souvent situé excentriquement.

Bien que dans la littérature plus récente on fasse une distinction entre leucocytes et lymphocytes, on peut se demander si cette distinction est suffisamment justifiée, c. à d. si elle correspond à des catégories fixes de globules blancs sanguins. Comme les dénominations leucocytes et globules blancs ne sont pas particulièrement recommandables, vu que ces globules ne sont pas plus blancs que beaucoup d'autres cellules, il semblerait préférable de désigner ces globules sous le nom de lymphocytes.

Plaquettes sanguines ou de *Bizzozero* (hématoblastes de *Hayem*), thrombocytes. C'est sous cette dernière dénomination qu'on désigne le plus souvent la plaquette sanguine dans la littérature récente, vu le rôle qu'on attribue à ces éléments dans la coagulation du sang. La constitution histologique et l'origine des thrombocytes sont du reste encore très controversées.

La disparition du noyau des globules rouges (mammifères) a été expliquée soit par l'expulsion, soit par la dissolution, soit par la dégénérescence chromatolytique. Pour *Giglio Tos* il s'agit d'une transformation chimique se traduisant par le fait que le noyau devient d'abord érytrophile et finalement homogène (La struttura e l'evoluzione dei corpuscoli rossi del sangue. Torino 1897). D'après *Maslow* le noyau disparaît par une espèce de désagrégation intra-cellulaire, ou il s'atrophie et perd l'affinité pour les matières colorantes (Arch. f. mikr. Anatomie, 51, 1898).

Tissu conjonctif. Cellules inoblastes donnant naissance aux fibres conjonctives ou fibres élastiques. Chondroblastes. — Un exemple démonstratif de cellules s'entourant d'une coque cartilagineuse est fourni par les cellules revêtant par places les tendons fléchisseurs des doigts (non ossifiés) des oiseaux passereaux.

Cellules géantes formatives donnant naissance à des cellules médullaires; il n'est pas établi avec certitude que les cellules géantes représentent uniquement des éléments destructeurs. On peut également citer des observations à l'appui des fonctions formatives de ces cellules (*Denys*. Quelques remarques sur la division des cellules géantes de la moelle. Anat. Anzeiger, 1888).

Cellules pigmentaires digitées: cette forme se distingue de la forme étoilée par le fait que les prolongements cellulaires sont plus courts et épais que dans la dernière variété et qu'ils se terminent par des extrémités en forme de doigt de gant ou même renflées. La variété plate de la cellule pigmentaire est représentée dans la lamina fusca.

Cellules ramifiées à prolongements filiformes: cette variété particulière et caractérisée par ses prolongements particulièrement grêles et longs se rencontre dans le tissu interstitiel des muscles chez la grenouille.

Cellules conjonctives chromophiles. Il s'agit des cellules qu'on trouve également dans le tissu interstitiel de la grenouille et qui se distinguent par le fait qu'elles fixent vivement à l'état frais le bleu de méthylène.

Cellules séro-adipeuses: dont le contenu graisseux a été résorbé par suite de dénutrition.

Cellules adipeuses à noyau central. Ces cellules se distinguent par le fait qu'elles sont infiltrées par de nombreuses gouttelettes graisseuses plutôt fines, et que lors même que le corps cellulaire est entièrement rempli de ces gouttelettes, le noyau n'est pas refoulé à la périphérie comme c'est le cas des cellules adipeuses ordinaires.

Cellules dites d'engrais. Cette dénomination impliquant une interprétation qui non seulement n'est pas établie mais contestée, on pourrait désigner ces cellules sous le nom de grando-plasmatiques pour les distinguer des cellules plasmatiques ordinaires.

Endothélium conjonctif. On pourrait donner ce nom aux cellules plates revêtant les espaces, fentes ou sinus lymphatiques du système conjonctif, pour distinguer ces cellules du revêtement des membranes séreuses et du système vasculaire ou lymphatique à paroi propre.

Tissu adipeux blanc et gris. Cette distinction se base sur le fait qu'on constate chez le rat blanc des îlots adipeux, de coloration grisâtre et ressemblant à du tissu glandulaire, et qui se composent de cellules adipeuses à noyau central mentionnées plus haut, c'est-à-dire renfermant de fines gouttelettes graisseuses.

Tissu conjonctif trabéculaire: formé de trabécules cloisonnant un espace renfermant une quantité plus ou moins grande de sérosité, comme le tissu trabéculaire sous-arachnoïdien.

Membranes vasculaires. Ces membranes se distinguent non seulement par leur riche vascularisation, mais encore par le fait qu'elles sont pourvues par places de plis ou de prolongements villeux très vascularisés et en rapport avec des revêtements épithéliaux: les villosités du chorion chez le fœtus; les plexus choroïdes de la pie-mère; la choroïde de l'œil.

Membranes enveloppantes viscérales, enveloppes des viscères (rein, rate, testicule).

Innervation du tissu conjonctif. Réseaux péricellulaires décrits autour des chromatophores (*Ballowitz*, *Eberth* und *Bunge*. Arborisations terminales constatées en connexion avec les tendons, Pelotons encapsulés (C. *Dogiel*, Ueber die Nervenendapparate in der Haut des Menschen. Zeitschr. f. wiss. Zoologie, 1903).

Membranes séreuses. Fossettes ou cavernes: on constate ces formations à la séreuse péritonéale dans la région prévertébrale de la grenouille; la couche conjonctive de la membrane se réfléchit dans ces fossettes renfermant des cellules granuleuses et plus petites que les cellules endothéliales avoisinantes.

Tissu cartilagineux. Fibres de la substance fondamentale: il s'agit des fibres isolées et non pas de la présumée texture fibrillaire de la substance fondamentale hyaline.

Faisceaux conjonctifs perforants du cartilage: existent dans la tête du fémur de la grenouille, autour du cylindre osseux qui pénètre dans le cartilage épiphysaire. Le côté externe de ce cylindre osseux est entouré d'un prolongement du périoste renfermant des vaisseaux sanguins. C'est à partir de cette couche conjonctive que de grêles fascicules de fibres conjonctives entourées d'espaces clairs se portent à l'extérieur en traversant la substance fondamentale du cartilage.

Fibro-cartilage d'insertion: couche fibro-cartilagineuse intermédiaire au niveau des insertions tendineuses et des ligaments fibreux.

Cartilages mixtes: renfermant à la fois du tissu cartilagineux hyalin et du tissu cartilagineux élastique ou fibreux.

Transformation pseudo-fibreuse du cartilage hyalin; n'est pas identique avec le fibro-cartilage, il s'agit plutôt d'une espèce de dissociation de la substance fondamentale.

Tissu chondroïde. Il s'agit d'un tissu apparemment intermédiaire entre le tissu cartilagineux et le tissu conjonctif. La substance fondamentale se rapproche de celle du cartilage hyalin; les cellules ressemblent aux cellules conjonctives ramifiées. L'existence dans ce tissu des espaces péricellulaires et des canalicules anastomotiques accompagnant les prolongements cellulaires rappelle la disposition qu'on trouve dans la cornée. Le dit tissu est représenté dans la tunique propre du labyrinthe membraneux des vertébrés inférieurs.

Ossification. Enchondrale néoplastique: s'accompagnant de résorption du cartilage et de néoformation du tissu osseux; enchondrale directe: consistant dans les transformations directes du tissu cartilagineux en tissu osseux, mode d'ossification discuté.

Ossification intra-membraneuse et fibreuse directe: Il y a à distinguer entre ces deux modes d'ossification et par conséquent entre les os qui en résultent. On pourrait désigner sous le nom de "métaplastiques„ les os conjonctifs résultant de l'ossification intra-membraneuse, alors qu'il y a des remaniements essentiels dans l'intérieur de la membrane respective. Les os conjonctifs "autoplastiques„ comprendraient ceux qui résultent de l'ossification fibreuse directe. Le processus histologique de l'ossification intra-membraneuse est tout à fait analogue à celui de l'ossification sous-périostique, avec cette différence que dans le premier cas l'ossification se passe dans l'épaisseur d'une membrane conjonctive (comme à la calotte crânienne), dans le second cas au-dessous d'une membrane conjonctive.

On désigne communément les os enchondraux sous le nom de "primaires„ et les os conjonctifs sous celui de "secondaires„. Dans l'un comme dans l'autre cas cependant, l'os est une formation secondaire, qu'il soit précédé par du cartilage ou par du tissu conjonctif.

Ossification centro- et téléodiaphysaire: pour spécifier l'ossification qui se passe d'une part au centre de la diaphyse, d'autre part au niveau du cartilage de conjugaison.

Points d'ossification. On pourrait préférer les expressions, foyers ou îlots d'ossification, vu qu'il ne s'agit pas d'un point. Quant à l'ossification qui se passe au niveau des cartilages de conjugaison, elle est étalée en surface et non pas circonscrite en point.

Amas et piles chondrocytaires. Les premiers s'observent au centre de la diaphyse; les seconds du côté des cartilages de conjugaison.

Moelle cartilagineuse: remplissant les espaces résultant de la fonte des capsules cartilagineuses.

Rainure d'implantation: Constriction circulaire à la limite des épiphyses et de la diaphyse et où les fibres du périoste pénétrent en partie dans le cartilage.

Fibres constitutives et perforantes (ossification, tissu osseux). On pourrait donner le nom de constitutives aux fibres faisant partie intégrante des lamelles osseuses (fibres de v. *Ebner*) pour les distinguer des fibres perforantes.

Cellules géantes dans l'ossification intra-membraneuse. On rencontre des cel-

lules géantes à noyaux multiples ou polymorphes dans la calotte crânienne des
fœtus humains, entre la couche fibreuse externe et les travées osseuses extérieures.

Bourrelets fibro-cellulaires sous-périostiques (poissons). Le tissu de ces bourrelets a été désigné par *I. Schaffer* sous le nom de "vesikuläres Stützgewebe,, tissu
de soutènement vésiculaire (Anat. Anzeiger, XXIII, 1903).

Tissu ostéo-cartilagineux (tissu osseux mixte). On pourrait donner ce nom aux
os représentés chez les vertébrés inférieurs et qui se composent de tissu osseux
englobant des îlots de cartilage. Ce tissu se distingue nettement de l'os enchondral
ordinaire des mammifères par le fait que dans ce dernier les îlots cartilagineux ne
renferment que de la substance fondamentale, alors que le tissu ostéo-cartilagineux
des vertébrés inférieurs contient du tissu cartilagineux complet (substance fondamentale et chondrocytes).

Tissu fibro-capsulaire propre de la chorde dorsale (poissons osseux). Sur la
coupe transversale, on constate dans ce tissu des travées séparant les cellules et
ressemblant à des capsules épaisses; mais il s'agit en réalité, comme on peut le re-
reconnaître sur la coupe longitudinale, des travées en forme de fibres rigides dont
l'agencement est longitudinal et plexiforme. Dans la zone moyenne ces travées sont
particulièrement épaisses.

Tissu lymphadénoïde. C'est à dessein que les cellules globuleuses principales
de ce tissu sont désignées ici sous le nom de lymphoïdes, vu les divergences qui se
sont manifestées dans la littérature plus récente par rapport à l'origine de ces cellules (epithélium lymphadénoïde?).

Les "Gitterfasern,, ont été signalées par *Oppel* dans la rate (Anat. Anzeiger, VI).

Tissu lymphadénoïde diffus: ne formant ni follicules ni cordons circonscrits.

Follicules crypto-bordants: entourant des cryptes épithéliaux.

Follicules parenchymateux: faisant partie des parenchymes (comme les follicules de la rate).

Follicules interstitiels: dans le tissu conjonctif interstitiel, souvent au voisinage des conduits excréteurs des glandes.

Système vasculaire. Endocarde: La couche "intermédiaire,, tranche assez
distinctement, au moins par places, sur les couches externe et interne de l'endocarde d'homme, et contient des éléments qui pourraient correspondre à des cellules
musculaires lisses.

La couche "sous-endothéliale,, est encore désignée sous le nom de "lamellaire,, et renferme des noyaux aplatis dans le sens de la surface.

Valvules: face axiale: dirigée du côté de l'orifice (ostium) limité par les valvules, par opposition à la face pariétale. La dénomination: face axiale qu'on trouve
dans quelques manuels prête quelque peu à l'équivoque, vu qu'on peut penser à la
face médiane passant par l'axe de la valvule. La couche "cellulo-fibrillaire,, des
valvules sigmoïdes se distingue, chez l'homme, par son aspect plus clair et la réduction de l'élément fibreux.

Artères. Il est indiqué de reconnaître à côté des types: élastique et musculaire
encore un type intermédiaire.

Artérioles précapillaires: il n'est peut être pas superflu de donner un nom
propre aux dernières ramifications artérielles précédant les capillaires.

Les terminaisons nerveuses sensitives des vaisseaux sanguins et lymphatiques ont été décrites en particulier par *Dogiel*, *Ruchmanow* (Anat. Anz. XIX, 1901)
et *Kytmanoff* (ibid. XIX).

Les cellules vasoformatives de *Ranvier* ont été aussi interprétées comme des produits de la régression du réseau vasculaire; comp. l'exposé de v. *Ebner* dans le traité de v. *Koelliker*, Tome III, p. 673.

Parenchymes lymphadénoïdes: Le classement de ces organes en paravasculaires et parépithéliaux paraît être justifié par des faits soit d'ordre morphologique, soit d'ordre histogénétique. Les ganglions lymphatiques surtout, mais aussi la rate, rentrent dans la première catégorie. Dans les ganglions lymphatiques, la substance folliculaire affecte des rapports particulièrement intimes avec les sinus lymphatiques et la circulation de la lymphe; dans la rate, on constate des rapports particulièrement intimes entre les éléments de la pulpe splénique et les éléments figurés du sang. Le développement de la rate est cependant encore incomplètement élucidé. A côté des auteurs qui assignent à cet organe une origine purement mésenchymateuse (*Laguesse, Nicolas*, Archives de Biologie XX, 1903, parmi les auteurs plus récents), il y en a d'autres qui font dériver cet organe de l'ébauche du pancréas (v. *Kupffer*, 1892).

Le thymus paraît au contraire rentrer tout naturellement dans la seconde catégorie d'organes lymphadénoïdes, vu que la première ébauche de ce corps est sans contredit d'origine épithéliale, et que dans l'organe formé on constate des îlots ayant tous les caractères d'épithélium. Les follicules des amygdales, de l'appendice iléo-cæcal, du cæcum ou de la région inférieure de l'intestin grêle contractent des rapports avec des diverticules épithéliaux partant de la surface de la muqueuse.

Cellules à hématolytes: On pourrait appeler de ce nom les cellules de la pulpe splénique renfermant des débris de globules rouges du sang.

Voies vasculaires de la pulpe splénique: voies intermédiaires entre les capillaires artériels et veineux, et qu'on envisage plus généralement comme des fentes lacunaires interceptées entre les cellules de la pulpe.

Cellules vasoendymaires fusiformes: cellules revêtant les capillaires veineux de la pulpe splénique, et qui se distinguent cependant des cellules endothéliales ordinaires.

Fibres élastiques transversales des ronces(pulpe splénique): Compar. v. *Ebner* dans le traité de v. *Kolliker*, 6e édit. Tome A, p. 279.

Thymus. Cellules thymiques à structure granulo-fibrillaire concentrique: Ces cellules ont ceci de particulier qu'on reconnaît dans leur intérieur des fibrilles qui se composent de granules et qui sont agencées d'une manière concentrique autour du noyau. Chez la grenouille, les dites fibrilles sont déjà visibles à un grossissement moyen. Les cellules peuvent renfermer deux noyaux; les fibrilles protoplasmiques se groupent dans ce cas autour de chacun d'eux. Dans le thymus du lézard, on constate des cellules analogues, bien que pas identiques. Ces cellules se distinguent par leur aspect luisant et l'agencement concentrique des granules protoplasmiques; elles peuvent renfermer deux noyaux et même plusieurs; on rencontre, de plus, des cellules de ce genre pourvues de prolongements.

Système tégumentaire. Vallécules: pour désigner les sillons séparant les crêtes dermiques.

Derme, reptiles. Lamelle dermique marginale: il s'agit d'une fine lamelle dermique située à la limite de l'épiderme et qui tranche par son aspect hyalin sur la couche dermique pigmentée sous-jacente. La couche fasciculée n'est pas partout également bien différenciée; la couche compacte ou lamellaire se compose de lamelles régulièrement disposées et tassées.

Plan squameux de l'épiderme: comprenant la couche renfermant les écailles.

Poches squamifères : pour désigner les sillons qui correspondent à la partie cachée des écailles ; plan du toit : comprenant la couche cutanée en dessus de l'écaille ; plan du lit squaméal : la couche cutanée située en dessous.

Les couches décrites se rapportent en particulier à la peau du lézard.

Lames dermiques intermédiaires (poissons osseux) : lames qui séparent les loges renfermant les écailles (squaméales).

Cellules granuleuses (Lamproie). On constate dans ces cellules un réseau fibrillaire terminal disposé autour du noyau et étant en connexion avec les prolongements intracellulaires (Compar. ma note : Beitrag zur Kenntnis der Körnerzellen des Neunauges. Anat. Anzeiger, XXV, 1904).

Glandes sébacées. Epithélium centro-acineux : pour désigner l'épithélium en dégénérescence graisseuse remplissant la région centrale de la vésicule ou du saccule glandulaire.

Epithélium sébacé à noyau central : pour distinguer l'épithélium des glandes sébacées proprement dites de l'épithélium d'autres glandes à sécrétion également sébacée, mais dont l'épithélium a la forme prismatique et renferme un noyau qui n'a pas de situation fixe.

Glandes sébacées annexes. On pourrait désigner sous ce nom les glandules ayant la structure des glandes sébacées, mais qui sont annexées à d'autres glandes. On en trouve un exemple dans les glandules sébacées des tétins de la chatte, glandules qui s'ouvrent dans les conduits excréteurs de la glande mammaire.

Glande uropygienne : La description se rapporte en particulier à la glande du moineau.

Mamelon glandulaire : visible à l'œil nu et renfermant les confluents et les conduits excréteurs de la glande.

Confluents sous-mamillaires : situés au-dessous de la région du mamelon ; confluents mamillaires : situés dans l'épaisseur du mamelon.

Les trois zones épithéliales décrites à l'épithélium du conduit glandulaire commun se succèdent de l'intérieur à l'extérieur. Il n'y a pas de démarcation tranchée entre ces zones qui correspondent aux changements successifs que subissent les cellules épithéliales.

Glandes cutanées du pouce (grenouille). Cloisons intra-glandulaires : à l'intérieur du sac glandulaire commun, et délimitant les diverticules glandulaires secondaires.

Glandes paracutanées. Il ne serait peut-être pas superflu de réunir sous une dénomination à part les glandes situées à la région de transition entre le tégument externe et les membranes muqueuses, telles que les glandes de Meibomius, les glandes circumanales ou celles du prépuce.

Ongles. Loge onguéale : on pourrait donner ce nom à la région renfermant la racine de l'ongle.

Lame recouvrante de la racine : repli cutané couvrant la racine de l'ongle.

Lame épidermique rétro-onguéale : remplissant la rainure onguéale et située en arrière du bourrelet onguéal (ongle fœtal).

Sillon intermédiaire : qu'on constate à la limite des zones moyenne et antérieure de l'ongle fœtal.

Poils. Plaque sous-papillaire : Epaississement bien accusé au-dessous de la région du col de la papille.

On divise communément les couches épithéliales entourant la racine en deux gaines : l'externe et l'interne. En se basant sur l'histogenèse du follicule pileux, on pourrait distinguer la gaine épithéliale externe de la racine sous le nom de gaine épithéliale folliculaire, et la gaine épithéliale interne ayant un développement propre — sous le nom de gaine épithéliale radiculaire.

Eminence myo-épithéliale (?). Bourgeon épithélial situé en dessous de la glande sébacée et qui paraît être en rapport avec la traînée cellulaire renfermant des noyaux aplatis et qui correspond au muscle redresseur du poil.

Poils à sinus vasculaires. La description se rapporte en particulier aux poils du chat. Tunique fibreuse engaînante de la glande sébacée; prolongement de la tunique fibreuse commune du follicule entourant vers l'extérieur la glande sébacée.

Piquants (hérisson). Stries longitudinales, visibles à la loupe à la surface des piquants.

Stries médullaires convexes; visibles dans la substance médullaire de la racine sur la coupe microscopique passant par l'axe du bulbe.

Epithélium du fond folliculaire; revêtant le fond du follicule et se continuant d'une part avec l'épithélium revêtant la papille, et d'autre part avec l'épithélium de la paroi folliculaire (ou gaine épithéliale externe).

Couche bulbaire sous-épithéliale; Cette couche, en contact immédiat avec l'épithélium du fond folliculaire, se distingue par son aspect plus hyalin et homogène du reste de la substance du bulbe du piquant.

Utricules sébacés folliculaires. La glande sébacée des piquants du hérisson se présente sous forme d'utricules isolées particulièrement grêles et allongées et se terminant par une extrémité renflée.

Plumes. Ame de la plume; cette dénomination, par trop poétique, pourrait être remplacée par une autre plus conforme à la structure de ce corps, p. ex. strie médullaire cornée (Markhornstreifen).

Prolongements papillaires intermédiaires; s'engageant entre les crêtes épithéliales.

Region génératrice de la hampe; Les couches sont comptées à partir de la papille. Couche alvéolaire; renfermant des cellules polyédriques-arrondies dont l'ensemble forme une trame alvéolaire.

Organe de la gustation. Pore gustatif externe et interne, en supposant à ce pore une certaine hauteur. On peut se demander s'il y a lieu de faire cette distinction.

Härchenkranz (couronne ciliée). Schwalbe a décrit aux cellules pariétales des gobelets gustatifs de fins prolongements formant par leur ensemble une espèce de couronne ciliée; il ne s'agit pas de cils des cellules centrales ou gustatives.

La division des cellules gustatives en cellules en bâtonnet et cellules en pointe n'est pas admise par tous les auteurs. Les cellules fusiformes (Spindelzellen) de Krause correspondraient aux Stäbchenzellen de Schwalbe.

Cupule nerveuse (Nervenschale). Nom donné par Key (1861) à l'extrémité évasée du nerf en rapport avec le disque gustatif (grenouille). Mentionnons encore la dénomination : Nervenkissen, coussinet nerveux, donnée par Engelmann à la partie plus dense du chorion papillaire en rapport avec le disque gustatif.

Pour ce qui concerne les terminaisons nerveuses (réseaux péricellulaires, terminaisons de continuité) et les catégories cellulaires qu'on peut reconnaître dans le disque gustatif de la grenouille, je renvoie à la thèse de Pépont; Des terminaisons nerveuses et des cellules de l'organe de la gustation de la grenouille. Lausanne, 1904, travail sorti de notre laboratoire.

Cellules ganglionnaires sous-épithéliales. L'interprétation de ces cellules est controversée; on les a aussi envisagées comme des cellules conjonctives (Ke-

(zinz), ou des cellules dérivant des gaines nerveuses (Scheidenzellen, v. *Ebner*).

Manteau nerveux (Mantelschicht): couche nerveuse décrite par *Niemack* (Der nervöse Apparat in den Endscheiben der Froschzunge. Anat. Hefte, 1892).

Plexus sous-gemmal capilliforme; décrit par *Lenhossék* (Anat. Anz. 1893) et *Dogiel* aux bourgeons gustatifs des poissons (Arch. f. mikr. Anat. 1897).

Organe de l'olfaction. Les appendices ciliés des cellules olfactives peuvent avoir plutôt la forme d'une pointe, p. ex. chez le rat blanc.

La structure annelée du prolongement périphérique des cellules de soutènement s'observe p. ex. chez le rat blanc.

Canaux latéraux (poissons). Enveloppe conjonctive: ce n'est pas une enveloppe dans le sens ordinaire du mot, mais une couche épaisse en forme de manchon et qui a une structure propre. L'agencement des couches se rapporte en particulier aux canaux de la *torpille*.

Appareil de l'audition. Canaux semi-circulaires: l'espace cavitaire cloisonné entourant les canaux membraneux est aussi désigné sous le nom d'espace 'péri-lymphatique'; cette dénomination prête cependant à l'équivoque et peut faire croire qu'il s'agit d'un espace entourant un lymphatique; ainsi l'on entend sous le nom d'espaces lymphatiques périvasculaires l'espace entourant les vaisseaux sanguins, sous le nom d'espace péricellulaire, on comprend ordinairement l'espace pouvant entourer certaines cellules.

Le tissu trabéculaire qui traverse l'espace cavitaire entourant les canaux semi-circulaires peut être très délié et se présenter sous forme d'un tissu réticulé à larges mailles irrégulières remplies de sérosité.

Calices nerveux; décrits par *R. Krause* à l'épithélium des crêtes acoustiques (Ergänzungsheft zu Anat. Anzeiger, 1896).

Couche fibro-hyaline de la bandelette sillonnée; occupe la région périphérique au pourtour du sillon spiral et de la région de la crête spirale; cette couche se distingue par son aspect plus hyalin de la couche principale ou fasciculée de la bandelette.

Membrane basilaire. Sur les coupes de cette membrane, on reconnaît deux couches limitantes plus claires, l'une au dessous de l'épithélium cochléaire, l'autre en rapport avec le revêtement de la face tympanique de cette membrane; dans la couche comprise entre ces couches limitantes, il y a des noyaux très aplatis.

Epithélium limitant interne: on pourrait donner ce nom à l'épithélium qui limite du côté interne la région des cellules ciliées internes, épithélium qui se distingue par plusieurs caractères de l'épithélium du sillon spiral interne.

Cellules intermédiaires (intercalaires) de la région des cellules ciliées internes; chez les mammifères, ces dernières cellules sont entourées de cellules à part à noyau basal.

Eminence nerveuse interne des cellules ciliées externes: on pourrait donner ce nom à une petite éminence granuleuse qui va se rendant à ces cellules du côté inférieur, au dessous de la région moyenne de la cellule, et à laquelle éminence on voit aboutir les fibrilles nerveuses ayant traversé la région du tunnel. Cette éminence granuleuse se continue dans la profondeur avec une strie granuleuse qu'on peut suivre jusqu'à la membrane basilaire. La dite strie paraît être tout à fait indépendante des cellules de Deiters, vu qu'on peut encore reconnaître entre la strie granuleuse la plus interne et la cellule de Deiters comme une couche plus claire;

cette dernière strie, n'étant pas placée entre les cellules de Deiters, a un trajet un peu ondulé.

Stries limitantes : On reconnaît entre les cellules de Deiters des stries intermédiaires d'aspect hyalin, et qui se terminent dans la profondeur par un renflement conique qui repose sur la membrane basilaire. Si ces stries limitantes correspondent ou non aux stries de Retzius, c'est une question qui n'est pas facile à résoudre par la méthode des coupes.

Épithélium limitant externe. De même que pour la région des cellules ciliées internes, on pourrait donner ce nom à l'épithélium qui limite du côté extérieur les cellules ciliées externes.

Revêtement cellulaire de la face tympanique de la membrane basale : Ce revêtement a tous les caractères d'un revêtement épithélial.

Ligament spiral; plan profond : dirigé du côté de la paroi osseuse ; plan superficiel : dirigé du côté de la lame basilaire.

Couche lacunaire ou vésiculaire de la bandelette vasculaire : on pourrait désigner sous ces noms la couche plus claire située entre la lame épithéliale et la couche conjonctive sous-jacente, et renfermant des cellules claires et des vaisseaux.

Crêtes acoustiques (oiseaux). La description se rapporte en particulier aux passereaux chanteurs. Les cellules en bouteille (ou en cruche) qui se trouvent au niveau des bourrelets latéraux des crêtes se distinguent, dans les préparations conservées dans la glycérine, par leur aspect à la fois opaque et luisant.

Limaçon (oiseaux). Bandelette vasculo-épithéliale : cette bandelette plissée et vascularisée remplissant la rampe vestibulaire contient deux espèces de cellules épithéliales : des cellules vésiculaires relativement volumineuses et des cellules notablement plus petites, granuleuses et ayant un reflet luisant dans les préparations examinées dans la glycérine.

Lames chondroïdes du limaçon : Ces lames se composent d'un tissu ressemblant au cartilage et sont traversées par des vaisseaux sanguins ; l'une d'elles renferme la loge du ganglion cochléaire, et est traversée par les fibres nerveuses se rendant à l'épithélium de la lame basilaire.

Renflement terminal du limaçon. A ce niveau, les lames chondroïdes finissent par se fusionner dans la région de la rampe tympanique, de manière à former une lame chondroïde unique dont la coupe ressemble à une nacelle ; il reste entre la lame basilaire et la lame chondroïde un espace comparable à un tunnel. Des fibres nerveuses émanant du ganglion cochléaire traversent la lame chondroïde pour se rendre à la tache nerveuse située dans le renflement terminal du limaçon.

Labyrinthe membraneux des *amphibiens*. La description se rapporte à la *grenouille*. Excavation cupuliforme des crêtes acoustiques : cette excavation, comparable à une cupule, reçoit la lame neuro-épithéliale de la crête. Pour éviter des confusions, il y a lieu d'ajouter que cette cupule n'a rien à faire avec la "cupula„ des auteurs.

Les dénominations des excroissances de l'utricule d'après *Retzius* sont ajoutées en parenthèse ; l'excroissance dite *algae* n'a cependant pas la forme d'une bouteille chez la grenouille.

Chez les *poissons osseux*, on constate au-dessus de la lame neuro-épithéliale des crêtes acoustiques un enduit de consistance gélatineuse et renfermant aussi des cellules desquamées et altérées ; c'est la cupula des auteurs, ne représentant pas en réalité un corps morphologique propre.

Des cellules granuleuses en forme de cruche se trouvent chez les poissons osseux en dehors de la région des crêtes acoustiques.

Oreille moyenne. Les données anatomiques, et notamment pour ce qui concerne les osselets, ont été laissées naturellement de côté. Quelques termes seulement servant de préliminaires aux descriptions histologiques ont été mentionnés.

Oreille externe. Îlots cartilagineux ramollis; on les constate dans le cartilage de l'oreille d'homme adulte.

Conduit auditif externe. Glandes sébacées à conduit évasé; chez l'homme également.

Appareil de la vision. Bourrelet cellulaire post-cornéen, qu'on constate p. ex. chez la perche à la face postérieure de la cornée dans la région de l'angle irido-cornéen.

Cellules visuelles à bâtonnet et à cônes. Région exo-limitante et endo-limitante; c'est pour désigner d'un mot les parties de ces cellules situées soit en dehors, soit en dedans de la membrane limitante externe.

Portion intermédiaire des bâtonnets et des cônes: on pourrait donner ce nom à la partie qui traverse la membrane limitante externe et relie le segment interne des bâtonnets ou des cônes au segment nucléé des cellules visuelles.

Cellules à bâtonnet des oiseaux: ellipsoïde cylindrique; le corps qu'on désigne communément sous le nom d'ellipsoïde a chez ces animaux une forme cylindrique.

Corpuscule bacilliforme des bâtonnets: en forme de grêle bâtonnet, et situé en dessous de l'ellipsoïde; à ce corpuscule fait suite une strie médiane (pigeon).

Cellules visuelles à cône: variété bacilliforme, se rapprochant de la forme bâtonnet; le segment externe est grêle et allongé; le segment interne aussi, très élizé, se rapproche bien plutôt de la forme cylindrique; la gouttelette colorée placée à la limite des deux segments dépasse même dans le sens de la largeur le diamètre du segment interne (moineau, pigeon).

Cônes doubles (oiseaux). Ces cônes sont hétéromorphes; seul le cône grêle contient une gouttelette colorée. Dans le cône épais, on constate de plus en dessous du corps ellipsoïde un autre corps, d'aspect homogène, de configuration elliptique allongée, — corps hyalin accessoire.

Cônes doubles (reptiles, lézard). De ces cônes, également hétéromorphes, seul le cône plus long contient une gouttelette colorée. Dans le segment interne du cône plus court, qui est aussi plus épais, il y a un amas assez gros de granules pigmentés, d'un jaune orange, et occupant la place de l'ellipsoïde. Comme chez les oiseaux on constate également dans le segment interne du cône plus épais, un corps hyalin profond qui s'étend jusqu'au voisinage de la région de la membrane limitante externe.

Les cônes doubles de la grenouille sont également hétéromorphes; la gouttelette huileuse des cônes est incolore.

Pour éviter des redites, les dénominations communes aux cellules visuelles des vertébrés ont été omises pour les oiseaux, reptiles et amphibiens.

Les dénominations relatives aux cellules visuelles des poissons se rapportent en particulier à la perche.

Aux cônes dissociés de la perche, on reconnaît assez facilement les fibrilles basales partant de l'extrémité profonde du cône élargie en forme de pied.

Les cellules jumelles à cône de la perche paraissent être homomorphes. Couche spongieuse externe de la rétine. Cellules à prolongements descendants; ces cellules sont aussi décrites par les auteurs avec la couche suivante (couche des grains externes).

Arbuscules vasculaires de la rétine. Les rameuscules artériels qui fournissent au réseau capillaire forment par leurs branches une figure tout à fait comparable à un arbuscule (chat).

Glandes tubulo-acineuses de la conjonctive. Ces glandes portent aussi les noms de glandes de Soppey ou de Krause.

Troisième paupière des mammifères. Eminences pigmentaires visibles déjà à l'œil nu à la troisième paupière du lapin, et se groupant à une petite distance à partir du bord libre. On trouvera une description détaillée du revêtement épithélial de la 3e paupière dans le travail de R. Koch sorti de notre laboratoire: Epithelstudien, Arch. f. mikrosk. Anatomie, Bd. 63, 1903.

Glandes de la 3e paupière (mammifères), homomorphes, comme chez le lapin, le mouton, le chat. Chez le veau, il y a à la région basale de la paupière un îlot glandulaire de structure différente, signalé par Peter.

Conduits excréteurs perforants: traversant la lame cartilagineuse.

(Glandes hétéromorphes) chez le hérisson, à lobules hétérogènes.

Autres glandes de la cavité orbitaire: Glande sous-orbitaire. Glande orbitaire externe (adparotidienne). Glande de Harder. On trouvera des données plus détaillées relatives à ces glandes et à leur classification dans mes travaux: Zur Kenntnis der Gland. infraorbitalis einiger Säugetiere. Anat. Anz. 1894. Drüsenstudien, I und II, Internat. Monatsschr. f. Anat. 1895 et Arch. f. mikrosk. Anatomie, 1900. On trouvera des figures explicatives ayant trait soit aux glandes soit à d'autres parties de ce rapport dans mon Atlas zur vergleich. Histologie der Wirbeltiere, 1894.

Glande sous-orbitaire accessoire (lapin). Il s'agit d'une traînée glandulaire située obliquement en dehors et en haut de la glande sous-orbitaire proprement dite, mais ayant la même structure.

Pour ce qui concerne la plupart des glandes de la cavité orbitaire, seules les particularités de structure ont été mentionnées, les dénominations ayant trait à la structure générale des glandes ont été omises pour éviter des redites.

Conduits exo-parenchymateux (ou exo-glandulaires): Cette dénomination pourrait être utile pour désigner les segments des conduits excréteurs situés en dehors du parenchyme glandulaire, vu que leur structure peut présenter quelques particularités. Ces canaux ne sont pas toujours terminaux, mais peuvent aussi s'aboucher de manière à former un seul conduit excréteur terminal.

La glande sous-orbitaire du rat blanc et la glande orbitaire externe (ou adparotidienne) du même animal s'ouvrent en commun à la région externe de l'orbite. La structure de cette dernière glande a des particularités propres communes en cela avec la portion séroalvéolaire de la glande sous-orbitaire.

L'embouchure de la glande de Harder ne se trouve pas toujours à la face interne de la troisième paupière (comme chez le lapin), mais peut se trouver aussi à la face externe de cette paupière (hérisson).

La structure hétéromorphe de la glande de Harder du lapin est beaucoup moins accusée que chez le hérisson et le porc, vu que les différences portent, chez le lapin, sur la structure de l'épithélium et non pas sur le type glandulaire.

Glandule accessoire. Il s'agit d'un petit îlot glandulaire annexé au conduit de la glande de Harder du lapin, et s'ouvrant dans ce conduit non loin de son embouchure. Cette petite glandule se distingue totalement par sa structure alvéolaire-séreuse de la glande principale.

THÈME 3 — ORIGINE, NATURE ET CLASSIFICATION DES PIGMENTS

(Les pigments cellulaires des Vertébrés)

Par M. le Dr. MARCK ATHIAS (Lisbonne)

Le nom de *pigment* sert à désigner toute une série de substances naturellement colorées, ayant comme caractère commun celui de donner des couleurs aux tissus et aux produits de sécrétion des animaux et végétaux [1].

Dans les tissus ces substances se présentent sous une forme figurée ou non figurée et sont tantôt contenues dans les cellules, tantôt en dehors d'elles, dans les espaces ou liquides intercellulaires. Dans les liquides de l'organisme, tels que la bile, l'urine, etc., les pigments se montrent toujours à l'état dissous.

Ces pigments peuvent être élaborés par l'organisme dans lequel ils se trouvent, ou bien y avoir pénétré du dehors; dans le premier cas, ils sont *intrinsèques*, dans le deuxième *extrinsèques*.

Le groupe des pigments renferme un nombre assez considérable de substances dont la composition chimique, pour beaucoup encore mal connue ou même tout à fait inconnue, est très différente; leurs fonctions, pour plusieurs d'entre elles encore ignorées, semblent être également très distinctes.

Les substances pigmentaires sont largement répandues dans la nature; les tissus végétaux ainsi que les animaux en sont plus ou moins abondamment pourvus.

Malgré le grand nombre de recherches dont les pigments ont été l'objet, il y en a beaucoup sur lesquels nos connaissances sont très imparfaites, surtout pour ce qui concerne ceux des Invertébrés. Il est impossible d'établir une classification chimique ou physiologique des pigments qui existent dans le règne animal, car la constitution et le rôle de plusieurs d'entre eux n'ont guère été étudiés d'une façon systématique; tout au plus en connaît-on les

---

[1] Nous ne parlons pas, bien entendu, de ces couleurs dites de *structure* dues à des interférences lumineuses et à des phénomènes de diffraction que présentent les téguments et leurs dérivés chez un grand nombre d'animaux et qui ont été très bien décrites par *Krukenberg* (Vergleichende ... einer vergleichenden Physiologie der Farbstoffe und der Farben — *Vergleichend-physiologische Vorträge* — Heidelberg, 1892) et plus récemment par *Mandoul* (Recherches sur les colorations tégumentaires — Thèse de la Fac. des Sc., Paris — 1903).

caractères physiques et la distribution. Les substances pigmentaires, sur lesquelles nous possédons actuellement plus de données certaines, sont celles qu'on rencontre chez les Vertébrés. Dans ce rapport, qui doit se limiter à présenter un tableau d'ensemble de nos connaissances actuelles sur l'origine, la nature et la classification des pigments, nous nous occuperons de ceux des Vertébrés, sans négliger toutefois de faire mention de ceux qui existent chez les Invertébrés.

Nous ne traiterons que des pigments physiologiques se présentant sous forme de particules dans l'intérieur des cellules, laissant complètement de côté tout ce qui a trait aux pigments du sang et autres liquides de l'économie et à la pigmentation pathologique.

Nous divisons notre rapport en trois parties. Dans la première nous décrivons les substances pigmentaires au point de vue de leurs caractères physiques et chimiques. Dans une seconde partie nous étudions leur distribution dans les différentes cellules de l'organisme où on les rencontre à l'état normal. La troisième partie est consacrée à la question de l'origine des pigments, au mécanisme de leur production.

I

Il est aujourd'hui admis par tous les auteurs que la plupart des pigments cellulaires figurés qu'on rencontre chez les Vertébrés constituent deux grandes groupes, deux familles naturelles: les *mélanines* et les *lipochromes* [1]. Mais, outre ceux-ci, il y a un petit nombre de substances pigmentaires spéciales, peu connues, qui n'existent que chez quelques espèces animales et qui ne rentrent pas dans ces groupes, telles que la *turacine*, la *turacoverdine*, la *coerubine*, etc.

1.° *Mélanines* — Ce sont des pigments de couleur brune plus ou moins foncée, parfois noirâtre, qu'on peut rencontrer dans de nombreux tissus, auxquels ils donnent une coloration brune ou noire. A l'état normal, sont pourvus de mélanine : la choroïde, l'iris, la peau, les poils, certaines régions du système nerveux, telles que le locus coeruleus et le locus niger de l'Homme, etc.; chez les Amphibiens et les Reptiles il y a aussi des cellules chargées de mélanine dans les organes internes, tels que le foie, le

---

[1] Voir à ce sujet : G. Bohn — L'évolution du pigment — Coll. Scientia, n° 11. Paris 1907.

péricarde, le mésentère, les gaines des nerfs et des ganglions, etc. Ce pigment existe également chez les Invertébrés; les organes de protection et de sécrétion de plusieurs Mollusques Céphalopodes, (Sèche, Poulpe, etc.) sont pourvus d'un pigment désigné sous le nom de *mélaïne*, qui se rapproche beaucoup du pigment choroïdien. A l'état pathologique il y a souvent production de mélanine dans les tissus où on n'en trouve pas normalement ou dans les néoplasies; les tumeurs mélaniques sont assez fréquentes chez l'Homme; le Cheval blanc est souvent atteint de tumeurs noirâtres, riches en mélanine.

Les mélanines ont, comme caractère distinctif important, l'inaltérabilité. Elles sont insolubles dans l'eau, l'alcool, l'acétone, le chloroforme, l'éther, le xylol, le toluol, l'acide acétique, les acides minéraux dilués, etc., ainsi que l'ont constaté de nombreux auteurs parmi lesquels, *Sieber, Horschfeld, Abel et Davis* [1], *Spiegler* [2], *Landolt* [3], etc., pour les mélanines normales, *Berdez* et *Nencki*, etc., pour les mélanines des tumeurs.

L'acide sulfurique concentré n'attaque pas la mélanine, à froid; l'acide chlorhydrique ne la dissout même pas à chaud. (*Berdez und Nencki, Rosenstad* [4], etc.); par contre l'acide nitrique la transforme en produits facilement solubles.

D'après *Landolt*, le pigment choroïdien se dissout rapidement dans un mélange de bichromate de potasse et d'acide sulfurique dilué.

Vis-à-vis des alcalis, les pigments mélaniques ne se comportent pas tous de la même façon. Quelques-uns sont facilement solubles; tels sont ceux des poils, de certaines productions pathologiques, etc.; tandis que d'autres, même à chaud et avec des alcalis concentrés, ne montrent qu'une faible solubilité. La mélanine de la peau, des plumes, des yeux et des tumeurs mélaniques du cheval ne se dissout que très lentement dans la potasse; la solution a une couleur brune et par les acides il s'y forme un précipité brun. D'après *Rosenstadt*, le pigment de l'épiderme et des poils de l'Homme et des Mammifères, de la Grenouille, des nœvi et

(1) J. *Abel* and H. *Davis*. — On the Pigment of the Negro's Skin and Hair. — The Journal of experimental medicine. — vol. 1, n° 2, 1896.

(2) E. *Spiegler*. — Ueber das Haarpigment. — E. *Hofmeister's* Beiträge zur chemischen Physiologie und Pathologie. — B. ..., 1903.

(3) H. *Landolt*. — Ueber das Melanin der Augenhäute. — *Hoppe-seyler's* Zeitsch. f. physiol. Chemie. — Bd. XXVIII. 1899.

(4) H. *Rosenstadt*. — Studien über die Abstammung und die Bildung des Haarpigments. — Arch. f. mikr. Anat. — Bd. 50, 1897.

des mélano-sarcomes n'éprouve aucune altération par la potasse et le sulfure d'ammoniaque.

Les mélanines se décolorent toutes par l'eau de chlore, l'eau oxygénée, l'acide sulfureux, le chlorhydrate d'aniline et l'alcool, le chlorate de potasse et l'acide chlorhydrique, l'ammoniaque, etc. Fondues avec la potasse elles dégagent une odeur de scatol ou d'indol.

Étant donnée leur faible solubilité, il est très difficile et même presque impossible d'obtenir des mélanines absolument pures, pour une analyse chimique rigoureuse; pour les extraire on est obligé d'employer des acides forts ou des alcalis, qui dissolvent bien d'autres parties des tissus, ce qui entache d'erreur les résultats. Néanmoins, les recherches entreprises par un grand nombre de chimistes ont démontré que les pigments mélaniques sont composés principalement de carbone, d'hydrogène, d'azote et d'oxygène; on y a rencontré parfois aussi du soufre et plus rarement du fer. Les proportions de ces différents éléments ne sont pas encore suffisamment connues, car les résultats des analyses, d'une même espèce de pigment, ne sont pas tout à fait concordants.

Nous allons passer en revue les principaux travaux publiés sur cette question.

Pigment de la peau et des poils. — Les études chimiques sur ce pigment ont porté, jusqu'à présent, sur la peau et les cheveux humains (*Floyd, Sieber, Abel et Davis*), les crins du Cheval (*Nencki et Sieber, Jones, Spiegler*), la laine des Moutons (*Spiegler*).

Les procédés mis en usage par ces auteurs pour isoler la substance pigmentaire sont différents. *Floyd* a fait la recherche du fer dans les cendres de la peau d'individus blancs et nègres, après l'avoir bien lavée à l'eau, à l'alcool et à l'éther; il a trouvé 2,28 % de fer dans la peau du nègre, moitié moins dans celle du blanc.

Sieber a extrait le pigment des cheveux en les faisant macérer dans la potasse caustique, après un traitement par l'alcool et l'éther et en précipitant ensuite la matière colorante par l'acide acétique. *Abel et Davis* ont mis en liberté le pigment de la peau et des cheveux en faisant agir, sur le tissu, de l'acide chlorhydrique à 5-10 %, pendant 10 jours, à froid, ou une solution à 5 % d'hydrate de potasse à chaud. Dans le premier cas, après avoir enlevé l'acide, la substance était macérée dans de la potasse à chaud pendant quelques heures pour dissoudre le pigment, qui était ensuite précipité par un mélange d'alcool et d'éther, séparé par filtration, redissous par de la potasse ou de l'ammoniaque, représenté par l'alcool-éther, et ainsi de suite. Dans le second procédé, le pigment, dissous par la potasse, est précipité par l'alcool, soumis à l'action de l'acide chlorhydrique dilué à froid, redissous par la potasse, et précipité de nouveau, après filtration, par l'acide acétique; le pigment est ensuite recueilli sur un filtre et bien lavé à l'eau et à l'alcool, dissous par de l'hydrate de potasse dilué, chauffé, précipité encore une fois par l'acide acétique, dissous par de l'ammoniaque, filtré et reprécipité par l'alcool et l'éther, et ainsi de suite, jusqu'à ce qu'il ne laisse que un ou deux pour cent de cendres. Le même procédé a été employé par *Jones* pour les crins du Cheval; en traitant les granules pigmentaires par la potasse caustique concentrée, il a obtenu un produit acide, *l'acide mélanique*, dépourvu de soufre et présentant les réactions de la mélanine. L'autre part *Spiegler* se sert du procédé suivant pour isoler le pigment des crins du Cheval noir et blanc et de la laine noire et blanche du Mouton: lavage dans une solution de carbonate de soude, dissolution par l'hydrate de potasse à 5 %; précipitation du pigment par l'acide chlorhydrique dilué et ébullition dans ce même acide dilué afin de dissoudre les substances protéiques mélangées au pigment; dissolution du résidu par de l'ammoniaque, nouvelle précipitation par l'acide chlorhydrique, ceci répété plusieurs fois; lavage du produit à l'alcool, sulfure de carbone et éther. Cet auteur obtient ainsi une poudre brun-noir ayant les caractères de la mélanine et qu'il nomme *acide du pigment (Pigmentsäure)*.

Les analyses de *Spiegler* l'ont conduit à donner deux formules empiriques, l'une pour les pigments des productions noires, l'autre pour celui des productions blanches; ce sont respectivement: $C^{30} H^{36} N^{8} SO^{12}$ et $C^{30} H^{38} N^{8} SO^{9}$. Il croit vraisemblable que les deux substances possèdent un noyau moléculaire identique et que les différences de coloration dépendent de l'existence d'un groupement chromogène.

PEAU ET CHEVEUX HUMAINS:

	C %	H %	N %	O %	S %	Fe %	Cendres %
Siebel	56,14	7,57	8,5		4,19	0	0,88
(cheveux)	57,19	6,57			2,71	0	0
Abel et Davis	61,83	8,86	17,01	20,70		traces	—
(épiderme du nègre)	53,56	5,11	15,47	23,33	2,53	traces	
(poils du nègre)	52,74	3,54	10,51	29,88		traces	
	50,06	5,15	12,87	23,85	1,77	traces	—

CRINS DU CHEVAL :

Stein	57,8	4,2	11,8	24,5	2,1	—	—	
Jones	58,14	3,52	13,18	—	0	—	0,44	} acide mélanique
	57,94	3,86	13,06	—	0	—	—	
Spiegler	59,49	3,87	11,18		5,43	traces	9,80	} acide du pigment
(cheval noir)	60,02	5,91	10,54		—	—		
(cheval blanc)	48,59	7,04	12,69		2,80	traces	16,28	
	48,51	7,06	12,38		—	—		

LAINE DES MOUTONS :

Spiegler	51,00	6,13	10,54		2,91	—	10,85	} acide du pigment
(laine noire)	50,91	6,15	10,31					
(laine blanche)	55,45	7,38	10,62		2,30	—	2,30	
	55,29	7,40	10,87					

Pigment choroïdien. — Ce pigment a été l'objet de nombreuses recherches, dont les plus importantes sont celles de *Scherer, Gmelin, Rosow, Sieber, Hirschfeld, Mays, Scherl et Landolt.*

D'après les analyses faites par *Scherer*, en 1841, le pigment choroïdien contient :

$$
\begin{aligned}
&C \ldots\ldots\ldots\ldots\ldots\ldots 57,90 - 58,07\ \% \\
&H \ldots\ldots\ldots\ldots\ldots\ldots\ 5,83 - 5,96\ \% \\
&N \ldots\ldots\ldots\ldots\ldots\ldots\ldots\ 13,77\ \% \\
&O \ldots\ldots\ldots\ldots\ldots\ldots 22,50 - 21,59\ \%
\end{aligned}
$$

Il a obtenu 9,80 % de cendres ; la recherche du soufre et du fer ne semble pas avoir été pratiquée par cet auteur.

La présence du fer a été constatée dans ce pigment par *Gmelin*, qui en a trouvé une petite quantité dans les cendres. Ces deux auteurs ont extrait le pigment par des moyens mécaniques ; le premier s'est servi du pinceau pour le séparer du tissu après avoir bien lavé celui-ci avec de l'eau pour enlever le sang ; *Gmelin* l'a simplement passé à travers une toile qui retenait les débris de la membrane.

Les analyses de *Rosow* ont donné le résultat suivant :

$$
\begin{aligned}
&C \ldots\ldots\ldots\ldots\ldots\ldots\ldots\ldots\ 54,29\ \% \\
&H \ldots\ldots\ldots\ldots\ldots\ldots\ldots\ldots\ \ 5,35\ \% \\
&N \ldots\ldots\ldots\ldots\ldots\ldots\ldots\ldots\ 10,18\ \% \\
&O \ldots\ldots\ldots\ldots\ldots\ldots\ldots\ldots\ 20,18\ \% \\
&S \ldots\ldots\ldots\ldots\ldots\ldots\ldots\ldots\ldots\ \ 0 \\
&Fe \ldots\ldots\ldots\ldots\ldots\ldots\ldots\ldots\ \text{traces} \\
&\text{Cendres} \ldots\ldots\ldots\ldots\ldots\ldots\ \ 9,59\ \%
\end{aligned}
$$

Le matériel pour ces analyses a été obtenu: 1° en faisant agir pendant 3 à 4 semaines de l'acide acétique concentré sur la choroïde, en lavant à fond le résidu et en le laissant sécher dans le vide; 2° en abandonnant le tissu à la putréfaction pendant une semaine, et recueillant ensuite les granules pigmentaires mis en liberté en les faisant passer à travers un linge; le produit a été traité par l'acide acétique, lavé et desséché dans le vide.

Mme *Sieber* a étudié le pigment de la choroïde du Bœuf; ce pigment a été extrait en le faisant d'abord passer à travers un linge et en chauffant le résidu sec jusqu'à l'ébullition pendant deux heures dans de l'acide chlorhydrique à 10 %, pour transformer les substances protéiques en produits solubles; il était ensuite recueilli sur un filtre, lavé et séché. Les résultats qu'elle a obtenus s'éloignent quelque peu de ceux des auteurs précédents; voici les chiffres qu'elle indique:

C.................	59,9 % —	60,34 %
H.................	4,61 % —	5,02 %
N.................	—	10,81 %
O.................	24,68 % —	23,89 %
S.................	0	—
Fe................	0	—
Cendres..........		2,13 %

Cet auteur n'a donc rencontré ni du soufre ni du fer; les cendres seraient constituées, en grande partie, par de la silice.

Hirschfeld, qui a analysé aussi le pigment de l'œil du Bœuf en employant un procédé semblable à celui de *Sieber*, avec cette différence qu'au lieu de le faire bouillir dans l'acide chlorhydrique il l'a laissé agir à froid, n'a pu trouver non plus du soufre ni du fer; dans les cendres il y aurait principalement de l'acide silicique. D'après *Mays*, le pigment choroïdien contiendrait une petite quantité de fer; *Scherl* n'en a pas constaté l'existence dans le pigment de la choroïde du Chien.

Mays a fait digérer le tissu pigmenté dans du suc pancréatique, qui n'attaque pas la matière colorante; *Scherl* s'est servi de l'acide nitrique à 1:10 en y laissant le tissu pendant 24 heures, a dissous ensuite le pigment dans une solution faible de bicarbonate de soude et l'a fait précipiter de nouveau par l'acide nitrique.

Bien plus récemment *Landolt* s'est aussi proposé de déterminer la composition élémentaire du pigment choroïdien de l'œil du Bœuf; l'extraction a été faite par le procédé suivant: la choroïde était détachée et le pigment enlevé sous l'eau au moyen d'un pinl'eau, et passé ensuite à travers un filtre en soie; le filtrat était additionné d'un égal volume d'une solution saturée de sulfate d'ammoniaque et le tout chauffé à 80°. Le pigment, qui se trouvait ainsi rassemblé, était alors recueilli sur un filtre et bien lavé à l'eau, à l'alcool et à l'éther. La substance colorante que l'auteur a obtenue par ce procédé était une poudre amorphe, brun-foncé, complètement insoluble dans l'eau, l'alcool, l'éther, le chloroforme, le benzol, le sulfure de carbone, l'acide acétique, l'hydrate de chloral.

Landolt a aussi cherché à voir si le pigment possédait ou non un stroma incolore et à l'en séparer; pour cela il a fait séjourner pendant plusieurs jours des choroïdes dans une grande quantité de pepsine et acide chlorhydrique, en plaçant le tout dans un bain de sable à 40°. De cette façon tout le tissu était digéré et le pigment seul tombait au fond du vase; il a été recueilli, lavé, convenablement traité et analysé. Le résultat a été négatif pour ce qui concerne l'existence d'un stroma de nature albuminoïde.

Voici d'après l'auteur les moyennes des chiffres auxquels il est arrivé dans ses analyses:

C	54,48 %	52,72 %	58,82 %
H	5,33 %	3,69 %	5,37 %
N	12,65 %	11,56 %	11,16 %
O	27,32 %	32,03 %	26,61 %
Le moins de	0,01 %	—	—
Cendres	1,9 %	—	—

Pigment des mollusques (mélanine) — Le pigment mélanique sécrété par différents Céphalopodes (*Sepia, Octopus*, etc.) et connu sous le nom de *noir de Sèche*, a été examiné au point de vue chimique par plusieurs auteurs; quoique les analyses qui ont été pratiquées soient déjà un peu anciennes, nous résumons dans le tableau ci-après les résultats des principales, avec l'indication du nom des auteurs:

	C	H	N	S	Fe
Desfosses et Variot	54,4	3,05	8,1	—	—
Gérot	53,6	4,02	8,6	—	—
	53,9	4,01	8,8	—	—
Nencki et Sieber	56,36	3,56	12,21	0,51	0
	56,31	3,65	12,44	0,52	0

Les analyses les plus complètes sont, ainsi qu'on le voit, celles de *Nencki* et *Sieber*, les seuls qui ont fait la recherche du fer et du soufre. Ils ont employé la méthode suivante: La glande a

été lavée à la potasse à 10 %; ensuite le pigment a été précipité
par l'acide chlorhydrique, redissous dans de l'ammoniaque et de
nouveau précipité; le produit obtenu (*acide de Sèche, Sepiasäure*)
a été lavé à l'eau, à l'alcool et à l'éther, et soumis alors à l'analyse.

Nous avons ainsi parcouru les principaux travaux faits sur la
composition chimique des différentes mélanines normales. D'après
ces travaux nous voyons donc que dans la constitution de ces pigments, il entre toujours du carbone, de l'oxygène, de l'hydrogène et de l'azote; ce sont des substances azotées. Les proportions
de ces différents éléments sont, en moyenne, les suivantes: $C = 55,43$
$H = 5,13$ $N = 11,53$ $O = 25,86$.

D'après *Hofmeister* le rapport atomique entre les trois com-
posants $N : H : C = 1 : 6 : 5$. En prenant les chiffres que nous avons
donnés, qui représentent les moyennes trouvées par les auteurs,
ce rapport sera: $N : H : C = 1 : 6,2 : 5,6$, qui se rapproche beaucoup
de celui qu'indique *von Fürth* [1] dans sa revue sur les pigments
mélaniques.

Le soufre et le fer n'entrent pas dans la composition de toutes les mélanines.

Pour ce qui concerne le soufre, il est des pigments, tels que
ceux de la peau et des poils des Mammifères, qui en possèdent
une assez forte proportion; en effet on en a trouvé jusqu'à 4,10 %
chez le nègre *(Sieber)* et jusqu'à 3,13 % dans les crins du Cheval
noir *(Spiegler)*; il est vrai que *Jones* n'en a point rencontré dans
ce même pigment, mais ce résultat négatif est dû peut-être à des
erreurs dans la méthode employée pour l'analyse et ne peut pas
infirmer les résultats positifs des autres auteurs.

Le noir de Sèche, d'après les analyses de *Nencki* et *Sieber*,
en est aussi pourvu. Par contre, dans le pigment choroïdien l'existence du soufre n'a jamais été constatée.

Quant au fer il n'a été rencontré qu'assez rarement dans les
pigments mélaniques normaux étudiés jusqu'à présent; il ne semble donc entrer que d'une façon exceptionnelle dans la composition de ces pigments et, quand il existe, il est toujours en très
faible proportion. Ce fait a une certaine importance au point de
vue de l'origine des mélanines, ainsi qu'on le verra plus loin.

Des études chimiques que nous venons de relater sommairement, il se dégage la conclusion que les pigments mélaniques

[1] von Fürth : Physiologische und chemische Untersuchungen über melanotische Pigmente
— Centralbl. f. allg. Pathol. und patholog. Anatomie. — Bd. XV — 1904.

constituent une famille naturelle de substances pigmentaires caractérisées par un certain nombre de propriétés physiques et chimiques bien définies; il y en a plusieurs variétés qui diffèrent entre elles notamment par la présence ou l'absence de soufre et de fer.

2° *Lipochromes* — Ces pigments présentent une couleur jaune, orangée, rouge ou vert-jaunâtre. Il sont caractérisés par un certain nombre de propriétés qui les distinguent bien nettement des pigments mélaniques.

Les lipochromes sont solubles dans l'alcool, l'éther, le chloroforme, la benzine, le sulfure de carbone, etc., c'est-à-dire dans les dissolvants des matières grasses; «ils possèdent, dit *Arm. Gautier* (1), les apparences générales des corps gras qu'ils colorent souvent dans l'économie». Avec le sulfure de carbone, ils donnent des solutions rouges. Ils ne sont pas détruits par la soude caustique bouillante, en solution aqueuse ou alcoolique. Avec l'acide sulfurique concentré et l'acide nitrique nitreux ils prennent une couleur bleue ou verte, quand ils sont à l'état sec; quelques-uns se colorent en bleu verdâtre par l'iodure de potassium iodé, d'autres ne changent pas de couleur. Ils se décolorent plus ou moins rapidement à la lumière.

Ces pigments donnent des spectres d'absorption qui varient avec la nature du milieu dans lequel ils sont en dissolution, et la concentration de celle-ci *(Krukenberg, Tudichum)*. Dissous dans l'alcool ou l'éther, ils présentent des bandes d'absorption dans le violet; dans le sulfure de carbone ces bandes se montrent le plus souvent déplacées vers le rouge; dans le chloroforme et les huiles, ces bandes se placent au milieu du spectre.

Les lipochromes sont assez abondants chez les Vertébrés surtout chez les Oiseaux, Reptiles, Amphibiens et Poissons. Le type des pigments de cette famille est la *lutéine* qui existe dans le jaune de l'œuf des Oiseaux et dans les corps jaunes de l'ovaire des Mammifères. On a rencontré chez des Oiseaux plusieurs pigments qui appartiennent au groupe des lipochromes; tels sont la *tétronérythrine de Wurm* ou *zoonérythrine de Bogdanow*, pigment rouge qui se trouve dans la crête du Coq des bruyères *(Wurm)*, le liseré rouge des yeux du Faisan, les plumes du Cardinal et du Flamant, et dont l'existence a été constatée aussi chez des Poissons et des Invertébrés (Mollusques, Crustacés, Echinoder-

---

(1) A. Gautier, Chimie biologique. Paris 1897.

mes et Coelentérés); l'*araroth* extrait par *Krukenberg* des plumes
rouges de certains Perroquets, la *psittacofulvine*, la *zoofulvine*
(pigment jaune), la *corioxulfurine* et la *picofulvine* (pigment vert)
isolés par le même auteur des plumes de différents Oiseaux; la *lipochrine* qui a été trouvée dans la peau des Salamandrines et des
Grenouilles; la *lacertofulvine* rencontré dans la peau de quelques
Lacertides (*Krukenberg*). Ces pigments existent également, en
plus ou moins grande abondance, dans les téguments des Reptiles,
Amphibiens et Poissons. La couleur rouge de la chair du Saumon
est due à un lipochrome dissous dans une huile qui imprègne les
fibres musculaires.

Ils constituent les sphères huileuses des cônes de la rétine,
découvertes par *Capranica* en 1877 et nommées par lui *lutéine*
et par *Kühne corpuscules de lipochrine*. Le *rouge rétinien, pourpre
rétinien* ou *érythropsine* découvert par *Boll* en 1876 qui imprègne
les articles externes des bâtonnets, paraît être aussi un lipochrome;
la partie des bâtonnets où il existe du rouge rétinien se colore en
noir par le tétroxyde d'osmium. Ce pigment jaunit et se décolore
à la lumière, et se recolore à l'obscurité; les acides, l'iode, la
chaux, etc., le *décolorent*. On en trouve encore en plus ou moins
grande quantité, dans les cellules nerveuses, notamment celles de
l'Homme et des Mammifères vieux.

Les lipochromes sont encore plus répandus chez les Invertébrés que chez les Vertébrés. On a décrit un grand nombre de
pigments de cette famille chez les Echinodermes, les Coelentérés,
les Crustacés et les Mollusques, en leur donnant souvent des
noms tirés de ceux du genre ou de l'espèce animale chez laquelle
on les a trouvés; tels sont: la *pentacrinine*, l'*ophiurine*, l'*astrogris-
cine*, l'*astroviolettine*, l'*astrociridine*, la *velelline*, l'*astroïdine*, la
pélagéine, la *rhizostomine* et bien d'autres qui ont été décrits
chez des Echinodermes et des Coelentérés. Chez les végétaux il y
a également un grand nombre de pigments qui appartiennent à la
famille des lipochromes.

Les lipochromes sont des substances hydrocarbonées; l'analyse élémentaire a démontré qu'ils sont constitués par du carbone,
de l'hydrogène et de l'oxygène.

D'après *Krukenberg* ces pigments ont une étroite parenté
avec la cholestérine, opinion qui a été soutenue plus récemment
par *Colle* (1903); peut-être en sont-ils des éthers.

Ces substances pigmentaires se rapprochent aussi par plusieurs autres caractères des corps gras; en effet, ils sont solubles

dans les dissolvants de ces derniers et comme eux ils réduisent le bioxyde d'osmium en prenant une coloration noire plus ou moins intense et se colorent en rouge par le Sudan III.

Tout porte donc à croire que les lipochromes sont des graisses imprégnées d'une matière colorante soluble et se présentant dans la plupart des cas sous forme de gouttelettes plus ou moins petites dans l'intérieur des cellules.

3.° *Autres pigments.* — La *turacine* est une substance rouge pourpre qui existe dans les plumes de quelques Oiseaux (Musophagidés, etc.); elle contient du cuivre et répond, d'après *Church*, (1870) à la formule: $C^{62} H^{65} Cu^2 N^2 O^9$. *Krukenberg* affirme qu'elle renferme du fer en assez grande quantité. Voici, d'après ce dernier auteur, les caractères de cette substance; elle est soluble dans l'eau pure, plus facilement dans l'eau alcalinisée et est insoluble dans les dissolvants des lipochromes. Les acides minéraux et quelques sels (alun, acétate de plomb, chlorure de chaux) la précipitent de ses solutions aqueuses. La turacine est très stable à l'action de la lumière et de la chaleur. L'acide nitrique fumant la détruit quand elle est sèche, à froid, en produisant une coloration noire. L'acide sulfurique concentré la transforme en *turacéine*, qui se colore en violet pourpre par les acides. Le spectre de la turacine ressemble beaucoup à celui de l'oxyhémoglobine, mais ne se modifie point par les agents réducteurs (acide sulfhydrique, sulfure d'ammonium), ni par l'action des alcalis forts. La turacéine présente deux bandes d'absorption, l'une large après la raie D, l'autre plus faible avant cette raie.

La *turacoverdine* a été trouvée à l'état naturel par *Krukenberg* dans les plumes de *Corythaeola cristata* et de *Corythaix alli-cristata* (Oiseaux de la famille des Musophagidés); la turacine exposée à l'air pendant longtemps à l'état humide, se transforme en turacoverdine. Celle-ci présente une couleur verte et se distingue de la turacine par son spectre d'absorption qui ne montre qu'une bande immédiatement avant la raie D. Elle ne contiendrait pas de cuivre, mais aurait du fer en quantité relativement grande.

La substance colorante sèche brunit par l'acide sulfurique concentré, à froid; l'acide nitrique, l'acide chlorhydrique et la soude concentrés ne l'attaqueraient pas ou très lentement. En versant une solution aqueuse de turacoverdine sur de l'acide sulfurique de façon à ce qu'ils ne se mélangent pas, celui-ci se colore en rouge violet près de la zone de contact.

La *zoorubine* de *Krukenberg* est un pigment rouge que cet auteur a extrait des plumes des Oiseaux du paradis, de quelques *Trogonides* (*Pyrotrogon diardi*), *Alectorides* (*Otis tarda*) et *Phasianides* (quelques variétés de *Gallus domesticus*), etc.

Cette substance offre les caractères suivants: elle est soluble dans les liquides alcalins, insoluble dans l'alcool, le chloroforme, les huiles, le sulfure de carbone. Les acides minéraux dilués la précipitent de ces solutions alcalines. A l'état sec, l'acide nitrique la fait pâlir, l'acide chlorhydrique la colore en violet foncé, l'acide sulfurique en bleu verdâtre. Si l'on verse une solution de zoorubine sur l'acide sulfurique concentré de façon à ce que les deux liquides restent séparés, celui-ci reste incolore, mais la solution, au contact de l'acide, prend une couleur rouge violacée, plus tard vert foncé. En acidifiant légèrement par l'acide acétique une solution de zoorubine, celle-ci prend une coloration rouge cerise par l'addition d'une trace d'un sel de cuivre.

Ce pigment ne contient ni du cuivre, ni du fer, ni du soufre, ni du manganèse; l'azote ne semble pas entrer dans sa constitution. Il ne donne pas de spectre caractéristique.

Zeyneck (¹) a isolé récemment des nageoires d'un Poisson téléostéen (*Crenilabrus*) une matière colorante bleue de nature albuminoïde, soluble dans l'eau, qui, précipitée par le sulfate d'ammoniaque et séchée, se présente en lamelles amorphes, raides. Cette substance donne au spectroscope une large bande d'absorption dans le rouge, mal limitée vers le jaune. Sa composition serait: C — 50,09 %; H — 6,82 %; N — 14,85 %; S — 0,62 %; O — 27,62 %; elle ne contient ni fer, ni phosphore, ni cuivre.

Cette matière s'altère rapidement sous l'influence des acides, des alcalis, de l'alcool et de l'eau bouillante. Ses solutions aqueuses ne coagulent ni par la chaleur, ni par l'acide acétique. Réaction de *Millon* négative. Par le chlore elle devient pourpre. La pepsine-acide chlorhydrique la digèrent promptement. Chauffée avec de l'acide chlorhydrique elle se décolore d'abord, puis devient d'un bleu-indigo plus intense que la teinte primitive et donne une spectre constitué par deux bandes qui occupent à peu près la même place que la bande large du carmin d'indigo du commerce.

(¹) Zeyneck — Ueber den blauen Farbstoff aus den Flossen des Crenilabres pavo — Zeitsch. f. physiol. Chemie — Bd. 36 — 1903.

II

Les pigments dont nous venons de décrire les principales propriétés, se trouvent le plus souvent contenus dans des cellules, sous forme de granules et de granulations *(chromochondres de Schneider* (¹)*)*, de grandeurs variables et de forme ordinairement sphérique, parfois allongée, anguleuse.

Au point de vue de leur pigmentation, ces cellules constituent deux groupes bien distincts: *cellules pigmentaires* et *cellules pigmentées*.

Les *cellules pigmentaires*, appelées aussi *chromoblastes, chromatoblastes, chromatophores* et *chromocytes*, représentent une espèce cellulaire déterminée dont la fonction principale est la fonction pigmentaire. Dans les *cellules pigmentées*, par contre, la pigmentation est accidentelle ou ne se montre qu'à une période plus ou moins tardive de l'évolution de l'élément; ce sont des cellules quelconques de l'organisme (épithéliales, nerveuses, glandulaires, musculaires ou autres) qui dans certains cas sont plus ou moins abondamment pourvues de granulations pigmentaires.

Nous allons décrire d'abord les cellules pigmentaires et ensuite nous jetterons un rapide coup d'œil sur la pigmentation de quelques-unes des cellules chez lesquelles ce phénomène se produit dans les conditions physiologiques.

Les *cellules pigmentaires* existent chez tous les Vertébrés. Elles sont très répandues chez les Reptiles, les Amphibiens et les Poissons, où on les trouve en abondance dans le derme. Il y en a également, en plus ou moins grand nombre, dans l'épiderme et dans les organes internes, tels que le péritoine, le péricarde, les méninges, le foie, la rate, les nerfs, les ganglions nerveux, etc. Les nerfs et les centres nerveux sont souvent entourés d'une couche de ces cellules, notamment ceux du sympathique qui se montrent sous l'aspect de cordons noirs (Grenouille, Crapaud, etc).

Les cellules pigmentaires sont souvent situées dans le voisinage des vaisseaux sanguins, qu'elles longent sur une plus ou moins grande étendue, en leur formant une sorte de manchon.

Ces cellules existent aussi dans la choroïde de tous les Vertébrés, où elles forment ce qu'on nomme le *pigment choroïdien*.

(¹) K. C. Schneider, Lehrbuch der vergleichenden Histologie der Tiere — Leipzig — 1902.

Chez l'Homme (à part l'organe de la vision) on rencontre des chromocytes chez les individus de race noire dont le derme en est plus ou moins abondamment pourvu.

Les cellules pigmentaires sont aussi très répandues chez les Invertébrés (Vers, Mollusques et Crustacés); elles atteignent, chez les Céphalopodes, des dimensions considérables.

Quel que soit le Vertébré (¹) où on les étudie, les chromocytes présentent un corps de forme arrondie, allongée, triangulaire ou étoilée, qui émet le plus souvent des expansions plus ou moins longues, fréquemment ramifiées; aussi bien le corps que les expansions sont remplis de *granules* de couleur jaunâtre, brune, parfois très foncée, presque noirâtre.

Souvent les expansions de ces cellules semblent fragmentées, c'est-à-dire qu'on voit des sortes de boyaux plus ou moins longs, quelquefois ramifiés, qui paraissent indépendants du corps cellulaire ou des autres expansions. Cet aspect est dû à ce que les granules de pigment manquent par places qui, n'étant pas colorées, ne sont pas visibles; l'étude des modifications des chromoblastes sous l'action de certains agents chimiques démontre qu'il y a continuité de protoplasma depuis le corps cellulaire jusqu'aux dernières ramifications des prolongements.

Les granules de pigment possèdent généralement une forme sphérique; tels sont les granules des chromoblastes des Vertébrés inférieurs, etc. Dans quelques cas leur forme n'est pas sphérique; dans les cellules pigmentaires de la rétine les granules de pigment ont la forme de bâtonnets à extrémités effilées (*fuscine de Kühne*). Les dimensions de ces granules sont également variables; le plus souvent elles ne dépassent pas un μ, mais il y en a de plus gros.

Dans la plupart des cas les granules de pigment des chromoblastes sont constitués par de la mélanine et ces éléments méritent bien le nom de *mélanocytes* qu'on leur donne souvent; quelques auteurs les nomment aussi *mélanoblastes*.

Chez les Vertébrés inférieurs, il y a cependant des chromocytes qui contiennent des lipochromes de couleur jaune orangée ou

---

(¹) Chez les Vertébrés et la plupart des Invertébrés il n'y a que des chromoblastes simples, c'est-à-dire formés d'une seule cellule; chez les Mollusques il existe des chromoblastes plus composés, pour lesquels [illegible] a proposé le nom de chromatophores (Marchand). Ils sont constitués par une cellule chromatique, remplie de pigment, limitée par une membrane mince sur laquelle sont insérés extérieurement des éléments très allongés, de structure [illegible], dépourvus de pigment, et qui, pour quelques auteurs, seraient de nature contractile [illegible], [illegible], plus clairs, de nature [illegible]. (Kerschner; Ballowitz, Rawitz; Solger, etc.)

rouge et qui se trouvent mélangés aux mélanocytes, dans un certain ordre.

Dans la peau de quelques Batraciens, la Rainette par exemple, il y a des cellules à pigment jaune et des cellules à pigment noir; mais c'est surtout dans la peau des Reptiles, particulièrement dans celle du Caméléon et du *Galeote versicolor*, que ces différentes sortes de chromocytes ont été rencontrées.

Keller (1) a rencontré dans le derme du Caméléon plusieurs variétés d'éléments pigmentaires. Il y a tout d'abord des cellules pigmentaires noires ou *mélanophores*, très nombreuses, ayant, lorsqu'elles sont bien étalées, un corps globuleux placé plus ou moins profondément, duquel partent vers la surface cutanée des expansions longues, ramifiées, qui se terminent à la limite entre le derme et l'épiderme par des extrémités renflées, ce qui leur donne un aspect qui rappelle celui des cellules de *Purkinje* du cervelet. Il y a encore des cellules qui présentent une forme semblable, beaucoup plus petites, qui n'existent que dans certains endroits et qui renferment un pigment rouge pourpre; il leur donne le nom d'*érythrophores*. Entre ces deux variétés il y aurait comme intermédiaire des cellules ayant dans leur intérieur des granulations brunes et rouges en proportions très variables. Entre les prolongements de ces cellules se trouvent deux autres espèces de corpuscules, qui constituent le pigment blanc ou jaune de *Brücke*: les *leucophores* et les *ochrophores*, qui contiennent respectivement des granules incolores (*guanine* donnant à la lumière réfléchie la couleur blanche) ou jaunes, qui auraient entre eux une étroite parenté. Il y a, finalement, les *xanthophores* qui sont remplis de gouttelettes graisseuses jaunes et de granules de la même couleur (lipochrome) et qui se trouvent à la limite entre le derme et l'épiderme, au-dessus des éléments précédents. Chez d'autres espèces de Reptiles (*Calotes jubatus, Lacerta*) *Keller* a trouvé des éléments pigmentaires semblables, à l'exception des leucophores et des érythrophores qui font défaut chez ces animaux.

Mandoul (2) décrit trois sortes de cellules pigmentaires dans la peau du *Galeote versicolor* (Reptile de Cochinchine): *noires, rouges et jaunes*; les premières sont assez profondément placées dans le

(1) R. Keller — Ueber den Farbenwechsel des Chamaeleons und einiger anderer Reptilien — Arch. f. d. ges. Physiol., Bd. 61, 1895.
(2) A. H. Mandoul — Recherches sur les colorations tégumentaires - Thèse de la Fac. des Sc., Paris — 1941.

derme et envoient des prolongements qui se ramifient immédiatement au-dessous de l'épiderme; les rouges, placés à côté d'elles, ont
une forme irrégulièrement arrondie; les jaunes, de forme également arrondie, mais plus régulière, occupent la région supérieure,
sous-épidermique.

Chaque cellule pigmentaire renferme un noyau avec de nombreuses granulations chromatiques, qui se trouve, d'ordinaire, au
milieu du corps cellulaire; ce noyau ne possède pas de pigment
et se montre, dans les préparations non colorées, comme une tache claire. Le noyau peut être multiple; *Solger* (¹) a trouvé chez le
Brochet des cellules pigmentaires pourvues de deux à six noyaux.

À côté du noyau on a constaté la présence, dans quelques
cellules pigmentaires, d'un centrosome et d'une sphère attractive.
Il y a déjà plusieurs années, *Solger* (²) en a vu dans des chromocytes de la peau de la région sus-orbitaire du Brochet (*Esox lucius*)
fixées après avoir placé l'animal à l'obscurité pendant une demi-
heure pour que le pigment se soit éloigné du centre du corps de
la cellule; pendant la division cellulaire cette sphère se dédouble.
Ce même auteur a vu, dans la région ethmoïdale de la Perche
(*Perca fluviatilis*), des cellules pigmentaires pourvues d'une sphère
d'attraction présentant la particularité curieuse de contenir en
son intérieur un tout petit amas de granulations de pigment entouré d'une zone claire et ayant au centre un espace clair où doit
être logé le centrosome.

Zimmermann a également mis en évidence la sphère d'attraction dans les cellules pigmentaires de différents poissons (*Sargus
annularis, Blennius trigloides, Fierasfer acus*, larve de *Trigla*);
cette sphère s'y présente comme un amas central dense de l'archoplasma, ovalaire, qui envoie des filaments plus ou moins nombreux, irradiés en tous sens; l'aspect de cette formation varie
d'une espèce à l'autre.

Keller a rencontré, dans les mélanophores du Caméléon et
de *Calotes jubatus*, une formation qu'il croit être une sphère attractive, se présentant sous la forme d'une tache claire, au milieu
de laquelle il y avait un petit corpuscule fortement réfringent, se
colorant intensivement et qui pourrait bien être le centrosome.

(¹) B. Solger — Zur Kenntnis der Pigmentzellen — Anat. Anz. — 83-9, 1891.

(²) R. Solger — Ueber Pigmenteinschlüsse in der Attraktionssphäre ruhender Chromatophoren
— Anat. Anz. — Bd. 9, 1891.

L'existence d'une sphère attractive a été encore démontrée par *Van der Stricht* [1] dans les cellules pigmentaires de la *lamina fusca* de l'œil du chat. Elle se montre comme une petite masse claire, à limites nettes, indiquées par des granulations pigmentaires, située à côté du noyau qui est excavé à ce niveau et la recouvre en partie; dans cette zone claire il y a des filaments très minces qui se prolongent parfois parmi les granulations pigmentaires et qui s'enchevêtrent et s'anastomosent en formant un réseau ou bien s'irradient autour d'un point central. La plupart des fois on ne voit pas de centrosome; rarement, il y a au centre de la sphère un tout petit corpuscule, à côté duquel il existe parfois un autre accessoire encore plus petit.

Plus récemment *Prowazek* [2] a constaté la présence de la centrosphère, avec une disposition radiée autour, dans les cellules pigmentaires de quelques Poissons osseux *(Trigla lineata, Crenilabrus griseus)*; au centre de la sphère il y aurait un petit amas de pigment. Dans les cellules pigmentaires jaunes, cet auteur a vu autour de la sphère un pigment rouge-orangé plus grossier.

La multiplication des cellules pigmentaires a été étudiée par *Flemming, Zimmermann, Nussbaum*, etc. Ces savants ont reconnu qu'elle se fait par mitose et que pendant celle-ci il se produit des modifications dans la disposition des granulations de pigment. C'est ainsi que *Zimmermann* a constaté, dans les cellules pigmentaires intra-épithéliales, que le pigment s'accumule à la surface au stade de peloton et qu'au stade de monaster il émigre vers l'intérieur, en se plaçant au milieu des chromosomes; finalement, il se dispose comme une sorte de cloison dans le plan équatorial de la cellule. Au moment où celle-ci va se diviser, l'ébauche de l'étranglement qui séparera les deux cellules-filles se montre sous forme d'une ligne claire qui partage en deux la cloison pigmentaire. Des constatations semblables auraient été faites par *Nussbaum* chez des embryons de Grenouille.

D'après *Flemming* la division du corps cellulaire succède tardivement à celle du noyau et ne se produit que lorsque celui-ci est au repos.

Van der Stricht n'a pas vu de signes de mitose dans les cellules pigmentaires de la *lamina fusca* de l'œil du chat; par con-

---

[1] O. van der Stricht — La sphère attractive dans les cellules pigmentaires de l'œil du chat — bibliog. anatom que — vol. III — 1895.

[2] S. Prowazek — Beitrag zur Pigmentfrage — Zoolog. Anzeiger, Bd. 23, 1900.

tre il a cru observer quelques rares divisions directes; la sphère
attractive se diviserait en même temps que le noyau.

L'un des caractères les plus remarquables des cellules pigmentaires ce sont les modifications qui s'y produisent et qui entrainent
des changements plus ou moins rapides dans la coloration des tissus. Parmi les Vertébrés c'est dans la peau des Reptiles, Amphibiens et Poissons que les chromocytes présentent au plus haut
degré cette propriété; les changements de couleur du *Caméléon*,
du *Galéote*, bien connus, sont en grande partie dus à ces éléments.
La peau des Grenouilles et des Crapauds montre également des
variations dans l'intensité de la coloration qui dépendent aussi
des cellules pigmentaires.

Une série de faits et d'expériences, déjà anciennes pour la
plupart (*Brücke, Wittich, Axmann, Hering, Vulpian, P. Bert,
Pouchet, Krukenberg, Leydig, Lode, Bimmermann, Fischel, Carnot*, etc. (¹), sur lesquels nous ne pouvons pas nous étendre ici, a
démontré que ces mouvements des chromocytes sont sous la dépendance du système nerveux. Aussi l'existence de nerfs se terminant sur ces éléments était depuis longtemps soupçonnée et
quelques auteurs avaient même décrit des fibres nerveuses qui seraient en rapport avec eux. *Leydig*, le premier, en 1873, a signalé
ce fait dans la peau de Batraciens et Reptiles. *Hermann* a constaté, au moyen du chlorure d'or, des nerfs en connexion avec les
cellules pigmentaires de la peau de la Grenouille. *Lode* a pu mettre en évidence, dans les nageoires de différents Poissons, des
nerfs allant aux chromatophores.

Mais ce ne fut que par l'emploi de la méthode *de Golgi* que
l'existence des nerfs des chromatocytes a pu être démontrée
d'une façon indubitable. *Ballowitz*, en 1893, ayant appliqué cette
méthode à la peau de Poissons (Brochet, Perche, etc.), a affirmé
qu'il y avait un rapport entre le trajet des nerfs et la sphère attractive des cellules pigmentaires; les fibres nerveuses chemine-
raient en spirale ou en anneaux de façon à entourer la sphère
d'attraction; de ces anneaux partiraient des fibrilles terminales
s'irradiant en partie sur le corps et en partie sur les prolongements
des cellules pigmentaires; quelques fibrilles passeraient à travers
le corps cellulaire et les prolongements.

(¹) Voir à ce sujet le mémoire de G. *Pouchet* — Les changements de coloration sous l'influence
des nerfs — Journ. de l'Anat. et de la Physiol. — t. XII — 1873 et la Thèse de P. *Carnot* — Recherches
sur le mécanisme de la pigmentation — Paris, 1896.

En 1895, *Eberth* et *Bunge* (1) ont étudié par le chromate d'argent les nerfs de la peau de la Grenouille et de différents Poissons (Cyprinus, Lota vulgaris); pour mieux les voir ils ont fait agir de l'eau de chlore pour décolorer le pigment. Ils ont pu voir alors, que la terminaison des nerfs a lieu par des divisions dichotomiques variqueuses et des bouts libres, avec des renflements, il y aurait souvent formation d'un réseau. Les fibres nerveuses sont appliquées sur les chromatophores sans présenter aucune continuité avec leur substance; il y en a qui longent les expansions de ces éléments et qui ou se terminent sur eux ou bien s'en vont ailleurs.

En quoi consistent les modifications que subissent les cellules pigmentaires? Cette question a été l'objet d'un certain nombre de recherches ayant pour but de voir si la cellule changeait de forme en rétractant ses prolongements et en en poussant d'autres, ou bien s'il n'y avait pas un simple déplacement des granules pigmentaires dans l'intérieur du protoplasma sans que la cellule modifiât sa forme. On sait, en effet, que si on examine les cellules pigmentaires de Batraciens soumis à l'influence de certains agents chimiques ou physiques, au lieu de ces éléments étoilés, pourvus de nombreux prolongements, on en voit qui ont l'aspect de boules beaucoup plus foncées, sans expansions; dès que cesse la cause qui avait déterminé ce phénomène, les chromocytes reprennent leur aspect primitif. On a pensé, alors, que ces éléments étaient doués de la propriété de rétracter leurs prolongements et d'en émettre d'autres. Les expansions des chromocytes seraient ainsi comparables aux pseudopodes des Amibes.

Ces mouvements ne sont pas admis par tous les auteurs; il y en a beaucoup qui inclinent à croire que les cellules pigmentaires ne rétractent pas leurs expansions, mais qu'il n'y a qu'un déplacement des granulations pigmentaires vers le corps de la cellule, qui devient ainsi plus foncé. La disparition momentanée du pigment des expansions les rend invisibles, de sorte que le retrait de celles-ci n'est qu'une apparence. Cette opinion est partagée dès longtemps par *Brücke, Virchow, Lister, Solger, Biedermann, Ballowitz, Zimmermann, Keller*, etc., dont les observations sont assez démonstratives.

(1) *Eberth and Bunge*—Die Endigung der Nerven in der Haut des Frosches— Anat. Hefte, Bd II —1895.—Die Nerven der Chromatophoren bei Fischen— Arch. f. mikr. Anat., Bd 46, 1895.

152   MARCE ATHIAS

Solger et *Biedermann* en examinant des cellules pigmentaires dites contractées de Poissons et Amphibiens, sur des coupes tangentielles de la peau fraîche, ont pu distinguer les prolongements dépourvus de granules pigmentaires partant du pourtour du corps cellulaire.

Ballowitz (¹) a fait chez des Poissons des constatations qui confirment celles des autres auteurs. Par la méthode de *Golgi* il est arrivé à imprégner des expansions non pigmentées des chromoblastes jusqu'à leurs ramifications les plus fines.

Keller (²) a pu voir également les expansions des mélanophores de la peau du Caméléon après le départ du pigment et est même parvenu à les colorer en jaune pâle par la méthode de *Biondi-Heidenhain-Dehors*.

Ces auteurs ont constaté, en outre, qu'il reste parfois des granules de pigment isolés ou en petits groupes par ci par là même dans les dernières branches des prolongements, après que la masse pigmentaire principale s'est rassemblée dans le corps de la cellule.

Carnot (³) a étudié les chromoblastes à l'état vivant dans la membrane interdigitale de la Grenouille et a suivi les modifications qu'il présente sous l'influence d'une injection de chlorhydrate d'aniline et de nitrite d'amyle, réactifs qui provoquent, le premier le retrait de ces cellules, le deuxième le retour à l'état d'extension. Dans ces conditions il a constaté que le plus souvent les nouveaux prolongements qu'on voit apparaître sont superposables à ceux qu'on a vu rentrer; mais il a aussi observé plusieurs cas où le nouveau prolongement ne partait pas absolument du même point que l'ancien et même qu'un prolongement rentré dans la cellule pouvait être remplacé par plusieurs prolongements, quand elle revenait à l'état d'expansion. D'après cet auteur il se produit tout d'abord un transport des granules pigmentaires à l'intérieur de la cellule, mais après le départ de ceux-ci, il y aurait une rétraction amiboïde des prolongements et si, lorsqu'ils se forment de nouveau, ils se superposent aux anciens, cela vient de ce que la voie est déjà tracée, la place libre et que le nouveau prolongement suit ainsi tout naturellement la route de l'ancien.

D'après les observations que nous venons de citer, il paraît bien

(¹) L. Ballowitz.—Ueber die Bewegungserscheinungen der Pigmentzellen.—Biol. Centralbl. t. IX, 1889.
(²) Keller, loc. cit.
(³) Carnot, loc. cit.

établi, malgré les doutes exprimés par quelques auteurs, que les changements d'aspect que nous offrent les cellules pigmentaires, du moins celles de la peau des Amphibiens et des Poissons, sont dus à une migration du pigment des expansions vers le corps cellulaire, plutôt qu'à des retraits et des allongements successifs de ces expansions, c'est-à-dire à des mouvements comparables aux mouvements amiboïdes.

Flemming (1) et *Rabl* (3) inclinent aussi vers cette façon de voir, contrairement à *Fischel* (2) qui admet la rétraction des prolongements des cellules pigmentaires de la peau de la larve de Salamandre.

Au sujet de la nature et de l'origine des chromocytes, bien des discussions se sont produites.

Quelques auteurs qui ont étudié spécialement les éléments pigmentaires de l'épiderme prétendent qu'ils ne sont pas de véritables cellules. C'est ainsi que *Schwalbe* pensait que les expansions ramifiées qu'ils présentent ne sont autre chose que les interstices entre les cellules épithéliales, qui seraient comblés par des granules de pigment. Au dire de *Kromayer* (4) le pigment de l'épiderme serait un produit de la destruction des fibrilles qui traversent les cellules épithéliales en les réunissant, fibrilles qu'il a étudiées d'une façon approfondie au moyen d'une méthode spéciale; dans cette hypothèse les chromocytes seraient tout simplement les granules dérivés de ces fibrilles, disposés en séries radiées autour des espaces laissés par les cellules épithéliales.

D'autres auteurs, par exemple *Riehl*, ont considéré les chromocytes comme étant des leucocytes chargés de granules colorés.

Renaut (5) pense aussi que les cellules pigmentaires ramifiées de l'épiderme sont des leucocytes sortis des vaisseaux par diapédèse et renfermant des granulations d'origine hématique. Dans le derme, ces leucocytes abandonneraient des granulations de pigment qui seraient fixées par les cellules conjonctives. *H. Rabl* (6) incline

(1) W. *Flemming* — Ueber den Einfluss des Lichtes auf die Pigmentirung der Salamanderlarve — Arch. f. mikr. Anat., Bd. 46, 1895.

(2) A. *Fischel* — Ueber Bräunung und Entwicklung der Pigmente — Arch. f. mikr. Anat., Bd. 47, 1896.

(3) H. *Rabl* — Pigment und Pigmentzellen in der Haut der Wirbeltiere — Ergebnisse d. Anat. u. Entwickel. — Bd. VI, 1897.

(4) F. *Kromayer* — Vergl. optische ... der Zelle in neuer Auffassung. Beiträge zur Pigmentfrage — Dermatologische Zeitschrift, Bd. IV — 1897.

(5) J. *Renaut* — Traité d'histologie pratique — Paris, 1899.

(6) H. *Rabl* — Ueber die chromatische ... des Pigments in der Haut der Larven der Urodelen Amphibien — Anat. Anz. — Bd. X, 1895, et bei ..., Ergebnisse d. Anat. und Entwickel. — Bd. VI, 1897.

aussi à croire que ces cellules pigmentaires intra-épithéliales sont des éléments migrateurs, du moins en partie; le pigment dont ces éléments sont chargés proviendrait de la destruction de globules rouges du sang (peau de larves d'Urodèles). Ces cellules épidermiques sont, pour cet auteur, bien distinctes des éléments pigmentaires du derme.

Pour ce qui concerne les chromocytes du derme, deux hypothèses principales se partagent depuis longtemps la faveur des histologistes et encore aujourd'hui aucune d'elles n'est définitivement établie sur des bases suffisamment solides pour faire rejeter complètement l'autre. Les uns admettent la nature mésodermique des chromocytes et en font une variété des cellules du tissu conjonctif. Pour d'autres ces cellules sont d'origine épithéliale; ce seraient des cellules épithéliales modifiées.

En tête des auteurs qui soutiennent la première théorie, nous devons placer *Ehrmann* (1). D'après lui, les chromocytes dérivent de cellules mésodermiques spéciales, les *mélanoblastes*, cellules bien distinctes des autres cellules du tissu conjonctif. « Sämmtliche Pigmentzellen des erwachsenen Thieres, dit *Ehrmann*, entstammen primären Melanoblasten, welche unter dem Ectoderm zuerst in der Umgebung der Hirnblase, aus dem Mesoderm entstanden sind ».

La nature mésoblastique de ces éléments est généralement admise par les histologistes. Nous citerons, parmi ceux qui partagent cette façon de voir, *H. Rabl, Rosenstadt, Kölliker* (2), *Mathias Duval* (3), *Prenant* (4), qui considèrent les cellules pigmentaires comme une variété de cellules du tissu conjonctif.

L'origine épithéliale des chromoblastes a été soutenue par quelques observateurs, notamment par *Kodis, Yarisch, Post*, etc.

D'après *Metchnikoff* (5) les éléments ramifiés qu'il désigne sous le nom de *pigmentophages*, dont l'apparition coïncide avec le blanchiment des cheveux et des poils, seraient d'origine épidermique; ils absorberaient le pigment des poils et le transporteraient dans le bulbe et le derme, jouant ainsi le rôle d'éléments phagocytaires.

(1) *Ehrmann* — Das melanotische Pigment und die pigmentbildenden Zellen des Menschen und der Wirbelthiere etc. — Bibliot. Medica. Cassel — Abt. D.H. H.6 — 1896.

(2) *A. von Kölliker* - Handbuch der Gewebelehre des Menschen, Bd. I, 1889.

(3) *M. Duval* - Précis d'Histologie - Paris, 1900 (2e éd.)

(4) *Prenant, Bouin et Maillard* — Traité d'Histologie, t. I — Paris, 1911.

(5) *E. Metchnikoff* — Sur le blanchiment des cheveux et des poils — Ann. de l'Inst. Pasteur — vol. XV — 1901.

Tout récemment la nature épithéliale des chromoblastes a été défendue assez énergiquement par *Loeb et Strong*, dans plusieurs travaux, dont les derniers datent de 1904 [1]. Les savants américains s'appuyent principalement sur les observations faites par eux au cours de leurs expériences de transplantation de fragments de peau chez le Cobaye et la Grenouille. Ils ont constaté que dans la régénération de la peau de la Grenouille les cellules pigmentaires de l'épiderme (qu'ils nomment chromatophores) se comportent d'une façon identique aux cellules épithéliales et non comme celles du derme qui se régénèrent beaucoup plus lentement.

Dans la peau du Cobaye en voie de régénération, les cellules pigmentaires offrent au début un aspect nettement épithélial. Il n'y aurait aucune disposition indiquant la migration de ces cellules du derme vers l'épiderme. Elles se reproduisent par mitose dans la peau en régénération, en plein épiderme, et avant que le tissu du derme sous-jacent se soit régénéré.

D'après *Lewis*, les cellules pigmentaires de la choroïde tireraient leur origine des cellules épithéliales pigmentées de la vésicule optique; elles seraient donc d'origine épithéliale. *Loeb* admet que les chromocytes du derme de la Grenouille et du Cobaye proviennent également des éléments épithéliaux, opinion qui avait déjà été émise par *Maurer* [2]. Il n'y a pas de faits assez démonstratifs pour que cette théorie puisse être acceptée plutôt que celle de l'origine mésodermique des éléments pigmentaires; *Loeb* luimême dit: «The question, however, can not as yet be regarded as decided». Des recherches plus étendues sont nécessaires pour trancher cette question.

Cellules pigmentées. — Dans presque tous les tissus et les organes du corps des Vertébrés il peut exister des cellules dont le cytoplasma se montre plus ou moins chargé de substances pigmentaires figurées. Ce sont les cellules de l'épiderme et de ses dérivés celles qui sont le plus généralement pigmentées dans toutes les classes des Vertébrés. Aussi cette pigmentation a attiré l'attention d'un grand nombre d'histologistes et a donné lieu à une foule de travaux, dont les plus importants sont ceux de *Kölliker*, *Ehr-*

---

[1] L. *Loeb and R. M. Strong* — On regeneration of the pigmented skin of the frog, and on the character of the chromatophores — The American Journ. of Anatomy — Vol III — 1904. — L. *Loeb* — The character of chromatophores — The Journ. of the American med. Assoc. — Vol XLIII, 1904.

[2] *Maurer* — Die Epidermis und ihre Abkömmlinge — Leipzig, 1895.

mann, *Maurer*, *Post*, *Rosenstadt*, *Rabl*, *Kromayer*, *Carlier*, *Grimm*,
Renaut, *v. Brunn*, *d'Evant*, etc. (¹)

Les cellules nerveuses sont aussi très fréquemment pigmentées, surtout chez l'Homme. L'existence de cellules ayant dans
leur corps des granules pigmentaires plus ou moins abondants, a
été constatée aussi dans la glande surrénale; le foie, le rein, la
moelle osseuse, le corps jaune, (*cellules à lutéine*), le testicule, les
ganglions lymphatiques, la muqueuse intestinale, le myocarde, le
sphincter papillaire des Poissons et des Amphibiens, la conjonctive, l'iris, les os, etc., etc.

Les leucocytes se montrent parfois aussi accidentellement
chargés de granules pigmentaires; on a observé ce fait, en dehors
de cas pathologiques (résorption de foyers hémorrhagiques, etc.)
dans la rate et la peau de la Salamandre (*Rabl*).

Nous ne pouvons pas, sans sortir des limites de ce rapport,
nous occuper en détail de la pigmentation des éléments de tous
les tissus; cette question a été traitée par de nombreux auteurs
dans des travaux spéciaux, dont les plus importants se trouvent
résumés dans les ouvrages d'Histologie, tels que ceux de *Leydig*,
de *Frey*, de *Kölliker*, de *Mathias Duval*, de *Prenant*, *Bouin* et
Maillard, de *Schneider*, etc., auxquels nous renvoyons le lecteur.
Nous dirons seulement quelques mots sur le pigment des cellules
nerveuses et des glandes surrénales dont la nature et la signification ont été l'objet de discussions dans ces derniers temps.

Les *cellules nerveuses* de l'Homme peuvent contenir deux sortes de pigments, ainsi qu'il a été démontré par les recherches déjà
anciennes de *Obersteiner* (1888) et confirmé par celles plus récentes de *Pilcz*, *Rosin*, *Marinesco*, *Olmer*, *Rothmann*, *Carrier*, *Mühlmann*, *Obersteiner*, *Athias* (²) etc. Ces deux pigments sont: un
pigment jaune clair qui se montre dans la plupart des cellules
nerveuses des individus âgés, et un pigment brun plus ou moins
foncé, parfois noirâtre, qui existe dans les cellules de certaines
régions du névraxe (*locus coeruleus* et *locus niger*) et dans quelques cellules des ganglions cérébro-spinaux et sympathiques,

(¹) On trouvera toutes les indications bibliographiques relatives au pigment de l'épiderme
dans : J. RABL (loc. cit.).
(²) *Pilcz* — *d'Evant* — Intorno alla genesi del pigmento epidermico — Atti d. R. Accad.
med.-chir. de Nap. di anno LVI, 1903.
Marinesco — Anatomie de cellule nerveuse — Lisboa 1906, et G. *Marinesco* — Recherches sur le pigment jaune des cellules nerveuses — Revue de psychiat. et de psych. expérimentale.
On y trouve toute la bibliographie de cette question.

Le *pigment foncé* se présente sous forme de granulations assez grosses, parfois irrégulières, distribuées dans toute l'étendue du corps cellulaire ou constituant des amas à la périphérie ou au voisinage du noyau. Il fait son apparition peu de temps après la naissance (2ᵉ et 3ᵉ année, *Pilcz*) et n'augmente pas en proportion avec l'âge. Sa solubilité dans la potasse, sa résistance aux acides et aux dissolvants des substances grasses, sa décoloration par le chlore naissant en présence de l'alcool, etc., font ranger ce pigment dans le groupe des mélanines. *Oliver* n'a pas pu y trouver du fer.

Quant au *pigment jaune*, il constitue des granules et des granulations de volume très variable qui s'accumulent tantôt dans un pôle de la cellule, très souvent près du cône d'origine de l'axone, tantôt aux deux pôles opposés du soma, tantôt autour du noyau ou à la périphérie, en formant un anneau incomplet ou un croissant. La quantité de ce pigment et le nombre de cellules qu'il envahit augmentent à mesure que l'individu avance en âge. Les importantes recherches de *Pilcz* ont montré qu'il fait son apparition vers l'âge de 2 ans dans les cellules du sympathique, de 6 ans dans les cellules de ganglions spinaux, de 7 à 8 ans dans les radiculaires de la moelle, après 20 ans dans les grandes pyramidales de l'écorce cérébrale. Quelques auteurs ont pu mettre en évidence, dans quelques cellules nerveuses, des granulations de même nature à un âge moins avancé; c'est ainsi que *Valente* en a vu dans les cellules des ganglions spinaux d'un enfant de 5 ans, *Mühlmann* dans des cellules nerveuses de nouveaux-nés de 3-4 mois; *Zappert* affirme même en avoir rencontré dans des cellules de la corne antérieure au 6ᵉ mois de la vie intra-utérine.

On peut rencontrer du pigment jaune dans un grand nombre de cellules nerveuses de l'Homme; il en est cependant quelques unes qui n'en présentent jamais ou seulement chez des individus très vieux et toujours en petite quantité. *Obersteiner* divise les cellules nerveuses, à ce point de vue, en deux groupes: *cellules lipophobes* qui, même chez des vieillards, sont dépourvues de pigment jaune ou n'en possèdent que très peu (cellules de *Purkinje*, cellules du noyau d'*Edinger-Westphal*); *cellules lipophiles* qui, à un âge peu avancé, sont richement pourvues de pigment (cellules radiculaires et funiculaires la moelle et du bulbe, cellules pyramidales, cellules des ganglions cérébro-spinaux et sympathiques, etc.).

Ce pigment jaune des cellules nerveuses présente quelques

propriétés communes avec les substances grasses, ainsi qu'il a été reconnu par *Obersteiner* en 1888 et confirmé par toutes les recherches poursuivies au cours de ces dernières années. En effet, il noircit par le tétroxyde d'osmium, se colore en rouge par le Soudan III et se dissout dans l'alcool, l'éther, le chloroforme, etc. *Olmer* l'a vu prendre une teinte bleue ou verte par l'acide sulfurique concentré. À cause de ces caractères, *Rosin* a cru devoir le ranger parmi les lipochromes, opinion qui a été acceptée *Bohn*, *Olmer*, *Rothmann* et nous-même.

Certains auteurs rejettent la façon de voir de *Rosin* et ne veulent même pas considérer les granulations jaunes des cellules nerveuses comme un pigment. Tels sont *Colucci*, *Marinesco*, *Carrier*, etc. Pour le premier de ces auteurs, il s'agit d'une dégénérescence spéciale des cellules nerveuses, à laquelle il donne le nom de *dégénérescence jaune globuleuse*.

Marinesco a publié sur la question une série de travaux très intéressants dans lesquels il s'efforce de démontrer que «le pigment jaune des cellules nerveuses ne mérite pas le nom de lipochrome, car s'il ne présente pas la réaction chimique de la lutéine (coloration bleue par l'acide sulfurique, etc.), au contraire de ce qui avait été constaté par *Olmer*. Pour le savant de Bucarest, ces prétendus granules de pigment sont des *granules et granulations d'involution*, qui n'auraient rien à faire avec un véritable pigment; ils seraient constitués par de la lécithine accompagnée, comme toujours, d'une substance grasse.

Une opinion semblable est soutenue par *Carrier*. Les granules foncés du *locus coeruleus*, du *locus niger*, etc., sont le pigment normal des cellules nerveuses; les granules jaunes seraient un produit de dégénérescence des éléments chromophiles et, peut-être, d'autres éléments constituants du protoplasma nerveux.

Lubarsch (1) et *Schob* (2), qui ont examiné les pigments qui se trouvent dans différents tissus de l'organisme humain, tels que le système nerveux, les muscles lisses, le foie, les reins, les glandes surrénales, les ovaires, le testicule, etc., aussi bien à l'état normal que dans des conditions pathologiques, sont arrivés à la conclusion que le seul pigment qui mérite le nom de lipochrome est la *lutéine* des cellules des corps jaunes, car ce serait le seul qui

(1) Lubarsch. — Ueber lutealähnliche Pigmente. — Zieglers Beitr. z. pathol. Anat. u. patholog. Anatomie, p. 22, 1902.

(2) E. Schob. — Zur Kenntniss der lutealähnligen Pigmente. — Virchow's Archiv, Bd. 177, 1904.

donnerait la réaction caractéristique avec l'acide sulfurique (coloration bleue) et la solution iodo-iodurée (coloration verte). D'autres pigments, parmi lesquels ceux des cellules nerveuses, se colorant en rouge par le Sudan et en noir par le tétroxyde d'osmium, sont bien de nature grasse, mais aucun d'eux ne peut être identifié aux lipochromes; ce seraient des pigments de déchet (*Abnutzungspigmente*), se trouvant en combinaison physique ou chimique avec une substance grasse.

A notre avis, il n'y a pas de raison pour ne pas considérer les granules jaunes des cellules nerveuses de l'Homme comme étant d'un pigment du groupe des lipochromes. Ils possèdent les propriétés physiques et chimiques des pigments de cette famille, étant comme eux solubles dans les dissolvants des matières grasses, réduisant le tétroxyde d'osmium, se colorant par le Sudan III. D'après *Olmer* ils prennent une couleur bleue ou verte par l'acide sulfurique, caractère qui a été nié par *Marinesco*, *Labarsch* et *Sehrt*; mais il nous semble que ces faits négatifs ne doivent pas faire rejeter une observation positive, sans que des recherches plus étendues soient entreprises pour vérifier de quel côté se trouve la vérité; ajoutons seulement que cette réaction ne se montre pas dans tous les lipochromes, ainsi que nous l'avons dit plus haut en parlant des propriétés chimiques des pigments de ce groupe.

Le pigment jaune se montre également chez des Vertébrés autres que l'Homme, mais sa présence est bien moins fréquente et jamais il n'y existe en quantité aussi considérable; *Rosin*, *Dexler*, *Rothmann*, *Olmer*, *Obersteiner*, etc. l'ont vu chez le Bœuf, le Cheval, le Singe, le Chat, etc. Nous en avons constaté l'existence, en quantité peu considérable, dans les cellules des ganglions spinaux du Chien, du Chat, du Lapin et du Cobaye, où il se montre sous forme d'un amas de petites granulations colorables par le tétroxyde d'osmium, situé d'ordinaire à la périphérie du corps cellulaire, souvent au voisinage du cône d'origine de l'axone. Nous avons observé qu'il prend une coloration noire, parfois bleuâtre par l'hématoxyline ferrique dans les pièces fixées au sublimé.

De même que chez l'Homme, le lipochrome est plus abondant chez les Mammifères vieux que chez les jeunes, ainsi qu'il résulte des études de *Dexler*, de *Rothmann* et d'*Olmer*.

Dans les cellules des ganglions spinaux et sympathiques des Oiseaux, *Timofew* a décrit un pigment jaune prenant une couleur rouge par les méthodes de *Oppel* et de *Mann* (safranine et bleu de Lyon).

Pugnat a signalé l'existence de granulations pigmentaires dans les cellules des ganglions de quelques Reptiles.

Chez les Amphibiens (Grenouille, Crapaud), les cellules des ganglions spinaux et sympathiques présentent très souvent des granulations jaunes ou orangées que nous avons vu se dissoudre dans l'alcool et noircir par le tétroxyde d'osmium. D'après *Böhler* ce pigment serait plus abondant en hiver qu'en été.

On n'a jamais constaté la présence de pigment dans les cellules du névraxe des Amphibiens adultes. Par contre, chez les larves de Grenouille, les éléments nerveux embryonnaires se montrent chargés d'un pigment brun, ayant les caractères des mélanines; ce pigment a été décrit par *Bataillon* et par nous. Au fur et à mesure que les larves se transforment en jeunes Grenouilles, les cellules nerveuses perdent le pigment, qui finit par disparaître; une fois la métamorphose terminée, elles en sont tout à fait dépourvues.

En ce qui concerne les Poissons, *Romano* a rencontré dans les cellules nerveuses du lobe électrique de la Torpille un pigment jaune ayant des propriétés qui le font considérer comme étant de nature grasse.

Le pigment des *glandes surrénales* est connu depuis longtemps, il a été décrit par *Simon, Leber, Hassal, Kölliker, Gandry, Gottschau, von Ebner, Hultgren et Andersson, Guieysse, Bernard et Bigard, Plecnik, Ciaccio, Mulon, Delamare, Diamare, Bonnamour, Celestino da Costa*, etc.

Ce pigment se présente sous la forme de granulations jaunes ou brun-jaunâtre et est inclus dans l'intérieur des cellules de la zone réticulée. Il est plus abondant chez l'Homme que chez les autres Mammifères, et sa quantité augmente avec l'âge [1].

Au sujet de la nature de cette substance pigmentaire, les auteurs ne sont pas d'accord. *Von Ebner* a constaté qu'il est peu soluble dans l'alcool et l'éther et qu'il résiste à l'action de la lessive de soude. D'après *Plecnik* les granules pigmentaires jaunâtres se colorent en noir par l'hématoxyline ferrique, en vert par le bleu polychrome de *Unna*; *Ciaccio, Diamare* et *Führmann* ont remarqué également que l'hématoxyline ferrique colore ce pigment. *Mulon*, qui a étudié à fond cette question chez le Cobaye,

---

[1] Celestino da Costa — As glandulas suprarenaes e suas homologas. Estudo citologico — Lisboa, 1905, qui contient toutes les indications bibliographiques relatives au pigment des glandes surrénales.

affirme que les granulations pigmentaires possèdent un substratum albuminoïde imprégné d'une matière colorante grasse (lécithine, lipochrome ou pigment ferrique). La réaction de *Lilienfeld* et *Monti* lui a révélé la présence de phosphore dans la graisse. Par le ferrocyanure de potassium, en présence de l'acide chlorhydrique, et par le sulfhydrate d'ammoniaque il a pu mettre en évidence du fer dans certaines granulations pigmentaires contenues dans les mêmes cellules que les granules de nature grasse. Finalement d'autres granules solubles dans la thérébenthine, l'éther, le chloroforme seraient constitués par du lipochrome.

Desmare n'a pas pu se convaincre de la présence du fer dans le pigment des surrénales et met en doute l'existence du lipochrome; pour lui il s'agit d'un pigment propre à la graisse de ces organes. Dans un travail postérieur à celui de cet auteur, *Mulon* insiste sur les caractères qui le portent à admettre que, dans les cellules des glandes surrénales, il y a des granules de lipochrome; ces caractères sont: la coloration qu'ils prennent à l'état frais par le tétroxyde d'osmium et le Sudan III, et la perte de leur coloration normale quand on les traite par des solvants des graisses (éther, cloroforme, xylol).

De nouvelles recherches nous semblent indispensables pour établir d'une façon précise quelle est la véritable nature du pigment des cellules de la glande surrénale.

III

L'origine et le mode de formation des pigments dans l'intérieur des cellules ont donné lieu à un grand nombre de recherches qui ont conduit leurs auteurs à formuler des hypothèses plus ou moins bien fondées surtout pour ce qui concerne les pigments mélaniques, desquels nous allons principalement nous occuper.

Deux théories, ayant toutes les deux de nombreux partisans et adversaires, ont été émises pour expliquer l'apparition des mélanines dans les éléments cellulaires, aussi bien à l'état normal que dans des conditions anormales, ou pathologiques. Pour les uns, les mélanines ne sont que des produits figurés résultant de la transformation de l'hémoglobine qui seraient absorbés tels quels par les cellules ou qui y pénétreraient à l'état de dissolution et y prendraient ensuite la forme granuleuse. Pour d'autres, les pigments mélaniques sont une élaboration, un produit du métabolisme cellulaire; ils seraient d'origine autochtone.

La *théorie de l'origine hématique ou hématogène* des pigments mélaniques, la plus ancienne en date, car elle a été formulée par *Virchow* en 1847, a été soutenue par une pléiade d'histologistes et d'anatomo-pathologistes, parmi lesquels les plus importants sont *Dressler, Langhans, Demiéville, Quincke, Nothnagel, List, Riehl, Meyersov, Koelliker, Duirck, Schmidt, Unna, Ehrmann,* etc., etc. Voyons sur quelles assises elle a été établie et quelle est la conclusion qui se dégage de l'examen des observations.

Un fait d'ordre anatomique qu'on a souvent invoqué à l'appui de d'origine hématique des pigments mélaniques est la présence de cellules pigmentaires au voisinage des vaisseaux sanguins, soit dans les conditions normales soit dans des cas pathologiques (*Demiéville, Ehrmann, Nothnagel, List,* etc.). En effet, on observe souvent cette disposition des chromocytes dans le derme des Amphibiens, par exemple, où ils sont en grande partie situés le long des vaisseaux (*Ehrmann*).

À l'état normal ce seraient les leucocytes qui, en se chargeant de globules rouges ou de pigments de ceux-ci dans l'intérieur des vaisseaux, en sortiraient et iraient porter le pigment aux tissus circonvoisins.

List affirme qu'il a pu voir dans les vaisseaux de la queue de larves d'Amphibiens (*Triton cristatus*), des formes de dégénération et de fragmentation des érythrocytes; desquels proviendrait le pigment qui abandonnerait les vaisseaux et passerait dans les tissus où il serait pris par des leucocytes et transporté par eux jusque dans les cellules épithéliales, par exemple.

Mais les cellules chargées de mélanine ne sont pas exclusivement situés près des vaisseaux; il est même fréquent d'en voir assez loin, éparses dans les tissus au milieu d'autres éléments anatomiques, sans affecter aucun rapport avec les vaisseaux sanguins (*Rosenstadt, Halpern*).

Rosenstadt [1] a cherché à voir des leucocytes pigmentés dans le sang des vaisseaux; il dit n'en avoir jamais vus, ni chez l'animal vivant ni dans des préparations sèches et fixées. Quant aux grains de pigment trouvés par *List*, il s'agirait de blocs d'hématine donnant la réaction du fer, qui n'auraient rien à faire avec la formation du pigment mélanique.

[1] R. Rosenstadt — Sind es über die Abstammung und die Bildung des Hautpigments — Arch. f. mikr. Anat., Bd. 50, 1897.

Ce qui montre encore que ce fait ne peut pas servir de base à cette hypothèse, c'est qu'il y a d'autres cellules pourvues de pigments, tels que les lipochromes et la guanine, qui, en aucun cas, ne peuvent être des dérivés de l'hémoglobine et qui néanmoins se trouvent près des vaisseaux (*Jarisch*); ces cellules existent en grand nombre dans la peau des Amphibiens.

D'après *Sieber*, dont la façon de voir est partagée par *Rosenstadt*, la disposition des cellules pigmentaires autour des vaisseaux peut être expliquée en admettant que, pour la formation de la mélanine, il est nécessaire des processus énergiques d'oxydation, qui doivent atteindre leur plus grande intensité au voisinage des vaisseaux sanguins. «Und wenn man sie, écrit cet auteur, auch in der Nähe der Blutgefässe findet, so wäre es viel plausibel das so zu erklären, das Pigmentzellen als Wanderzellen die Neigung haben, dort sich anzuordnen, wo für sie, wie es in der Nähe der Blutgefässe thatsächlich der Fall sein muss, die Ernährungsverhältnisse am günstigsten sich gestalten.»

Les partisans de la théorie de l'origine hématique de mélanines ont trouvé une preuve en faveur de leur opinion dans les résultats auxquels est arrivé *Langhans* (1870) qui a étudié la résorption des extravasats sanguins. Cet auteur, ayant introduit sous la peau d'un animal de petits caillots sanguins, a constaté qu'il se produit autour d'eux une accumulation de cellules contractiles qui absorbent les globules rouges qui sont en contact avec elles. Ceux-ci présentent alors les changements suivants: leur couleur devient plus foncée et ils prennent une teinte brunâtre; cette coloration n'est pas persistante et bientôt les globules se montrent jaunâtres ou rouge jaunâtres; ils donnent toujours la réaction de *Perls* pour le fer. Plus tard cette couleur devient jaune rougeâtre, rouge, rouge-brun; il se produit alors une destruction des globules, qui se divisent en un grand nombre de corpuscules irréguliers. Ensuite les dimensions de ces granules diminuent jusqu'à ce qu'ils ne soient plus reconnaissables et la pigmentation semble diffuse. La résorption peut se produire si vite qu'au bout de 3 à 4 semaines on ne trouve plus trace de pigment.

Quincke a injecté du sang de Chien dans le tissu cellulaire sous-cutané; il a trouvé ensuite des granules brun jaunâtres, la plupart contenus dans les cellules du tissu conjonctif ou les cellules migratrices. *Ehrmann* a fait des constatations semblables à la suite de contusions.

Schmidt a placé sous la peau de Grenouilles et de Lapins

de petites plaques de moelle de sureau imbibées de sang d'un animal de même espèce et a observé que la formation du pigment débute par la mise en liberté de l'hémoglobine, dont les gouttelettes sont entourées par des leucocytes, dans l'intérieur desquels se passent les autres transformations. Le pigment ainsi formé, dépourvu de fer, se montre alors sous forme de petits granules de couleur jaune d'or et fortement brillants, contenus dans des cellules ou libres dans les mailles de la moelle de sureau. Ces expériences montrent qu'il se forme un pigment aux dépens de l'hémoglobine.

Un résultat semblable a été obtenu par *Carnot* (¹) qui a suivi les modifications que subit le sang dans le tube digestif de la Sangsue et constata qu'il se transforme en granules de pigment sous l'action des sucs digestifs.

Mais aucun de ces faits ne prouve que la mélanine soit d'origine hématique, car il n'est guère démontré que le pigment qui résulte de la destruction des hématies soit bien de la mélanine.

D'après *Rosenstadt*, qui a répété les expériences de *Langhans* et en a confirmé les résultats, les granules colorés qui proviennent de la destruction des globules rouges sont un dérivé de la matière colorante du sang, mais ne sont pas du tout du pigment mélanique; l'aspect de ces granules, leur forme souvent anguleuse, leurs altérations ultérieures, la diminution de leur volume sont autant de faits qui les éloignent des véritables granules de mélanine. Ce que *Langhans* a pris pour la formation du pigment n'est, en somme, que le processus de résorption des caillots sanguins. De même pour ce qui concerne les observations des autres auteurs (*Quincke, Schmidt, Carnot*); les pigments qu'ils considèrent comme étant de la mélanine sont des matières colorantes d'origine hématique qui figurent comme pigments tant qu'elles ne sont pas complètement résorbées.

Vis-à-vis des réactifs, un pigment d'origine nettement sanguine, tel que celui de la *sarcomatosis cutis*, se comporte d'une façon tout à fait différente de la véritable mélanine; en effet, au contraire de celle-ci, il se dissout dans l'acide chlorhydrique concentré et dans l'acide sulfurique, tandis qu'il n'est pas attaqué par la potasse et le sulfhydrate d'ammoniaque (*Spiegler*).

(¹) P. Carnot.—Recherches sur le mécanisme de la pigmentation.—Thèse de la Faculté des Sciences, Paris 189?. Cet auteur donne des indications bibliographiques assez complètes relatives à cette question.

Les observations que nous venons de rapporter ne prouvent donc pas, en définitive, que les granules de mélanine qui existent dans les chromocytes et les éléments pigmentés soient réellement des produits d'origine hématique.

Ehrmann (¹) l'un des plus grands défenseurs de la théorie de l'origine hématique de la mélanine, apporte comme preuve de sa façon de voir, des observations qu'il a eu l'occasion de faire au cours de ses remarquables recherches sur la pigmentation des œufs et des embryons d'Amphibiens. Ce savant divise les œufs de ces Vertébrés en deux groupes: les œufs originairement pigmentés, tels que ceux de *Rana temporaria et esculenta, Siredon pisciformis, Bufo, Pelobates, Triton taeniatus, Hyla arborea*, etc., et des œufs non originairement pigmentés, qui comprennent ceux de *Salamandra maculata, Triton taeniatus*, etc.

Dans les œufs originairement pigmentés, le pigment, qui existe alors qu'ils sont encore dans l'ovaire, dérive, d'après *Ehrmann*, du sang maternel.

Les œufs non pigmentés dès leur origine évoluent sans former de substances colorantes; les phases de morula, blastula, gastrula, les feuillets du blastoderme et les ébauches des tissus sont dépourvus de pigment. Celui-ci ne fait son apparition chez les embryons qu'après le sang; la formation des cellules pigmentaires est en rapport avec celle des vaisseaux sanguins. Comme dans le premier cas, le pigment serait de provenance hématique, mais au lieu de tirer son origine du sang maternel, il la tirerait de celui de l'embryon.

La formation de ce pigment a lieu, d'après *Ehrmann*, dans des cellules spéciales appartenant au feuillet moyen, les *mélanoblastes*, qui ne sont identiques ni aux cellules du tissu conjonctif, ni aux leucocytes, ni aux cellules épithéliales. Le matériel avec lequel se forme le pigment est de l'hémoglobine, qui existe très diluée dans la lymphe et les sucs des tissus; par des processus vitaux des mélanoblastes, cette hémoglobine serait transformée en pigment mélanique. Formée tout d'abord dans les couches sous épidermiques, la pigmentation envahirait ensuite les éléments épithéliaux.

Scherl (²) partage l'opinion de *Ehrmann*; en poursuivant des

<hr>

(¹) Ce savant a publié plusieurs travaux sur le pigment rétinien et la question de l'origine de la mélanine; le plus récent est celui déjà cité plus haut, qui fait partie de la collection «Bibliotheca medica» Cassel, 1896.

(²) J. Scherl. Einige Untersuchungen über das Pigment des Auges. — Arch. f. Ophthalmol. — Bd. 39, 1893.

études embryologiques chez des Vertébrés de différentes classes, il aurait constaté que l'apparation du pigment de l'œil est en rapport avec le développement de l'appareil circulatoire; ce pigment ne serait autre chose qu'un dérivé, pourvu de fer, de l'hémoglobine qui sortirait des vaisseaux à l'état de dissolution, serait entraînée par le suc des tissus et se transformerait peu à peu d'abord en petites gouttelettes sphériques, ensuite en granules; les cellules épithéliales seraient une sorte de magazin de ces granules pigmentaires.

Le rapport entre l'apparition du sang et la formation du pigment, admis par *Ehrmann et Scherl*, ne peut être accepté sans réserve, car il y a des observations qui montrent qu'il n'existe pas; telles sont celles déjà anciennes de *Kosoto* (1863) et les plus récentes (1895) de *Winkler*. Ces deux auteurs ont pu trouver chez des embryons de Poissons, obtenus par fécondation artificielle, du pigment noir dans la peau, alors que les globules sanguins étaient complètement décolorés. Il en serait de même chez les embryons des Vertébrés (*Winkler*).

Un certain nombre de faits d'ordre anatomo-pathologique est souvent invoqué en faveur de l'origine hématique de la mélanine. Nous citerons, comme étant l'un de ceux qui pour quelques auteurs (*Ehrmann*, entre autres) a le plus de valeur, la formation de pigment brun ou noir dans les globules rouges des paludéens. Ce pigment, dont les caractères le font rapprocher de la mélanine, résulterait de la destruction des globules envahis par l'Hématozoaire; ceci plaiderait donc en faveur de la formation de la mélanine aux dépens d'hémoglobine.

Cette façon de voir est combattue par plusieurs auteurs qui inclinent à considérer ce pigment comme n'étant pas formé par la destruction des globules, mais plutôt comme un produit de l'activité du parasite. *Rosenstadt* fait remarquer que le pigment en question se comporte vis-à-vis des réactifs chimiques d'une manière semblable au pigment noir d'autres Invertébrés, chez lesquels l'hémoglobine manque complètement; par la réaction de *Perls*, cet auteur a pu constater qu'il est dépourvu de fer.

Ce qui semble prouver que la formation du pigment est bien due à l'activité propre du parasite et non pas exclusivement au fait de la destruction du globule, c'est que chez les Mammifères, aussi bien que chez les Oiseaux infectés par des Hématozoaires (*Plasmodium, Piroplasma, Proteosoma, Halteridium*), il se forme du pigment dans les globules envahis, alors que chez les Reptiles et les Batraciens on ne constate la présence d'aucun pigment dans les globules où il y a des parasites (*Drepanidium, etc.*)

S'il ne s'agissait, dans le premier cas, que d'un produit de transformation de l'hémoglobine, on ne pourrait pas comprendre pourquoi dans le deuxième il ne se forme pas de pigment, puisqu'il y a également destruction partielle du globule sanguin. L'activité du parasite doit, par conséquent, prendre une large part à cette formation, et le pigment malarique ne peut pas être regardé comme résultant uniquement de la destruction du globule. *Ich glaube vielmehr*, dit *Rosenstadt*, dass wir es hier mit einer besonderen Eigenschaft dieser Protozoën zu thun haben, melanotischen Pigment selbständig zu erzeugen.

Pour quelques auteurs, le pigment malarique n'a aucun rapport avec la mélanine; d'après *von Fürth* [1] les pigments qui, dans la malaria, apparaissent dans le sang et les organes sicherlich mit den echten Melaninen weder in physiologischer noch in chemischer Hinsicht irgend welche Aehnlichkeit besitzen und zweifellos hämatogenen Ursprungs sind. Dieselben Pigmente entstehen durch die Lebensthätigkeit Malariaplasmodien innerhalb der roten Blutkörperchen und Abblassen derselben auf Kosten des Hämoglobins. Comme on voit, la nature du pigment des paludéens n'est pas définitivement élucidée et son mode de formation est encore discuté. Toutefois, sa resistance aux réactifs chimiques, tels que les acides forts, le font rapprocher des pigments mélaniques.

Mais il n'y a pas dans le fait de l'apparition de ce pigment dans les globules rouges infectés par des parasites une preuve que la mélanine soit tout simplement un produit de la transformation de l'hémoglobine, comme le veulent plusieurs auteurs; il nous semble qu'on doit plutôt y voir un produit d'excrétion du parasite, résultant de son métabolisme. Le parasite vivant dans l'intérieur des hématies, se nourrit forcément aux dépens de l'hémoglobine et autres substances qui s'y trouvent, mais malgré cela le pigment qu'il élabore n'offre pas les caractères des pigments véritablement hématiques; il est dépourvu de fer, quoique le corps du parasite soit tellement imbibé d'hémoglobine que toute sa masse bleuisse lorsqu'on le traite par le ferrocyanure de potassium et l'acide chlorhydrique (*Rosenstadt*).

---

[1] v. von Fürth — Loc. cit.

D'autres faits anatomo-pathologiques qui ont été regardés comme des preuves à l'appui de la théorie de l'origine hématique de la mélanine ont moins de valeur, à ce point de vue, que celui dont nous venons de parler; aussi pour ne pas allonger outre mesure ce rapport nous les passons sous silence.

On a aussi invoqué, comme témoignant de l'origine hématique des mélanines, l'existence du fer dans la composition de quelques-unes d'entre elles. Mais, ainsi qu'il a été dit plus haut, le fer n'est pas un élément constant dans les pigments de cette nature, et par ce fait tombe l'un des arguments des partisans de la théorie.

Mais si la présence du fer dans quelques pigments mélaniques n'est pas une preuve de leur origine hématique, peut-on considérer son absence dans plusieurs de ces pigments comme étant absolument opposée à cette provenance? Évidemment non, car il est des dérivés de l'hémoglobine qui sont dépourvus de fer; telle est l'hématoporphyrine.

Ce qui dans la composition chimique des mélanines ne cadre pas avec son hypothétique origine hématique est la présence du soufre, plus fréquente que celle du fer. Aucun des dérivés connus de l'hémoglobine ne contient du soufre et il serait difficile de comprendre de quelle façon cet élément aurait été introduit dans le pigment, si celui-ci n'était qu'un simple produit de transformation de la matière colorante du sang.

De tout ce que nous venons de dire il ressort nettement que l'hypothèse de l'origine hématique de la mélanine n'est pas en parfaite harmonie avec les faits observés et que ceux qui semblent l'appuyer sont passibles d'une interprétation bien différente de celle qui leur a été donnée tout d'abord et qui cadre avec la *théorie de l'origine autochtone.* Cette théorie fut posée en 1864 par *Ritter,* à la suite d'études faites sur les cellules pigmentaires de la choroïde; plusieurs auteurs l'ont ensuite défendue et elle compte aujourd'hui un grand nombre d'adeptes; citons, parmi eux, *Mertsching, Ketterer, Kromayer, Kaposi, G. Schwalbe, Bataillon, H. Rabl, Reinke, Fischel, Abel et Davis, Carnot, Rosenstadt, Loeb, Landolt, Prowazek, d'Evant, Spiegler, Dacceschi,* etc.

Plusieurs faits militent en faveur de la théorie de la formation autochtone des pigments mélaniques. En ce qui concerne les pigments cutanés, qui ont toujours été un objet d'étude préféré par les auteurs qui ont voulu résoudre le problème de la formation du pigment, il y a un certain nombre d'observations qui démontrent nettement que les cellules épidermiques élaborent elles-mêmes leur pigment. Telles sont celles de *Retterer* (¹) qui datent de 1886, de *Jarisch, Carnot, Maurer, Rosenstadt*, et celles bien plus récentes de *d'Evant* (²) qui montrent que les cellules de l'épiderme peuvent présenter du pigment alors que dans le derme il n'existe pas le moindre granule coloré, ce qui prouve que le pigment des cellules épidermiques ne provient pas du derme, au contraire de ce qui était admis par *Aeby, Riehl, Kœlliker, Ehrmann, List, Minot*, etc.

D'Evant a constaté que, dans plusieurs cas, l'épithélium tégumentaire est fortement pigmenté, tandis que le reste du corps est absolument incolore (*Aplysia, Pleurobranchus*), aussi bien chez des embryons que chez des animaux adultes. Etant donnée l'activité chromogène du sang, ce fait ne serait pas suffisant pour exclure l'origine hématique du pigment épidermique, mais, dit l'auteur, "si domanda: perché le cellule connettivali, pure irrigate dal medesimo liquido, pure a contlato con gli amebociti migranti non ne assumono, non se ne appropriano? non ne prendono gli altri elementi nervosi, muscolari, ecc. del medesimo organismo?" Le même fait a été observé par l'auteur chez les embryons de plusieurs Vertébrés et Invertébrés (*Equus, Caria, Mus, Rattus, Rana, Bufo*).

Il est également intéressant de rappeler que les larves de certains Téléostéens, auxquelles on a donné le nom de *Leptocéphalides* (parce qu'on en faisait un genre distinct), sont absolument transparentes et possèdent un sang tout à fait incolore; malgré cela, il y a dans la peau de ces larves des cellules étoilées renfermant un pigment noir (*Carus, Peters, Günther*, etc.

La formation autochtone du pigment dans les cellules des bourgeons des cheveux et des poils a été bien établie par les recherches de *Schwalbe* (³) et de *Post* (⁴) qui ont étudié, le premier le renouvellement du poil blanc d'hiver de l'Hermine, le second le renouvellement des cheveux et des cils chez l'enfant nouveau-né.

(¹) *Ed Retterer* — Article «Pigments» du Dictionnaire encyclopédique des Sc. Méd. de Dechambre — 2ᵉ sér. XIX, p. 25, 1886.

(²) *E. d'Evant* — loc. cit. Dans ce travail on trouve résumées la plupart des recherches antérieures sur cette question.

(³) *J. Schwalbe* — Ueber den Farbenwechsel winterweisser Thiere — Morpholog. Arbeiten — Bd. II, 1893.

(⁴) *H. Post* — Ueber normale und pathologische Pigmentirung der Oberhautgebilde — Virchow's Archiv — Bd. 135, 1893.

Schwalbe a constaté que, à aucune époque de l'année, le derme et les tissus sous-jacents de la peau du dos ne contiennent du pigment, ainsi que la papille et le follicule conjonctif des poils; malgré cela, au printemps, où il se produit le renouvellement des poils, ceux-ci se montrent pigmentés. Le pigment, n'étant pas venu du derme où il n'y en a point, doit être évidemment élaboré par les cellules épithéliales. Les recherches de *Post* mènent à une conclusion identique.

Dans les plumes des Oiseaux les études de *Klee*, *Kohl* [2], *Rosenstadt*, etc., ont démontré que le pigment a aussi une formation endogène dans les cellules épithéliales, tout comme dans les poils des Mammifères.

De même que les cellules épithéliales, les cellules du tissu conjonctif (derme, choroïde, péritoine, etc.) sont capables d'élaborer des substances pigmentaires par l'activité propre de leur protoplasma. Ceci est admis actuellement par un grand nombre d'auteurs, parmi lesquels nous pouvons citer *Reinke*, *Fischel*, *Galeotti*, *Rosenstadt*, *Carnot*, *van der Stricht*, *Mathias Duval* et *Prénant*. D'après ce dernier savant, la formation du pigment dans les cellules pigmentaires doit être considérée comme un véritable acte glandulaire. «La cellule pigmentaire extrait du sang, dit-il, par un acte véritablement sécrétoire, et fixe sur ses plasmosomes et ses granules la substance nécessaire pour faire un produit spécial, le pigment mélanique. De là devient vaine et inexacte la distinction de deux théories, autogène et hématogène, de la pigmentation... Il faut dire que les cellules pigmentaires élaborent elles-mêmes une matière qu'elles empruntent au milieu, selon la règle imposé à tout élément glandulaire.»

Les expériences de greffes de peau pigmentée, pratiquées par *Kurz*, *Carnot et Deflandre*, *Kromayer*, *Loeb*, *Dieulafé et Mandoul*, chez l'Homme et d'autres animaux (Cobaye, Grenouille), ont fourni l'une des meilleures preuves de la formation autochtone des pigments mélaniques dans les cellules épidermiques. Ces expériences ont montré que des lambeaux de peau pigmentée, greffés sur de la peau blanche d'un animal de même espèce ou d'espèce différente, persistent et peuvent même envahir la région blanche voisine sur une étendue plus ou moins grande. Par contre, les greffes de peau blanche sur fond noir, sont assez rapidement envahies

---

[2] H. Kohl — Über die Entstehung des Pigments in der Epidermoidzellen der Batrachien — Verhandl. d. deutsch. Zoolog. Gesellschaft, t. IV, 1894.

par la pigmentation et finissent par disparaître en peu de temps. «En transplantant une cellule noire, écrit *Carnot* dans son important travail déjà cité, nous avons transplanté la propriété chromogène; si la cellule fabrique son pigment, toutes les cellules qui descendent de la cellule mère en fabriquent aussi; l'extension de la tache marque exactement l'extension de cette descendance. La surface noire indique le terrain occupé par les cellules dérivées des cellules greffées.

«Même en admettant que la cellule noire ne fabrique pas son pigment, on est alors forcé de dire qu'elle présente une affinité particulière pour les granules pigmentés qui lui sont apportés; cette affinité, propriété cellulaire transmissible à la postérité, nous permet la même assimilation de la surface noire avec la descendance de la greffe. Et plus loin: «On ne peut invoquer une infiltration des cellules blanches par les granules pigmentaires, car au moment où une tache noire reste stationnaire, une limite fixe s'établit, sans infiltration progressive des cellules blanches voisines». «Une cellule blanche peut donc rester au voisinage des noires sans s'infiltrer de pigment».

De ses études sur la transplantation de lambeaux de peau d'un animal à l'autre, chez le Cobaye et la Grenouille, et sur la régénération de la peau pigmentée, *Loeb* (1) conclut en disant: «The pigment originates in the epidermis, and the production of melanin is a peculiarity of certain epithelial cells which preserve this function if they are transplanted to a place where formerly nonpigmented cells were present».

Ces citations suffisent pour montrer l'appui que la question des greffes de peau pigmentée a apporté à la théorie de l'origine autochtone des pigments mélaniques.

S'il était nécessaire d'invoquer d'autres arguments d'ordre anatomo-physiologique pour servir de base à cette théorie, nous dirions que l'absence de ces pigments chez les albinos est un fait qui ne peut être expliqué qu'en admettant cette façon de voir; en effet, le sang de ces individus n'est-il pas aussi riche en hémoglobine que celui des individus normaux? Les cellules ne vivent-elles pas, chez les premiers, dans un milieu qui doit être identique à celui dans lequel se trouvent les cellules des seconds? néanmoins les cellules des albinos ne présentent pas un pigment qui, s'il

____

(1) L. Loeb — loc. cit. : Journ. of the med. Assoc., 1904.

n'était qu'un produit de transformation de l'hémoglobine y étant pénétré passivement, aucune raison n'existerait pour qu'il y soit totalement absent.

Il y a encore une question que nous ne croyons pas devoir passer sous silence et qui constitue une preuve d'une grande valeur à l'appui de la théorie dont nous nous occupons; nous voulons parler des *mélanines artificielles*, sur lesquelles nous ne pouvons dire ici que peu de mots.

Les intéressantes recherches de *Schmiedeberg, von Fürth, Chittenden, Albro, Rosenfeld, Ducceschi, Samuely* [1], etc., ont établi qu'en traitant à chaud par des acides, chlorhydrique, sulfurique, nitrique, etc., des substances protéiques incolores, telles que la séro-albumine, l'albumine de l'œuf, la fibrine, la caséine, la kératine, la tyrosine, etc., on obtient des produits ayant des propriétés identiques aux mélanines naturelles.

Ces *mélanines artificielles*, comme on les désigne, sont constituées par les mêmes éléments que les mélanines naturelles, dans les proportions suivantes, en moyenne: C — 54.83; H — 5,695; N — 9,655; S — 4,145. Comme on voit, ces chiffres se rapprochent beaucoup de ceux trouvés dans les mélanines naturelles et que nous avons indiqués dans la première partie de ce rapport. Comme celles-ci, les mélanines donnent de l'indol et du scatol sous l'action de la potasse caustique.

Les recherches chimiques poursuivies depuis une dizaine d'années sur les mélanines et leur production artificielle, conduisirent à admettre l'existence d'un *groupement chromogène de la molécule protéique*; ce fut *Neuki* le premier qui, en étudiant les produits de la digestion pancréatique, a mis en évidence la signification si importante de ce groupement, qui dans des conditions normales ou pathologiques aurait le principal rôle dans la production des pigments mélaniques. Les substances protéiques incolores, aussi bien que la matière colorante du sang, renferment, au dire de ce savant, un groupement chromogène qui serait la substance mère et de l'hématine et des mélanines.

Les mélanines naturelles seraient, d'après quelques auteurs, produites par des processus d'oxydation du groupement chromogène de la molécule protéique (*Samuely, Landolt*, etc). Ces pro-

---

[1] On trouvera tous les détails sur cette question, ainsi que la bibliographie, dans les excellentes pages de von Fürth (*Arbeiten* et du D. *Ducceschi — Sulle melanine — Archivio di histologia*, vol. I, fasc. ... — 1904).

cessus oxydatifs se dérouleraient avec la participation d'un ferment, la *tyrosinase*, dont l'existence a été reconnue par *Bertrand* chez des végétaux et par *ceux Fürth et Schneider, Przibram, Gessard* (1), etc. chez des animaux, Invertébrés (Insectes, Sèche) et Vertébrés; ces recherches démontrent que ce ferment se trouve dans l'organisme notamment aux endroits où il y a formation physiologique ou pathologique de mélanine.

Au dire de *Loeb*, la mélanine des chromatocytes dérive des substances protéiques de la cellule et ne peut pas être produite directement de l'hémoglobine par les raisons suivantes, que nous transcrivons intégralement et qui résument assez bien l'état de la question :

«1. — The sulphur content of the melanin is very large.

2. — From the melanin decomposition products can be obtained similar to the ones obtained from the melanoïdins, which themselves can be produced with the aid of acids from proteid substances.

3. — Tyrosin, a radical, present in cell proteids, can, with the aid of an oxydative ferment tyrosinase, be transformed into substances similar to the melanin of sepia, and similar, probably, to the melanins of vertebrates. It is therefore not unlikely that the production of the pigment of the chromatophores is due to a fermentation causing oxydative and condensation processes in certain decomposition products of cell proteids.»

Nous ne pourrons nous étendre davantage sur ces questions si hautement intéressantes sans dépasser les limites d'un rapport strictement anatomique; nous n'avons voulu qu'effleurer ce sujet et faire entrevoir, d'une façon sommaire, la contribution que les études chimiques peuvent apporter à la connaissance de l'origine si controversée des mélanines.

Passons maintenant à l'examen d'une autre question qui est non moins intéressante et qui est du domaine exclusif de la cytologie; c'est le mécanisme de la formation des granules pigmentaires dans le protoplasma cellulaire.

Voici les résultats obtenus par quelques-uns des principaux histologistes qui se sont occupés de cette question; on verra qu'ils ne sont pas toujours d'accord et même qu'il y a parfois des divergences assez considérables.

---

(1) C. Gessard — Tyrosinase animale — C. R. de la Soc. de Biol., t. LIV — 1902.

L'un des premiers à attirer l'attention sur ce problème fut *Reinke* [1], qui en étudiant les cellules pigmentaires du péritoine de la larve de Salamandre, a constaté qu'il y a des cellules remplies de corpuscules incolores en bâtonnets, prismes et blocs de différentes grosseurs, ayant des reflets métalliques, et des cellules présentant des granules sphériques de couleur verdâtre ou brune, plus ou moins foncée; entre ces deux sortes d'éléments, il a trouvé des formes intermédiaires contenant, à côté des corpuscules incolores, des granules faiblement colorés, en proportions variables. Chez les adultes, il a vu que les cellules à grains incolores avaient disparu. De ces faits, *Reinke* a conclu que les granules pigmentaires sont précédés d'un stade incolore et que le pigment se forme peu à peu.

Gaboffi, qui a étudié les cellules pigmentaires du péritoine d'un Amphibien jeune *(Sperlepes)*, a confirmé l'existence d'un stade incolore dans la formation du pigment. Il a rencontré, à côté des granules pigmentaires, des granules incolores se colorant intensivement par les teintures (fuchsine) et ayant une distribution semblable à celle des premiers. Une observation semblable a été faite par cet auteur dans des cellules épithéliales des larves de Triton.

Fischel [2] retrouve les deux espèces cellulaires décrites par *Reinke*, mais il n'admet pas qu'elles soient identiques et qu'il y ait des formes de transition entre l'une et l'autre. D'après lui, le pigment se montre tout d'abord sous forme d'une substance claire, et c'est par une sorte de transformation spécifique ou par addition d'une substance colorée qu'il prend sa leur couleur foncée, mais il ne croit pas que ce stade non pigmenté soit primitivement cristallin.

L'opinion de *Reinke* est acceptée par *Lubarsch* [3]; le pigment provient, pour lui, d'une formation cristalline non pigmentée. Il a trouvé des formes de transition entre les unes et les autres cellules dans le péritoine de la Salamandre.

Le même rapport entre les cristalloïdes et les granules pigmentaires existe, d'après *Lubarsch*, dans les cellules interstitielles du testicule de l'Homme. Cet auteur affirme que là où les cristal-

[1] *Reinke* — «Zellstudien. Ueber Pigment, seine Entstehung und Bedeutung. Arch. f. mikr. Anat. Bd. 45, 1894.

[2] A. *Fischel* — Zur Pigmentforschung — Anat. Anz., Bd. XII, 1896.

[3] O. *Lubarsch* — Zur Frage der Pigmentbildung — Anat. Anz., Bd. XIII.

loïdes abondent il n'y a que de rares granules de pigment ou même pas du tout, tandis que là où les premiers manquent, les derniers sont en grand nombre. Avant la formation du pigment, les cristalloïdes se diviseraient en fragments de formes différentes et ensuite en sphérules et grains non pigmentés; ce serait à ce moment que le pigment ferait son apparition sous forme de granules dont quelques-uns se coloreraient encore par les anilines acides.

D'après *Prowazek* [1], il y a dans le protoplasma des cellules épithéliales de la larve de Salamandre, avant l'apparition du pigment, des corpuscules qu'il nomme *plastides pigmentaires* colorables par le rouge neutre.

En étudiant la peau d'individus ayant des éphélides, sur des fragments fraîchement excisés des endroits où il y avait des taches pigmentaires jaunâtres et noires, *Törner* [2] a constaté la présence d'une substance jaune, aussi bien dans des cellules dermiques que dans les cellules épidermiques (cellules basales, réseau de *Malpighi* et parfois dans la couche cornée); cette substance, soluble dans l'alcool et le chloroforme et prenant une teinte grise par le tétroxyde d'osmium, ne peut être vue que sur des coupes faites par congélation et montées dans la glycérine. D'après cet auteur les granulations pigmentaires foncées, qui seraient moins nombreuses là où la substance jaune est plus abondante, résulteraient de la transformation de celle-ci.

Avant de se montrer sous forme de granules plus ou moins noirâtres, le pigment cutané serait donc une substance jaune, amorphe, fluide, infiltrant les cellules et ne prenant qu'ultérieurement la forme granuleuse.

Quelques auteurs ont fait jouer au noyau un rôle plus ou moins important dans la production du pigment. C'est ainsi que *Ritter* a pensé que les granules de pigment choroïdien étaient dus à une cristallisation, dans le cytoplasma, d'une substance dissoute dans le noyau. Pour *Merkaching* et *Kodis*, le pigment des cellules épidermiques et des cheveux aurait son origine dans la destruction du noyau. D'après *Jarisch*, ce serait de la chromatine nucléaire que proviendrait le pigment.

---

[1] *Prowazek* — Loc. cit.
[2] H. *Törner* — Beitrag zur Kenntnis des Pigmentes — Dermatologische Zeitschrift, Bd. XII, H. 6, 8, 1905.

Les résultats des recherches de *Bataillon* [1], sur les métamorphoses des Batraciens anoures, parlent dans le même sens. En effet, cet auteur a constaté qu'à l'époque de la métamorphose les phénomènes d'histolyse sont accompagné de modifications nucléaires, notamment une émission de *boyaux et balles chromatiques*, qui se transformeraient en granules de pigment dans le cytoplasma. Ce phénomène a été observé dans la peau, les muscles, le système nerveux, les glandes sexuelles, etc. Le noyau serait ainsi le centre de la pigmentation.

Ce pigment s'amoncelle dans les tissus en voie d'histolyse; sa production est extraordinairement accentuée pendant la métamorphose. Tout le pigment aurait d'après *Bataillon* la même origine chromatique nucléaire chez les Batraciens; des cellules amiboïdes, s'emparant des granules de pigment deviendraient des cellules pigmentaires.

La participation de la chromatine du noyau à la formation du pigment a été plus récemment soutenue par *Bohn* [2], qui attribue à ce fait une grande importance théorique.

On a même décrit du pigment dans le noyau, contrairement à *Ehrmann* qui affirmait que le noyau de certaines cellules n'en contenait jamais. *Leydig* signala ce fait dans les cellules pigmentaires du *Rhodeus amarus*; *Maurer* dit en avoir vu dans l'intérieur du noyau des cellules épidermiques superficielles du *Pleurodeles*, et le considère comme un produit de dégénérescence. *Ajello* en décrit dans les cellules hépatiques et rénales du Lapin empoisonné par le phosphore, l'arsénic, le bismuth, le sublimé, etc.

Rosenstadt aurait rencontré du pigment dans le noyau des cellules de la membrane clignotante de la Grenouille. On a fait une constatation semblable dans des cellules des mélanosarcomes (*Lukjanow, Steinhaus*).

Mais ce petit nombre de faits isolés ne mène à aucune conclusion relativement à l'origine nucléaire du pigment, car on pourrait aussi bien admettre son passage du noyau dans le cytoplasma que l'hypothèse inverse; ou bien il s'agit tout simplement d'une dégénérescence pigmentaire du noyau se produisant rarement dans des conditions particulières.

Tout ce que nous venons de dire relativement à l'origine et au

---

[1] E. *Bataillon* — Recherches anatomiques et expérimentales sur les métamorphoses des Batraciens anoures — Thèse de la Faculté des Sciences, Paris, 1891.
[2] G. *Bohn* — L'évolution du pigment — Paris, 1901.

mode de formation des pigments se rapporte essentiellement aux
mélanines. Pour ce qui concerne les lipochromes, la question n'a
jamais donné lieu à tant de discussions, du moins ceux des Vertébrés. Les auteurs qui s'en sont occupés les regardent comme étant
soit des matériaux de réserve soit des produits de déchet élaborés
dans le protoplasma cellulaire. Comme étant probablement des substances de réserve doit-on considérer les lipochromes des œufs,
des corps jaunes, des glandes surrénales et des amas graisseux,
tels que le corps adipeux des Amphibiens et l'organe de l'hiber-
nation des Mammifères hibernants.

Le pigment jaune des cellules nerveuses représente vraisemblablement un produit de dégénérescence de certaines parties du
cytoplasma, peut-être des éléments chromophiles.

Les lipochromes semblent, du moins dans certains cas, pouvoir se transformer en mélanines, qui en seraient alors des dérivés azotés; c'est ce qui paraît résulter de quelques travaux récents, tels que ceux de *Loisel* (1), de *Vörmer* (2), etc.

Ces recherches méritent d'être poursuivies et leurs résultats
ont besoin d'être confirmés avant d'être acceptés définitivement.

Quant aux causes qui dans les conditions physiologiques dé-
terminent la formation des pigments, elles sont très nombreuses;
signalons, comme en étant les plus fréquentes, la lumière, la chaleur, l'humidité, la nourriture, les excitations de toutes sortes, etc.,
dont l'influence sur la pigmentation est connue depuis longtemps et
a été démontrée par une foule d'observations. Nous ne pouvons
pas examiner en détail la façon dont ces différents facteurs agis-
sent en produisant ou en faisant varier la pigmentation des tissus, car une telle étude nous ferait sortir des limites que nous
avons imposée à ce rapport, dans lequel nous nous sommes proposé de résumer en un tableau d'ensemble ce qui concerne les
pigments cellulaires des Vertébrés en nous plaçant à un point de
vue purement anatomique.

---

(1) G. Loisel — Les pigments élaborés par les femelles — C. R. de la Soc. de Biol., 1904.
(2) Vörmer — Loc. cit.

PREMIER — CLASSIFICATION, ORIGINE ET ROLE PROBABLE DES LEUCOCYTES, MASTZELLEN ET PLASMAZELLEN

Par M. le Dr. G. LOVELL GULLAND
M. A., B. Sc., M. D., F. R. C. P. E

*Physician to the Children and Royal Victoria Hospitals, Assistant Physician
to the Royal Infirmary, Edinburgh*

I — VARIETIES OF LEUCOCYTES

It is impossible in the space at my disposal even to enumerate, much less to summarise, the literature which has appeared in recent years with regard to the varieties of leucocytes. I shall best serve the purpose of this report if I shortly recapitulate the points upon which all observers are agreed, and then discuss more fully those other matters about which there is as yet want of agreement.

There is now an almost complete consensus of opinion that there are at least four different series of leucocytes, and possibly a larger number. Ehrlich's classification of the granules still holds good to a very great extent, and Wolff's discovery of the azurophil granules in lymphocytes has given a fresh importance to Ehrlich's original views.

The two series of leucocytes about which there is least difficulty are 1. the eosinophil, or coarsely granular oxyphil, leucocytes and 2. the neutrophil, or finely granular oxyphil, cells. These are now known to start as leucocytes of the myelocyte form, that is cells generally of large size with a rounded pale staining nucleus and granules of the typical character in the cell body. In both these series the myelocytes are found normally only in the bone marrow, and perhaps in the case of the eosinophils to a certain extent in connective tissue, thymus, lymphatic glands and elsewhere, though it is doubtful whether they multiply in these situations to any very great extent. In pathological conditions myelocytes of both types may be found, not only in the marrow but in all the hæmopoietic organs, including the liver. This myelocyte form divides by mitosis; the resulting cell is rather smaller than the mother myelocyte but otherwise similar in character. It grows by enlargement both of the nucleus and of the cell body.

and its nucleus may remain rounded, especially in cases where the cell finds rapidly increases in size, or may become indented, kidney-shaped, and ultimately horse-shoe-shaped, and even ring shaped, though the last two forms are more characteristic of the neutrophil series than of the eosinophil. Most of the ripe eosinophils have a nucleus, in shape very like a pair of spectacles and only rarely does the nucleus assume a more polymorphous character. On the other hand, the nucleus of the neutrophil cell may, as is well known, assume almost any shape, and it has moreover a tendency to be made up of knobs of chromatin joined together by narrow bridges. I would remark, however, that our ordinary methods of film preparation make the narrowness rather more marked than it should be. Wet preparations made by my sublimate-alcohol-ether method, or in other ways, show a much more compact nucleus, as a rule, with thicker bridges between the knobs.

I have elsewhere shown in detail that this progression from the rounded form to the polymorphous nucleus is in full accordance with M. Heidenhain's [1] law as to the relative behaviour of nucleus and centrosomes in leucocytes and free cells generally. His conclusions, which I have amply confirmed and verified [2], are that the cytoplasm consists of a ground substance in which are embodied radii which have their centre in the centrosomes, astrosphere or attraction sphere. When the cell is in a state of rest the pull of these radii tends to bring the astrosphere to the centre of the cell. The usual obstacle is the nucleus, and in cells with a small amount of cytoplasm, for example the small myelocytes resulting from mitosis, the pull is not strong enough to bring this about. As the cytoplasm increases in amount, the pull becomes stronger and the nucleus is pushed to one side of the cell and ultimately deformed, becoming first oval and eccentric, then kidney-shaped and finally horse-shoe-shaped. At this stage the astrosphere comes to rest in the centre of the cell. These forms are quite commonly seen in every marrow. In some cells the cytoplasm grows out of proportion to the nucleus, and the astrosphere thus reaches the centre of the cell without causing any nuclear deformation. Many of the large myelocytes have this shape.

[1] M. Heidenhain, Arch. f. mikr. Anat. Vol. 43, 1894.
[2] Quart. Journ. of Physiol. 1895.

We have been accustomed to consider that after a cell with
a horse-shoe-shaped, or ring-shaped, nucleus begins to move, the
nucleus moves with it and may be secondarily deformed, and the
more amoeboid the cell the greater is the deformation likely to be.
For this reason the nuclei of the neutrophil polymorphous form
were supposed to be so much more deformed than those of the
eosinophil polymorphous form, because they are more actively
amoeboid. But a very acute paper by Pappenheim (¹) puts this
process in another light and gives a much better explanation. He
points out that polymorphism of the nucleus is not an expression
of the power of locomotion, nor of active kinetic locomotion, as
on the one hand mononuclear cells may also be amoeboid and
remain mononuclear during that process. Such cells are the mast-
cells of connective tissue, the primary wandering cells, the small
lymphocytes of the blood and others. On the other hand, polymorphous nuclei remain polymorphous when the cell is entirely
at rest, as in the ordinary neutrophils. The myelocytes are also
mobile, but the changes in the nucleus produced during their
movements are quite different from polymorphous nuclei. Polymorphism is really an internal plastic process, the expression of a
change in the internal structure of the cell, and really a process
of ripening. He agrees with the observations of M. Heidenhain,
which I have already cited. I would be inclined to go a step further and to consider that the nucleus becomes polymorphous in
order that the cell may become more actively amoeboid. There is
ample evidence that the power of amoeboid movement lies in the
cytoplasm, and that the nucleus is passive, and indeed except for
its relation to the life of the cell, rather a hindrance to movement. Therefore the more the nucleus is broken up into lobes with
narrow bridges between them, the easier will it be for the cytoplasm to drag it through narrow openings.

Pappenheim also considers that these changes of plastic ripening cannot be turned back, and that though in suppuration and,
for instance, in sputum, one often finds mononuclear neutrophil and
eosinophil forms, these are easily distinguishable from normal
mononuclear forms or myelocytes.

In these two granular series it is to be noted that only the
final polymorphonuclear forms are to be found in the blood in

---

(¹) Pappenheim. Folia Haem. 1907.

normal conditions. All the precursors of that stage are found normally only in the marrow, with the possible exceptions in the case of the eosinophils already noted. It is now fully agreed that a demand for polymorphs of either of these series in the blood or in the tissues results in an increase in the number of myelocyte forms in the marrow, and if the demand for cells is sufficiently great, results in an increase in the amount of functional marrow. Muir's [1] researches, in particular, in regard to the neutrophils, and those of others in regard to the eosinophils may be quoted with regard to this point.

With regard to the basophil series the evidence is not quite so complete. These forms are very scanty in either normal or pathological blood, with the single exception of splenomedullary leukaemia and a few other conditions in which experimentally it has been shown that they can be increased.

The form occurring in the blood is a polymorphonuclear one whose nucleus has very much the shape of that of the neutrophil polymorph, but is invariably very faintly stained. The granules are, of course, basophil and metachromatic and vary considerably in size and in the number which are present in each cell. Normally these cells number only about 5 % of leucocytes, and even in leukaemia they hardly ever rise above 5, or at the outside 10 %. Their myelocyte form is scanty in the bone marrow, but presents exactly similar characteristics to those already described in the other series, with the exception that it shows basophil granules instead of the other. These granules differ more in size than do those of the neutrophil myelocytes, but do not vary so much as in the polymorpho-nuclear basophil form. These basophil myelocytes occur with fair frequency in the blood in leukaemia, as Scott [2] has recently again demonstrated.

It is very difficult to know just what is the relation of this basophil series to the mast-cells of connective tissue, but I prefer to leave the consideration of this question until the relation between blood cells and connective tissue cells comes to be discussed.

Of late years an enormous amount of work has been done in regard to the relationship of the so-called hyaline cells to one

---

[1] Muir, Journ. of Path. & Bacter, and Trans. Path. Soc. London, Vol. 5?, 1902.
[2] Scott, Journ. of Path. and Bacter. 1906.

another and to the other blood cells, and so many are the views which have been expressed that it is impossible to take them all up, and I propose simply to relate the conclusions to which I have myself come, and to point out their difference from those of some other observers.

I regard the whole of the hyaline series—large lymphocytes, small lymphocytes, large mononuclears, and so-called transitionals as belonging to one large class which may be called lymphocytes, lymphoid cells or lymphoidocytes as may hereafter be found most desirable. The reasons on which I base this view are as follows:

1. Since Wolff discovered the azurophil granules in lymphocytes, I have made countless observations on their incidence in normal and abnormal conditions and I have found them in every form of the cells under discussion from the smallest lymphocyte to the largest mononuclears and transitionals and sometimes as numerous in the former as in the latter. The ordinary dry method is not altogether satisfactory for showing them, because as has been shown, they are probably to a certain extent soluble in water and they always shrink considerably in dry films. The method which I have found most satisfactory for demonstrating them is to drop a film of blood on a cover glass, before it is dry, into a weak solution of Wright's stain in methyl alcohol, and to leave the cover glass there for any length of time up to half an hour; then remove the cover glass, allow it to dry, and mount in balsam. If the stain is sufficiently diluted with methyl alcohol there is no precipitate on the surface of the film and the granules are exceedingly well brought out and are found to be larger, to be more numerous in the cells, and to be found in a larger proportion of cells than in dry films.

Pappenheim believes that these granules are not homologous with the granules of the neutrophil and eosinophil series, but that they are in some way a secretion product, and that they are contained in the meshes of the reticulum. It is extremely difficult to be sure whether this is the case or not, for a preparation which shows the granules well, never shows the reticulum of the cytoplasm satisfactorily. Wright's stain, or any of the stains which contain azur, do not bring out the reticulum nearly so satisfactorily as Jenner's stain does, but I have sometimes seen appearances which made me think that these granules, like those of the other series, are situated at nodal points on the reticulum. Further, I have often observed them in the small pseudo-podia which are thrown out by the small and large lymphocytes in blood. This is presumably more likely to occur if they are integral parts of the reticulum than if they are secretion granules.

2. Schridde [1] has devised a new method by which another series of granules are brought out in lymphocytes. He fixes in formol-Müller-osmium and stains with anilin water and acid fuchsin. With this method the eosinophil granules are dark red, the neutrophil a pale bluish red, and those of the lymphocytes a yellowish crimson. They are obviously not the same granules as those which are stained with azur as they are in the shape of thick rods, lie close to the nucleus and are midway in size between the granules of the two other series. It will of course be obvious from the nature of the stain that these granules must be faintly oxyphil. These granules are found in all the varieties of lymphocytes.

3. It has now been definitely shown that all these cells down to the smallest lymphocytes are capable of movement, though it is, of course, the larger cells of the class which move more actively by reason of their large amount of cytoplasm.

4. The cytoplasm of all these cells is basophil—intensely so in the smaller members of the series, less so in the larger. At Oxford in 1904 [2] I went very minutely into this point and showed that the reason for this difference between the large and small cells is that the strands of the reticulum are not only thicker, but much more tightly packed together in the small and large lymphocytes than in the mononuclears and transitionals, but that every gradation could be found between the terminal members of the series in this respect, and that it was quite common to find great variation in the character of the reticulum in different parts of the same cell, especially frequently in the cells which stand intermediate between the large lymphocyte and the large mononuclear.

5. Every trasition can be found between the round nucleus of the large lymphocyte and the most polymorphous nucleus of the transitional, and it will be found that the nucleus passes through exactly the same series of changes that has already been described in discussing the eosinophil and the neutrophil series, and the relation between the nucleus and the astrosphere is as

[1] Schridde, Zentral. f. Physiol. Vol. 19, 1905.
[2] Gulland, Brit. med. Journ. Sept. 1904.

constant as in them. The fact that the nucleus does not advance further in polymorphism is probably associated with the fact that these cells are not so amœboid as the members of the neutrophil series. I have never seen anything whatever which would lead me to suppose that there was any relation between the so-called transitionals and the polymorphonuclear neutrophils.

6. The difference in size in the cells is of course of no importance. It seems to me that the increase in size in the large mononuclears and transitionals is due largely to the taking up of fluid, as the strands of the reticulum are often widely separated and these cells are obviously soft as may be seen by the way in which they are indented in films by the red corpuscles. Many of the degenerated lymphocytes in films have the appearance of mononuclears and transitionals. It is, of course, quite well known that both these larger members of the series are found in lymph glands and also in lymph from the thoracic duct and large lymph vessels.

Beattie ([6]), among others, has observed many transitional forms between the different members of the series. Houston ([7]) believes that in normal blood it is fairly easy to distinguish between the different forms, but that this is not the case in some pathological conditions.

We are on more difficult ground when we attempt to trace exactly the relationship between the different members of the series, because this has lately been the subject of a heated discussion between Türk and Pappenheim ([8]). Pappenheim, as is well known, regards the large lymphocyte as the mother cell which produces all other forms — red corpuscles, the cells of the granular series, and the different forms of lymphoid cell; and he regards the small lymphocyte as being older than the large cell and a riper form. This is, of course, absolutely correct as regards the reproductive history of the cells, because there is no doubt that small lymphocytes are always produced by the mitotic division of the large forms, and this occurs in lymphatic tissue throughout the body and in marrow. But he appears to consider that the small lymphocytes, when they are once formed, are not capable of further development, but that they become destroyed in blood or tissue

([6]) Beattie, Brit. Med. Journ., Sept. 1914.
([7]) Houston, Brit. Med. Journ., Sept. 1910.
([8]) Folia Hæmat., 1908.

in the same way that polymorphs are. This conclusion I am very
unwilling to accept, for both in normal and pathological bloods and
in lymphatic tissue everywhere, one finds countless cells which
it is impossible to place with certainty in one or the other cate-
gory, and it is difficult to see whence they are derived unless it
is from the growth of small lymphocytes, and their conversion
into larger cells. He cites in support of his view the analogue of
the transformation of large megaloblasts into small normoblasts,
but this is really beside the mark, because the ultimate end of the
red cell is a non-nucleated non-amoeboid corpuscle which has
ceased to be a cell, and this cannot be said of the lymphocyte in
which, when degeneration does take place, the nucleus is the last
part to disappear.

It seems to me much more probable that the ranks of the
large lymphocytes are reinforced from their smaller congeners,
and that thus development from the large lymphocyte may take
place along two lines, ending in the one case in a large mononuclear, and in the other in the so-called transitionals. In the
former instance the protoplasm increases in amount more rapidly
than the nucleus does; the strands of the cytoplasm are much
more widely separated and from the large size of the cell the
astrosphere is able to lie in its centre without deforming the nucleus to any great extent. In the other case the nucleus increases
in size more rapidly than the cell body and in accordance with
Heidenhain's law becomes first indented, then horse-shoe-shaped,
and ultimately assumes the more markedly polymorphous forms
which are found in the transitionals of the blood.

That is to say that the large mononuclears are homologous
with the largest myelocytes of the neutrophil and the eosinophil
series, and the transitionals are homologous with the polymorphonuclear members of the two series.

I should not like it to be understood that these two sub-
series of lymphocytes are strictly separate from one another. It
seems to me that within different series change of circumstances
may result in alteration of the relations between nucleus and cell
body, and that therefore a large mononuclear may conceivably be
transformed into a transitional, and possibly the converse may
also hold. I have already noted, however, that many of the most
degenerated lymphocytes seem to be mononuclears and transitionals.

It is very difficult to find any terms which can be used in

stead of the objectionable terms «large mononuclear» and «transitional». Pappenheim's proposal of «Splenocyte» is unsatisfactory for many reasons. In the first place because there is no evidence whatever that these cells are formed specially in the spleen. In fact, our researches on that organ [1] went to show that the lymphocytes which are formed in the spleen are retained entirely or almost entirely in the organ and do not pass into the blood at all. And, in the second place, there are many observations on record where the numbers of these cells in the blood remained unchanged after splenectomy. For example, Houston [2] quotes a case of splenectomy where the proportion of large mononuclears was very distinctly increased, and Crescenzi's [3] observations go to show the same thing. I would submit that this is one of the points which may well be discussed by the Congress.

II. — RELATION BETWEEN BLOOD LEUCOCYTES AND CONNECTIVE TISSUE LEUCOCYTES

It seems to me that the proper way to approach the question of the relation between blood leucocytes and the so-called plasma cells, and eosinophil and basophil cells which are found in connective tissue, is not to attempt to investigate them from the side of inflammation, in which of necessity the conditions are obscured by the degeneration of cells and regeneration of fibrous tissue, but to look at the question rather from the broader phylogenetic point of view.

It is of course a commonplace that the lymphocytes are the least differentiated of the leucocytes, that they are found in many forms of lower animals where the cells of the granular series do not occur at all, and that they are the first cells to appear in the mammalian embryo (Browning [4] and others). They are moreover the most ubiquitous of the leucocytes. They are found in all parts of the ordinary lymphatic apparatus, in the blood and in the bone marrow, and in all these situations all the forms which I regard as belonging to the lymphocyte series may be found — some preponderating in one situation, some in another. They are definitely

[1] Paton, Garland and Fowler, Journ. of Physiol., 1903.
[2] Houston, Brit. Med. Journ., Sept. 1904.
[3] Crescenzi, Lo Sperimentale, 1904.
[4] Browning, Journ. of Path. & Bacter., 1905.

amœboid and they move from place to place even though their movement be comparatively slow. It is further known that, in addition to the ordinary lymphatic tissues and that of the alimentary and respiratory tracts, there are numerous small lymphomata situated round arteries and in various other positions, and it is also known that at need fresh lymphatic glands may arise, either out of these smaller lymphomata or, apparently, without their presence.

Schridde [1] has shown that his oxyphil granules are present in plasma-cells as well as in ordinary lymphocytes. Therefore I should regard all the ordinary plasma-cells as lymphocytes which are normally present in connective tissue wherever it is situated, and which ultimately are to be traced back to blood lymphocytes; though in all probability, one would have to go back many generations to trace the relationship. That is to say, lymphocytes are ubiquitous throughout the body because of their comparatively undifferentiated and phylogenetically primitive character. When inflammation takes place it depends, of course, largely on its type whether the neutrophils appear in the neighbourhood or not. In acute bacterial infections they of course do so, but in some chronic conditions they may be supplied in small numbers or not at all. The source of the lymphocytes which appear in inflammatory conditions may be partly from the blood, partly from all such lymphocytes or plasma-cells as are to be found within a reasonable radius from the source of irritation.

There seems to me to be no necessity to call in the assistance of endothelial cells to add to the supply. It is well known that these cells may act as phagocytes, and that they may on occasion become cubical or even cylindrical in character, and that they may possibly be cast off. I have never had any difficulty in distinguishing these cells from tissue lymphocytes and it is probable that the cast off cells rapidly degenerate. I have had very many opportunities of examining such cells in pleural effusions and in that situation, where the problem is not complicated by other factors, there is no difficulty whatever in distinguishing between the two kinds of cell.

To quote Muir: [2] «The spherical form and phagocytic function represent very primitive properties in the process of evolution and

---

[1] Schridde, Anat. Hefte, 1905.
[2] Muir, Brit. Med. Journ. Sept. 1904.

hence it is not surprising that cells of different classes should revert to a former state existing before specialization and differentiation occurred. Some have endeavoured to make a point of the mitotic figures which are often to be seen in endothelial cells in the neighbourhood of inflammation, and have suggested that these result in the formation of plasmacells or tissue lymphocytes, but it seems to me much more probable that these cells are an important source of fibroblasts which have nothing to do with the lymphocytes and have a different function.

I suggested some time ago that the collections of lymphocytes round the respiratory and alimentary tracts may have to do with the fact that these cavities are inhabited normally by attenuated and non-virulent organisms and that possibly the lymphocytes are adapted and sufficient to keep these in check, and that their relatively small percentage in the blood is due to the fact that they do multiply so easily in connective tissue so that the blood protection can easily be reinforced from that source.

The series which is phylogenetically next in age to the lymphocytes is the eosinophil series, and one finds that these cells appear in many cold-blooded animals and that they occur in mammalian embryos at a date not very much later than the lymphocytes, but long before the neutrophil series. These also are cells which are not adapted to meet acute infections. They seem to have a special relation to the toxins of parasites such as filaria, trichina, and many others, and possibly also to metabolic poisons such as that concerned in the production of some forms of asthma. They are not quite so ubiquitous as the lymphocytes, but they are certainly found with great frequency in connective tissue without any very evident reason for their presence, and it seems probable that they may multiply in these situations, from the fact that myelocyte forms are often found. They are probably produced mainly in the bone marrow, because it has been shown that in cases where there is a marked blood eosinophilia the number of myelocyte forms in the marrow is very greatly increased; but they seem capable of considerable adaptation to other conditions and in cases where the marrow is rendered unsuitable for their proliferation, as in some lymphatic leukaemias, they are found in numbers in the spleen, liver and elsewhere—sometimes in company with neutrophil myelocytes, but much more frequently, and apparently earlier, without them.

With the neutrophils the case is very different. These are

cells which in one or other of their forms—because of course their actual form varies greatly in different animals, and perhaps in talking of the mammalia generally, it would be better to use the term *oxyphil*, rather than neutrophil—are confined to warm blooded animals.

Muir has pointed out that this is due to the fact that organisms multiply much more rapidly in the tissues of warm blooded animals than they do in the tissues of cold blooded animals, and that therefore this special class of cells has been differentiated to defend the body against them, and that the phenomena of leucocytosis in warm blooded animals and the exceeding rapidity of its occurrence has to do with their urgent need of protection. Neutrophil cells are not found in the tissues under normal conditions. They appear there only in response to chemotactic stimuli and either perish there or return to the blood when the need for them is past. These cells are produced only from the neutrophil myelocytes in the marrow and even under very markedly pathological condition it is rare, except in splenomedullary leukæmia, to find them in the spleen and liver.

It is exceedingly difficult, however, to know just what should be said about the relation between the basophil cells of blood and those of connective tissue—partly because of their rarity in the blood, and partly because in connective tissue they assume so many different forms in different animals, while on the other hand, in those animals in which basophil cells appear in the blood, the blood cells are almost always closely similar.

A good many years ago I examined the connective tissue in a great many animals with a view to investigating these cells and found all gradations from the small, almost lymphocyte-like cells in the rabbit, to the huge mast-cells of the rat and others. Further, these cells differ immensely from one another in the shape of their cell body and in the staining of their granules. (In some the metachromasia is very much more marked than in others). There is no doubt that the mast-cells of connective tissue are amoeboid, and therefore *a priori* they must be related to leucocytes; but it seems to me that they are leucocyte forms which are apparently differentiated from residence in connective tissue, and it may possibly be the case that the comparatively few basophils which are to be found in the bone marrow and in the blood are really «escapes» from these connective tissue cells, and that these blood cells have become altered by their change of habitat. Some change there certainly must be because the myelocyte forms which are found in marrow are different, not only as regards their shape, but as regards the metachromasia of their granules from the myelocyte forms which one sees in the connective tissue of lymph glands, for instance. In the marrow cells the granules are small, different in size and are often scattered somewhat scantily in the cell body. In the myelocyte in lymph glands, on the other hand, the granules are large and densely packed. Of course another explanation is that the two really represent totally different cells which have nothing in common but the basophilia of their granules. They seem to be associated with inflammatory conditions, especially of a chronic kind, but their exact relation to these processes has not yet been made out.

These basophil cells are always scanty in the blood except in splenomedullary leukaemia, and Pappenheim declares that a very large proportion, if not all, of the basophils found in leukaemias are lymphocytes which have undergone a mucinoid degeneration. His own observations, however, with regard to the basophil leucocytosis produced by phrynotoxin [1] might have led him to another view.

To sum up. Lymphocytes of the blood, marrow, and tissues are members of one series of closely related and interchangeable cells which represent the primitive wandering cells and which occur everywhere throughout the body. Eosinophils, though less widely distributed, have a great power of adapting themselves to many conditions throughout the body, due to the fact that they also are comparatively undifferentiated. Neutrophil cells are essentially connected with the resistance to infection in warm blooded animals and are therefore confined to the marrow and blood, and do not appear in connective tissue unless called there by chemiotaxis. We have not yet sufficient information to dogmatise about the relationships or function of the basophil or mast-cells.

III. — The relation of leucocyte forms to one another.

From what has just been said with regard to the ancestral character of the lymphocyte and from all that is known of its history, it is obvious that it is the primary form of all leucocytes.

[1] Pappenheim : Folia Haem., 1906, 12.

so far at least as embryonic life is concerned. An immense amount of discussion has raged over the question as to whether the same can be said of lymphocytes in post-embryonic life — whether they form an absolutely independent series, or whether the other series spring from them. From everything that is known with regard to the facts of chemiotaxis and leucocyte response, I think one must conclude that for practical purposes, the different series are kept apart in adult life. Under ordinary conditions certainly mitotic reproduction of myelocyte forms is quite sufficient to supply ordinary needs.

Much has been written about the occurrence of eosinophil and neutrophil myelocytes with basophil cytoplasm and these have constantly been quoted as transitions from lymphocytes to the other forms. I think it would be impossible for us to deny the possibility of such a thing occurring. What has happened in embryonic life may, under certain conditions, occur again. The existence of pernicious anaemia is a sufficient answer to the objections to this view, but it must also be remembered that in judging of the nature of these cells, all young cells tend to have basophil cytoplasm and these forms may be simply freshly formed myelocytes.

IV.—THE RELATION OF LEUCOCYTES TO RED CORPUSCLES

If one goes far enough back in embryonic life, one reaches a stage at which there are no true leucocytes and no true nucleated reds but only undifferentiated cells which may become either one or the other, and in this sense it is possible to say that leucocytes and red cells start from a common origin. One set of these cells acquire or manufacture haemoglobin in their cytoplasm and become the megaloblastic precursors of ordinary red cells; the other set do not come to contain haemoglobin and become the precursors of the leucocytes (cf. Bryce [1]). The former cells multiply in mammalian embryos with extraordinary rapidity, while the latter remain almost stationary in number for a long period. It is thus easy to find stages in development at which the nucleated red cells outnumber the leucocytes in the embryonic body by thousands to one, and where the red cells are actively

---

(1) Bryce, Trans. Roy. Soc. Edinb. 1905.

dividing, while the leucocytes are not observed to be doing so. It would seem absurd at such a stage to talk of the derivation of red cells from leucocytes, and if this is the case at so early a stage of development, when both sets of cells are comparatively undifferentiated, it would seem still more idle to suppose that in adult life there can be relationship between the two. No author has attempted to connect any series of leucocytes with red cells other than the lymphocyte, and Pappenheim is at the present day the principal upholder of the view that the megaloblast or large nucleated red is derived from the large lymphocyte found in the marrow. As I understand him, his grounds for this view (¹) are that the cytoplasm of both sets of cells is basophil, that Saxer in embryonic lymph-glands and Bonnet-Grimberg in lymph-glands in anaemic states found that nucleated reds were formed from large lymphocytes, that in spleen in amphibia, and in the human subject in intoxications and in various forms of anaemia and leukaemia erythroblasts are produced. Pappenheim considers that in these cases the glands and spleen are subjected to a functional stimulus or a myeloid metaplasia which causes the large lymphocytes to resume an embryonic function which had fallen out of use. This hypothesis is brought forward in order to meet Türk's objection that red corpuscles are not normally produced in lymph-glands from large lymphocytes. I would point out, however, with regard to the various points mentioned, that all young cells tend to be basophil, erythroblasts among the rest, and that there is a long distance to travel from the lymphocyte to the megaloblast judging by microscopic appearances alone. In the former the nucleus contains one or more large nucleoli and widely spaced chromatin network, the cytoplasm is markedly reticular and intensely basophil, and centrosomes can in most examples be seen in the resting condition in favourably placed cells. In the latter the chromatin of the nucleus is closely woven, and does not contain nucleoli of the type seen in the lymphocytes; though the cytoplasm is basophil, it is not reticular but homogeneous, and to my eye at least there is never any difficulty in distinguishing it by the tone of colour alone from that of the lymphocyte, while it is always much greater in amount relatively to the nucleus than that of the cell which Pappenheim calls the large lymphocyte;

---

¹ Pappenheim, Folia Haem. vol. iv.

the centrosomes are not visible in nucleated reds in the resting condition.

As regards the lymph glands and spleen, in my own studies on developing lymph-glands [1] I never came across any appearance which even suggested the development of nucleated reds from lymphocytes, and on that and all the other conditions which Pappenheim cites there is the fallacy that nucleated reds are present in the blood and may therefore easily appear from that source in the spleen and in the capillaries of lymph-glands. I am fresh from a minute and prolonged study of all the organs in a large series of cases of pernicious anaemia [2] and leukaemia (about to appear in *Journal of Pathology*) and in no case and in no organ have I found evidence that red cells were being formed from leucocytes. One fails indeed to see why they should be supposed to be so formed. If you grant that erythroblasts can and do multiply by mitosis, which nobody doubts, and if they have a suitable locus for development as they have in the bone marrow, there is no reason whatever to suppose that their activities require to be reinforced by the lymphocytes under ordinary conditions. The conditions in lymphatic leukaemia alone might be cited as a sufficient argument against Pappenheim's view. I have gone over many marrows in this condition in acute cases in which the red count had fallen steadily as the white count rose. These marrows had undoubtedly been subjected to the functional stimulus of which Pappenheim speaks and were full of large lymphocytes, but I had often to search long and carefully before I could find a nucleated red of any kind. The lymph-glands in these cases were either normal or infiltrated with lymphocytes, but contained no nucleated reds outside the blood vessels. Surely in these cases where the patients were dying of anaemia, if in any, the hypothetical transformation of lymphocytes into erythroblasts ought to have been going on? But I could never see the slightest evidence of it, indeed the lymphocytes were often much too busily employed in devouring red cells to have any time to spare for the making of them!

Pappenheim raises one point, however, which is difficult to meet. He recalls Neumann's observations on the formation of bone with marrow spaces containing erythroblasts in the senile ossi-

[1] Galland, Journ. of Path. and Bacter. 1891.
[2] Galland and Goodall, Journ. of Path. and Bacter. 1905.

fication of the cartilages of the larynx, and declares that in such situations the erythroblasts must arise *de novo*, as there are more in the circulating blood. He considers of course that they arise from large lymphocytes. I am not prepared, however, to grant that this is the only possible explanation. We know practically nothing of the mechanism by which nucleated reds are prevented from appearing in the general circulation, and it seems to me possible that in some unknown way they may be drawn into the circulation under special circumstances—such as the formation of new bone. I have been much struck of late with the comparative frequency with which nucleated reds do appear in the blood without special anæmia or other marked call upon them. One case in particular I may cite: a tubercular pericarditis in an adult in which the red count was 5,200,000 per cmm. haemoglobin 102 p. c. The red corpuscles showed no change of importance, and yet the nucleated reds were sufficiently numerous to be demonstrated with ease in each film to a large class of students, and many of these erythroblasts had not pyknotic nuclei, but showed the active type. The marrow showed no increase in erythroblasts beyond the normal. Other similar cases that I have seen make me believe that if we looked for them, we should find nucleated reds in the blood more often than we do.

V.—SPECIAL POINTS

There are certain points which must be dealt with as regards the behaviour of different classes of leucocytes. *First* the much vexed question of the *source of the lymphocytes in the blood.* I have been led to take an interest in this from the experiments which I have made with other observers as regards digestion leucocytosis [1]. In animals we found that the rise was due largely to an increase in lymphocytes which was constant, and to a rise also in the polynuclears which was not so constant but might reach a higher figure. We succeeded in eliminating the intestinal mucous membrane, the spleen and the mesenteric glands as causes of this increase, and Goodall and Paton [2] have since shown that the source of these lymphocytes is the bone marrow. Their experiments prove that the actual number of lymphocytes passing

[illegible footnote citation]

into the blood from the thoracic duct is comparatively small — much smaller than one would have expected; and that it in no way accounted for the very great increase of lymphocytes in the blood. On the other hand, the blood coming from the marrow was shown to be very much richer in lymphocytes and in polymorphs during digestion.

Many other observations are now on record which go to prove that the thoracic duct is not an important source of lymphocytes in the blood though of course it undoubtedly does carry a certain number thither. The experiments of Crescenzi ([1]) are of great value in this respect. After splenectomy and drainage of the thoracic duct, it was found that the lymphocytes dropped rapidly for the first day or so, as one often finds to be the case after an operative procedure in animals. But after one to four days the lymphocytes returned to the normal point or rose above it. Crescenzi considers that this is due to a direct passage of lymphocytes into the blood from the lymphatic tissue, because he found that the marrow histologically showed no compensatory proliferation and that there was no new formation of collateral lymph paths; but it seems to me that his experiments show that the marrow was in reality producing lymphocytes actively all the time, and of course no compensatory change was necessary.

The large mononuclears and transitionals showed no constant change after these operations. They were sometimes increased, sometimes diminished. Our own experiments on the function of the spleen showed pretty definitely that that organ was not an important source of lymphocytes and the experiments of Azzurini and Massart ([2]) have confirmed this.

Further, there is now no doubt whatever that a large number of lymphocytes are actually present in the marrow. The observations of Pappenheim, Price Jones ([3]), Longcope ([4]), and my own repeated observations have put this beyond doubt. Longcope found in the marrow, under normal conditions, 22 to 32 per cent of lymphocytes, while the myelocytes were from 55 to 60 per cent. Again there are certain diseases where there is a marked chemiotactic passage of lymphocytes into the blood from the marrow — in

([1]) Crescenzi, La sperimentale, 1904.
([2]) Azzurini and Massart, Lo Sperimentale, 1904.
([3]) Price Jones, Brit. Med. Journ. Feb. 1908.
([4]) Longcope, Centr. f. Bacter. u. Paras. 1905.

whooping cough and small-pox in particular, and possibly in typhoid also.

I have discussed this question very fully in a recent paper on lymphatic leukæmia. From what we now know of the amœboid powers of lymphocytes, it seems to me that Ehrlich's view of their passive appearance in the blood must be given up.

Second : Weidenreich (¹) has lately revived the old view that *the eosinophil granules are related to and derived from hæmoglobin* mostly because he had found eosinophils in hæmolymph glands where destruction of red corpuscles was going on. I had thought that this view was long since given up. Ascoli (²) has answered Weidenreich, and Pappenheim (³) has pointed out that eosinophils are found in lower animals which have no red corpuscles or haemoglobin-containing plasma. Further, the staining of eosinophil granules is not by any means identical with that of red corpuscles. It is only when eosin is used that the two really resemble one another, and with almost all the other acid stains there are great differences in tint. Red corpuscles, when they are destroyed, or possibly even in the healthy condition, are taken up by lymphocytes and by endothelial cells and not by eosinophils. Further, it is quite easy to lake red corpuscles without dissolving eosinophil granules.

Third. One of the most important pieces of work which has appeared in recent years with regard to neutrophil leucocytes is contained in the series of papers published by *Arneth* (⁴). His primary contention is that with regard to a number of infectious diseases and general conditions much more information can be got by observing the kind of neutrophil leucocyte which is in excess than from the total leucocyte count. He considers that the normal leucocyte count in a healthy man is about 6000 and regards everything over 8000 as a leucocytosis. In this I am inclined to agree with him. I think that the number of 7000 usually given is too high. I have repeatedly observed healthy people with 6000.

He divides the neutrophil leucocytes found in normal and

(¹) Weidenreich, Folia Haemat. 1904 and 1905 ?

(²) Ascoli, Folia Haemat. 1904.

(³) Pappenheim, Folia Haemat. 1905, 3

(⁴) Arneth, Die neutrophilen weissen Blutkörper bei Infektionskrankheiten, G. Fischer 1904
     Münch. med. Woch. 1904 n° 45
     Zeits. f. klin. Med. Vol. 54, 1904
     Arch. f. Gynäk. Vol. 54, 1904

abnormal blood into five classes, the essential principle of classification being the character of the nucleus. The first class consists of two sub-classes: (a) Leucocytes with a plump, rounded or slightly indented nucleus with few «chromatic bodies»—what are generally called myelocytes. (b) Of the same kind of leucocyte with a simple nucleus but with a deeper indentation. In normal blood these are few in number or are absent.

The second class consists of those leucocytes which have a nucleus consisting of two main masses, the arrangement of which may vary in different cases, and these he divides into three sub-classes according tho these slight differences. These are also very few in number in normal blood.

The third class consists of those cells with three lobes in the nucleus, again with three sub-classes, and these constitute the majority of the neutrophil cells in normal conditions, about 48 per cent.

The fourth class contains the cells with four lobes in the nucleus and numbers about 23 per cent; whilst the fifth with five lobes or more, numbers only four per cent.

Arneth finds that the individual differences in healthy people are comparatively slight, and that these percentages are fairly constant.

In pathological conditions the ripe cells, that is to say those in which the nucleus is most broken up, are the first to disappear from the blood, until in extreme cases they have disappeared almost entirely and only the young forms, that is to say those with simple nuclei, remain. He classes the possible changes which may take place in the number and variations of these cells under six heads:

    I. Hyperleucocytosis (a) Iso- (b) Anisohyperleucocytosis
    II. Normoleucocytosis (a) Iso- (b) Anisonormoleucocytosis
    III. Hypoleucocytosis (a) Iso- (b) Anisohypoleucocytosis.

An isoleucocytosis is the case where the proportions of the five classes mentioned above are not altered however much the total number of the leucocytes may be changed. The anisoleucocytoses include those cases where the proportions of the different classes are altered. The severest form which one can meet with in an infection is an anisohypoleucocytosis, that is, a diminution in the total number with alteration in the proportions of the different classes; next an anisonormoleucocytosis; then an anisohy-

perleucocytosis, whilst the most favorable condition that can be
met with in an infection is an isohyperleucocytosis — that is, a
condition where the number of leucocytes is increased and the
proportions of the different classes remain approximately as in
normal blood.

Arneth finds that the clinical course does not always exactly
match the blood change, as sometimes a severe blood change may
be present with slight symptoms, and conversely; and sometimes
also very severe changes disappear. But as a general rule he regards marked changes in the neutrophil picture as associated with
a severe clinical condition. Anisohypoleucocytosis is found in severe fatal pneumonias, is constant in typhoid and measles, and
frequent in varicella and mumps; also in severe blood poisonings,
septic diphtheria, miliary tuberculosis, in sepsis with organisms
in the blood, acute rheumatism, foudroyant appendicitis and in
smallpox in the initial and eruptive stages. Arneth believes that
the point in common in all these conditions is that the cause of
the disease is circulating in the blood and inducing a destruction
of the cells; whilst in cases where only the toxins circulate in the
blood, without the actual presence of organisms, hyperleucocyto-
sis occurs. The pushing of the blood picture to the left, as Arneth
phrases it, that is the appearance of the young forms of the first
and second class in the blood, Arneth explains by the destruction
of leucocytes by the organisms. The ripe cells of the three last
classes are the first to be destroyed, because they furnish the most
effective antitoxins. He points out also that normally there must
be a breaking down of ripe elements in the blood in order to form
defensive substances and possibly such other bodies as precipi-
tins. When the blood returns to normal after an infection, there
is often at first a pushing of the blood picture to the right, that
is to say there are more ripe neutrophils than normal; and then
again to the left, so that there may be a series of balancing movements before equilibrium is reached.

Since the publication of Arneth's first papers, he has repeated his observations in different conditions. He has experimented
on rabbits, and finds that their pseudoeosinophils do not react
to stimuli in quite the same way as neutrophils, but he gets the
same results as regards the shape of the nucleus. In cachectic
conditions such as cancer, he finds that there is no change in the
neutrophil picture peculiar to the cancer itself. The changes which
occur, and are thereafter often very marked, are due to such com-

plications as bacterial infection and so on, and he has worked out the changes in puerperal leucocytosis, in tuberculosis, both miliary and chronic, and in other conditions. According to him, the essential change in an infection is a primary leucolysis varying in amount according to the cause of the infection, its degree of severity and the resistance of the individual; and following this, a reaction and the sending out of, first of all, all available ripe forms, and when these are exhausted, of the younger forms to take their place. Of course the two conditions very often go on side by side; where the infection persists leucolysis goes on along with reaction, and the actual number of cells in the blood, and their variety, will depend on the relation between these two factors.

While there is very much in this that has long been known and has been put forward, especially perhaps by Muir, Arneth differs from all his predecessors on these lines by endeavouring to reduce the proportion of leucocytes to actual figures and by trying to draw conclusions from these. As might be expected, his observations have attracted very widespread interest, and a number of other papers confirmatory and condemnatory have appeared on the subject. Of the latter may be cited that of Hiller [1], who makes many objections to Arneth's observations, some of them accurate enough, but affecting trivial points such as the presence or absence of the chromatic bodies, which Hiller — and I agree with him — regards as artefacts. He does not, however, succeed in impugning, to my mind, Arneth's main propositions; indeed with these he declares himself very largely in agreement. Hiller is a scholar of Grawitz, and therefore regards as possible the transformation of small lymphocytes into neutrophils, which I entirely agree with Arneth in regarding as impossible. Grawitz is of course a pronounced unitarian, and therefore does not consider that the change in shape of the nucleus can be regarded as of much importance, and Hiller echoes this view.

Pappenheim has replied to Hiller's paper, but most of the points which he makes have already been discussed in regard to the question of change in shape of the nucleus, and need not here be reverted to. Arneth's [2] reply to Hiller mainly consists of a restatement of his views, and is of value inasmuch as in it be

<hr>

[1] Hiller, Folia Haem. 19?? ?
[2] Arneth, Folia Haem. 19?? ?

clears away several points, such as the size of the cell, the presence of chromatic bodies and so on, which had rather tended to obscure his first observations.

My own feeling is that Arneth has made out an excellent case and that his classification of the changes which occur in pathological conditions will probably stand, though it is quite likely that alterations may be made in detail, and that his proportions of neutrophils under normal conditions may be found to be too rigidly drawn; indeed some observers have already shown that this is the case. We have always been accustomed to regard the presence of myelocytes in infections as indicating a severe type, and Arneth's observations are really the application of this general rule, and the putting of it on a sound basis.

Fourth: Functions of Leucocytes. — Nothing very new has been made out with regard to these. Arneth's view that the neutrophils break down to form antitoxins is plausible, but there is no definite proof that they actually do this. Grawitz [6] and Askanazy [7] have recently discussed this subject. Grawitz expresses the view that leucocytes produce defensive substances to resist foreign bodies and bacteria, but that they also are concerned in absorption, transport, assimilation of fat, glycogen, iron and proteids and that they further produce ferments. Of these last Askanazy shows that they give rise to the fibrin ferment, and also to a diastatic and proteolytic ferment. This of course is all in addition to the well known glycogen reaction. The actual purpose of the glycogen which appears in the neutrophils in certain inflammatory conditions etc. is not yet definitely known. It appears certain however, that it is not a degenerative change, but is associated rather with protection. The glycogen seems to be taken up in the blood and carried to the point which is threatened by organisms and possibly may there serve to nourish fibroblasts and other young cells.

Nothing very special has been added to our knowledge of the glycogen reaction since I wrote on the subject in 1911 [8].

[6] Grawitz, [illegible].
[7] Askanazy, [illegible].
[8] Gulland, Proc. Med. [illegible].

CONTENTS

THÈME 7 — MÉTAMÉRISATION EMBRYONNAIRE ; SON IMPORTANCE AU POINT DE VUE DE L'ANATOMIE COMPARÉE

Par M. le Prof. LOUIS ROULE (Toulouse)

Cette question est très vaste ; elle met en cause toute l'embryologie. Aussi un rapport détaillé serait-il trop étendu. Même en limitant ce sujet aux Vertébrés, ainsi qu'il semble dans un Congrès de Médecine, ce rapport demanderait des pages nombreuses, et courrait pourtant le risque de se trouver incomplet. Ce sujet est traité, du reste, et de manière satisfaisante, dans les Revues annuelles, que tout morphologiste est habitué à manier. En conséquence, il suffit de mentionner ici les quatre points principaux, qui paraissent au rapporteur primer les autres, et sur lesquels une discussion pourra s'engager de façon utile. Le rapport, en un cas pareil, se doit borner à servir d'amorce et de guide à la discussion.

1. *De la valeur morphogénétique de la métamérisation embryonnaire.* — La métamérisation embryonnaire paraît équivaloir, dans l'ontogénèse, à une représentation phylogénétique, plus ou moins modifiée, de dispositions ancestrales caractérisées par une métamérisation très accentuée. Elle ne semble pas correspondre à une disposition de tectogénèse, qui, propre à l'embryon, serait privée de toute signification phylogénétique.

2. *De la valeur phylogénétique de la métamérisation embryonnaire des Vertébrés.* — La métamérisation embryonnaire des Vertébrés leur paraît propre, en raison de ses caractères spéciaux, relatifs à sa limitation à certaines parties du mésoblaste, d'autres

parties se trouvant exclues, ou se bornant à recevoir l'empreinte et l'impulsion venues des premières. Elle se rapproche, pourtant, de celle des Annélides, permettant ainsi de trouver quelque affinité entre les deux groupes. Les Vertébrés doivent se prendre ici comme joints étroitement aux *Prochordata* et *Archichordata*.

3. *De l'origine de la métamérisation des Vertébrés* — La musculature semble la première, dans la phylogenèse, comme dans l'ontogenèse, à subir la différenciation en métamères. Sans doute convient-il d'y reconnaître une liaison avec la forme allongée des Protovertébrés, et avec leur existence pélagique active. Les centres nerveux et les organes des sens ne viendraient ici qu'en seconde ligne.

4. *De l'évolution de la métamérisation chez les Vertébrés* — La métamérisation paraît s'être exercée sur le tronc d'abord, et n'avoir gagné l'extrémité antérieure du corps que par la suite. Ses effets se modifient, quant à la tectogenèse, suivant deux impulsions complémentaires: a) la céphalisation, coalescence qui aboutit à la délimitation d'une tête formée par l'union étroite de deux parties de provenances différentes (l'extrémité antérieure, les premiers segments du tronc); b) l'amplification prise par les membres pairs chez les Vertébrés supérieurs. C'est en cela notamment que l'embryologie vient en aide à l'anatomie comparée, en permettant de retrouver, sous une conformation unitaire d'apparence, les vestiges d'une structure métamérique plus profonde et plus ancienne.

THÈME 2 — DÉFINITION, STRUCTURE ET COMPOSITION DU PROTOPLASME

(Definition, Chemistry and Structure of Protoplasm)

Par M. le Prof. GUSTAV MANN

(M.D. Edinburgh, D.Sc. Oxon, Physiology of Laboratory, Oxford.)

HUGO V. MOHL [1] described in 1844 the «primordial utricle» as a membrane composed of a nitrogenous compound lying on the inner side of vegetable cell-membranes, and also stated that it occurred in the Conferva without a nucleus, and that it persisted in chlorophyll-containing cells after the nucleus had been absorbed. The observations no doubt led him to the theory expressed

---

[1] H. Von Mohl: Botanische Zeitung, 1844, pp. [illegible].

in 1846 [1] that «the semi-fluid, nitrogenous substance contained in the cell ... is the presence of the solid constituents found subsequently in a developing cell, and that it supplies the material for the formation of the nucleus and the primordial utricles. This physiological consideration led him to introduce the word protoplasma.

Protoplasm is therefore, according to v. Mohl's definition, the mother-substance of the cell membranes and of the nucleus. That this conception is diametrically opposite to the one held by me will be shown later, and will, I hope, excuse me for having included the nucleo-proteids in my discussion.

Before attempting to give a definition of the word protoplasma, it is my intention to outline in the first instance our chemical and physico-chemical knowledge regarding the units out of which we believe protoplasm to be built up [2].

In protoplasm we have certain organic units which have received a great deal of attention, and also inorganic constituents which are greatly neglected. However much from a purely chemical point of view the isolation of the organic constituents is desirable, we should never forget, as I pointed out in 1902 [3], «that so-called pure ash-free albumins (proteids) are chemically inert, and, in the true sense of the word, dead bodies.

For descriptive purposes Proteids (Protein-Substanzen; Substances albuminoïdes) may be divided into three groups.

1. **Albumins** which occur in nature as «native albumins». They include the «albuminoïds» substances which form the supporting or connective tissues of the animal body.

2. **Proteids proper**, which are combinations of the native albumins with such other organic compounds as sugars or radicals containing phosphorus or iron.

3. **Derivatives** of the natural albumins and proteids, which retain in their chemical configuration the characteristics of albuminous substances, and are represented by the albumoses, peptones, peptids, and other compounds. These bodies are met with in nature as products of digestion and metabolism, but they may also be obtained artificially by hydrolysis of the more complex albuminous substances.

[1] Ibid., 1846, pp. 73, 74.

[2] The author has given full references in his *Text book on the Chemistry of Proteids*, Macmillan & Co., 1906, p. 6xx.

[3] Mann, *Physiological Histology*, 1902, pp. 2, 21, 224, 328, 345, 348.

On subjecting these compounds to the action of acids or alkalies, or to certain ferments acting preferably either in acid (pepsin) or alkaline (trypsin) solutions, they are broken up into smaller units called albumoses and peptones. On still further dissociating these latter we arrive at a number of substances known as amino-acids, characterized by the presence of one or more carboxyl-groups (CO.OH) and one or more amino-groups (NH₂), attached to a carbon chain. According as to whether the NH₂-radical is attached to the first, second, third... carbon-atom next the carboxyl-group we speak of α, β, γ... amino-acids.

$$
\begin{array}{lll}
\alpha\text{-amino-acid.} & \beta\text{-amino-acid.} & \gamma\text{-amino-acid.}
\end{array}
$$

Now most amino-acids derived from protoplasm are α-amino-acids and are characterized by a sweet taste, a characteristic which led to the simplest of all amino-acids, namely amino-acetic acid, so abundant in gelatine or glue, receiving the name of sweet-glue or glycocoll. In addition to α-amino-acids there are also found certain bitter amino-acids which are β-compounds, such as the amino-valerianic acid formed during the autodigestion of the pancreas (Levene) and probably also tryptophane. There are no γ-acids present in protoplasm.

Enumeration of the Primary Dissociation-Products

*(The numbers marked with a * have their constitutional formula given hereafter.)*

I. **Albumins**, as occurring in the cytoplasm

A. OPEN-CHAIN AMINO-ACIDS.

1. α mono-amino-mono-carboxylic acids.

*1. amino-acetic or Glycocoll	$C_2H_5NO_2$
2. amino-propionic	$C_3H_7NO_2$
amino-butyric	$C_4H_9NO_2$
3. amino-valerianic	$C_5H_{11}NO_2$
4. amino-iso-butyl-acetic	$C_6H_{13}NO_2$

b. mono-amino-mono-carboxylic hydroxy acids.

*5. amino-hydroxy-propionic or Serin	$C_3H_7NO_3$
6. amino-tetra-hydroxy-caproic	$C_6H_{13}NO_6$

(c) mono-amino-di-carboxylic acids.

  *7. amino-succinic or Aspartic acid $C_4H_7NO_4$
   8. amino-glutaconic $C_5H_7NO_4$

(d) mono-amino-di-carboxylic hydroxy acids.

  *9. amino-hydroxy-succinic $C_4H_7NO_5$
  10. amino-hydroxy-suberic $C_8H_{15}NO_5$

II. (e) diamino-mono-carboxylic acids.

  *11. diamino-propionic $C_3H_8N_2O_2$
  *12. diamino-caproic or Lysin $C_6H_{14}N_2O_2$
  13. guanidin-amino-valerianic $C_6H_{13}N_3O_2$

(f) diamino-mono-carboxylic hydroxy acids.

  14. diamino-trihydroxy-dodecanoic $C_{12}H_{26}N_2O_5$

(g) diamino-di-carboxylic acids.

  *15. diamino-glutaric $C_5H_{12}N_2O_4$
  16. diamino-adipic $C_6H_{12}N_2O_4$

(h) diamino-di-carboxylic hydroxy acids.

  *17. diamino-di-hydroxy-suberic $C_8H_{16}N_2O_6$
  18. diamino-hydroxy-sebacic $C_{10}H_{20}N_2O_5$
  19. caseinic acid (?) $C_8H_{16}N_2O_6$
  20. caseinic acid (?) $C_{15}H_{15}N_3O_5$

A. OPEN-CHAIN COMPOUNDS.

Glycocoll or Amino-Acetic Acid, $C_2H_5NO_2$

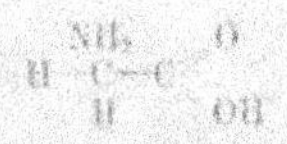

$$\begin{array}{ccc} & NH_2 & O \\ H - & C - & C \\ & H & OH \end{array}$$

Serin, $C_3H_7NO_3$ is α-amino-β-hydroxy-propionic acid.

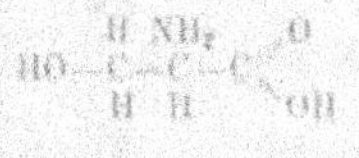

$$\begin{array}{cccc} & H & NH_2 & O \\ HO - & C - & C - & C \\ & H & H & OH \end{array}$$

Aspartic Acid, $C_4H_7NO_4$

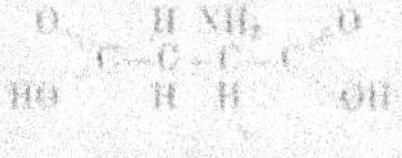

$$\begin{array}{cccc} O & H & NH_2 & O \\ C - & C - & C - & C \\ HO & H & H & OH \end{array}$$

Amino-hydroxy-succinic Acid, $C_4H_7NO_5$

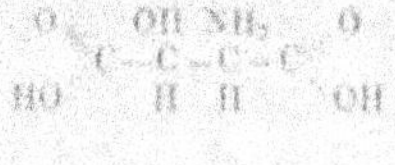

$$\begin{array}{cccc} O & OH & NH_2 & O \\ C - & C - & C - & C \\ HO & H & H & OH \end{array}$$

Diamino-Propionic Acid, $C_3H_8N_2O_2$

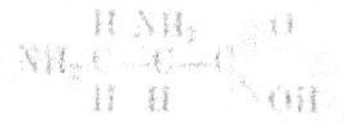

$$NH_2-C-C-C\begin{smallmatrix}H & NH_2 & O\\ & & \\H & H & OH\end{smallmatrix}$$

Lysin, $C_6H_{14}N_2O_2$.

$$NH_2-C-C-C-C-C-C\begin{smallmatrix}H & H & H & H & NH_2 & O\\ & & & & & \\H & H & H & H & H & OH\end{smallmatrix}$$

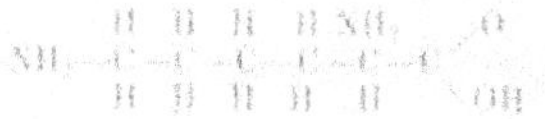

Diamino-glutaric Acid, $C_5H_{10}N_2O_4$.

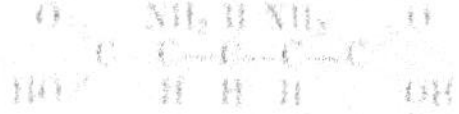

$$\begin{smallmatrix}O & & NH_2 & H & NH_2 & & O\\ C & -C-C-C-C & \\HO & & H & H & H & & OH\end{smallmatrix}$$

Diamino-dihydroxy-suberic Acid, $C_8H_{16}N_2O_6$.

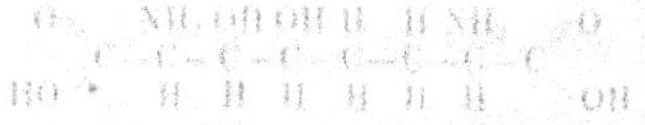

$$\begin{smallmatrix}O & & NH_2 & OH & OH & H & H & NH_2 & & O\\ C-C-C-C-C-C-C-C \\ HO & & H & H & H & H & H & H & & OH\end{smallmatrix}$$

Suberic acid is $COOH(CH_2)_6 COOH$.

B. RING-COMPOUNDS.

B. RING-COMPOUNDS.

$$\begin{array}{ccc} HC=CH & N=CH & \begin{smallmatrix}CH\\HC\diagup\;\diagdown CH\end{smallmatrix}\\ HC\quad CH & HC\quad CH & HC\quad CH\\ NH & NH & CH\\ \text{Pyrrol} & \text{Imidazol} & \text{Benzol} \end{array}$$

a. Pyrrolidin-carboxylic Acid, or Prolin, $C_5H_9NO_2$.

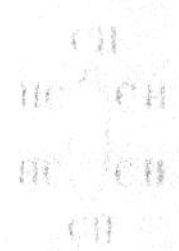

$$\begin{smallmatrix}H_2C-CH_2\\ \\ H_2C \quad CH\cdot COOH\\ \\ NH\end{smallmatrix}$$

Histidin.   Arginin.   Phenyl-Alanin. Tyrosin.

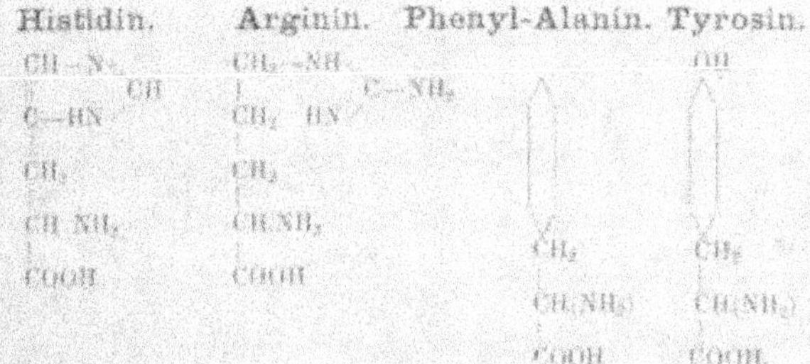

Tryptophane, or indol-amino-propionic acid $C_{11}H_{12}N_2O_2$

Tryptophane (Ellinger).   Tryptophane (Hopkins).

C. AMMONIA.

(m) ammonia.

  27. ammonia. NH_3.

D. THIO-AMINO-ACIDS.

(n) diamino-di-thio-di-carboxylic acid.

  *28. cystin $C_6H_{12}N_2O_4S_2$.

Cystin. $C_6H_{12}O_4N_2S_2$

S.CH_2—CH.NH_2—CO.OH   CH_2.NH_2—CH.S—CO.OH

S.CH_2—CH.NH_2—CO.OH   CH_2.NH_2—CH.S—CO.OH

A cystin or Protein-cystin   B cystin or Stone-cystin
(α-amino-β-thioglyceric acid   (β-thio-β-amino-glyceric acid
 disulphide.)   disulphide.)

II. Nucleo proteids, as occurring in the nucleus.

*(a) pyrimidin-derivatives.

 *1. 2-6 dioxy-pyrimidin or Uracil.
 *2. 2-oxy-6 amino-pyrimidin or Cytosin.
 *3. 2-6 dioxy-5 methyl pyrimidin or Thymin.

(b) purin-derivatives.

 *4. 6 oxy-purin or Hypoxanthin $C_5H_4N_4O$.
 *5. 2-6 dioxy-purin or Xanthin $C_5H_4N_4O_2$.
 *6. 6-amino-purin or Adenin $C_5H_5N_5$.
 *7. 2-amino-6-oxy-purin or
  Guanin $C_5H_5N_5O$.
 *8. guanylic acid $C_{10}H_{14}N_5O_9P$.

(c) laevulinic acid.

$$CH_3.CO.CH_2.CH_2.COOH \qquad C_5H_8O_3.$$

(d) metaphosphoric acid. $\qquad HPO_3.$

(e) pentose. $\qquad C_5H_{10}O_5$

Pyrimidin and its derivatives.

Purin and its derivatives.

Purin, the mother-substance of these 'xanthin-bases,' contains a pyrimidin-remainder: the meta-di-azin and the imido-azol radical.

The following formulæ are arranged in this order:

purin -oxy-purins -amino-purin -amino-oxy-purin

III. Haemo-proteids, as occurring in blood.

Haemoglobin

methyl-propylpyrrol or haemopyrrol

haematinic acid anhydrid

Haemoglobin derivatives.

IV. Glyco-proteids, pronounced acids containing no phosphorus.

   (*a*) Mucins: The arrangement of the carbohydrate radicals in the molecule is unknown. One of the secondary dissociation product is:

     glucosamin $C_6H_{11}(NH_2)O_5$.

   (*b*) Mucoids: The most characteristic substance is Chondroitinsulphuric acid or «Chondro-sulphuric acid» of unknown constitution, which contains sulphur in combination with an aminated polysaccharid.

V. Phospho-glyco-proteids: contain phosphorus and a laevorotatory polysaccharid «sinistrin» of unknown constitution.

VI. Albuminoids. The nature of these bodies makes their investigation exceedingly difficult, and they owe their characteristics either to a preponderance or absence of some of the aminoacids given above.

The Colour Tests.

None of the colour tests given by protoplasm are characteristic of it as such, as each test only indicates the presence of one or other of the radicals enumerated above. Thus the biuret-reaction, according to Schiff, is given by all compounds in which two $CONH_2$-groups are linked either to a carbon-atom or to a nitrogen-atom or directly to one another, and which therefore correspond to one of the three following types:

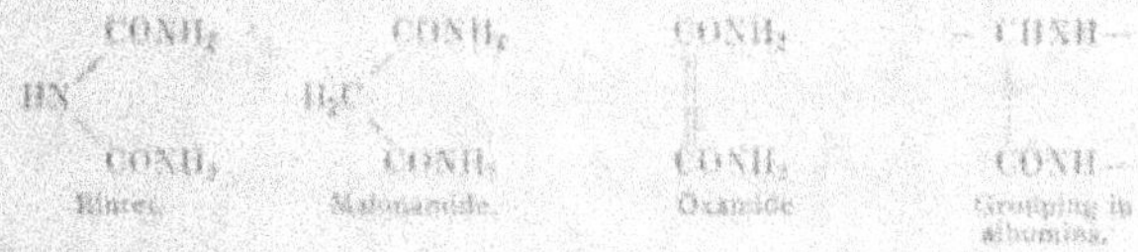

One of the $CONH_2$-groups may also be replaced by a CH_2NH_2-group or a $CSNH_2$-group.

Of these compounds oxamide may occur normally in gelatine (Kutscher and Schenck), while the grouping figured above is contained in all albumins. Millon's reaction shows the presence of tyrosin, as the latter is the only oxyphenyl-compound found in protoplasm. The xanthoprotein reaction indicates the presence of aromatic radicals, and is given especially well by tryptophane. The latter also gives the Adamkiewicz-Hopkins-Cole reaction with glyoxylic acid, and Rhode's reaction with aromatic aldehydes in the presence of sulphuric acid, while its derivatives give further the so-called pyrrol-reaction. Ehrlich's diazo-reaction indicates histidin, if tyrosin be absent; while the test of Molisch is an index to the carbohydrate radicals, as is also the glucosamin-test of Ehrlich. The black or brown colour obtained by boiling albuminous compounds with a lead salt and soda solution demonstrates the presence of sulphur.

Having described the dissociation-products it is possible to isolate from protoplasmic bodies, we have next to consider how they are linked up amongst themselves and also to such other radicals as iron and phosphorus.

The Linking of Protoplasmic Radicals.

Schützenberger [1] advanced, in 1875, the view that albumins ought to be considered as derivatives of urea, $NH_2 - CO - NH_2$, and of oxamide, $NH_2 - CO - CO - NH_2$, but this would only account for the guanidin-remainder, $- CNH \cdot NH_2$, occurring normally in arginin. The conception of Nasse, that albumins are built up as esters, containing the grouping $- C - O - C -$, will also only account for a small percentage of the total amount of albumin, for radicals containing the alcohol-group OH, such as serin, tyrosin, oxyprolin, and the diaminoxycarboxylic acids, are but few. For these reasons Hofmeister advanced in 1892 the theory that albumins are linked up according to the general formula:

$$-CH \begin{vmatrix} \\ \end{vmatrix} -NH-CO-x-NH-CH \begin{vmatrix} \\ \end{vmatrix} -CO-NH-$$

He based his view partly on the fact that this grouping occurs in argmin and in leucin-imide:

$$
\begin{array}{ll}
CH_2\ NH\ C\ NH_2\ NH_2 & C_5H_9 \\
(CH_2)_2 & CH \\
CH\ NH_2 & NH\ CO \\
CO\ OH & CO\ NH \\
& CH \\
& C_5H_9 \\
\text{Argmin} & \text{Leucin-imide}
\end{array}
$$

and partly on the fact that according to Löw and Schiff, relatively little NH_2 is present in albumins, judging by the amount of the nitrogen which is split off, and the ease with which the biuret-reaction can be prevented on subjecting albumins to the action of nitrous acid.

Hofmeister illustrated his theory by the following example in which leucin and glutaminic are linked together:

$$
CO\ -\!\!\!|\!\!\!-\ NH-CH-CO\ -\!\!\!|\!\!\!-\ NH-CH-CO\ -\!\!\!|\!\!\!-\ NH-
$$

$$
\begin{array}{ll}
C_5H_9 & (CH_2)_2 \\
 & CO\ OH \\
\text{Leucin} & \text{Glutaminic acid}
\end{array}
$$

In this compound the radical

$$
\begin{array}{l}
-CH-NH- \\
| \\
CO-NH-
\end{array}
$$

occurs, which is also met with in the following compounds giving the biuret reaction, namely,

$$
\begin{array}{lll}
CH_2\ NH_2 & CH_2-NH(CH_3) & CO\ NH_2 \\
CH_2\ NH_2 & CO-NH_2 & CH\ NH_2 \\
 & & CH_2 \\
 & & CO\ NH_2 \\
\text{Glücinamide (Schiff)} & \text{Sarcosin-imide (Schiff)} & \text{Aspargic acid amide (Eiched)}
\end{array}
$$

Phosphorus which was just now alluded to in connection with glutaminic acid, is one of the most characteristic constiments of nuclei as has been shown by Macallum's microchemical tests.

Burian [1] points out that purin-bases (see p. 207) must be preformed in the nucleic acid molecule, as they are very readily separated from the nucleic acid remainder. They are liberated partially by heating nucleic acid to 60°, and completely by boiling the same for ten minutes in water or by dilute acids; this fact, along with the observation that nucleic acids do not give the diazo-reaction described above, led Burian to assume that the purin-bases are linked to the remainder of the nucleic acid molecule by the No. 7 nitrogen.

As nucleic acids are further very resistant to caustic potash, and in this they resemble other organic phosphoric-acid amides, there probably exists in nucleic acids a direct union between the phosphorus of the nucleic acid remainder and the No. 7 nitrogen of the purin-base. The union of guanin in nucleic acid would therefore be represented by the formula

$$
\begin{array}{c}
HN\!-\!CO \\
\mid \qquad \mid \qquad\quad \mathrm{P\equiv} \\
NH_2\!-\!C \quad\; C\!-\!N \\
\mid \qquad\quad \diagdown \mathrm{CH} \\
N\!-\!C\!-\!N \diagup
\end{array}
$$

Hofmeister's so-called theory has been confirmed by the synthetic researches of E. Fischer and Curtius, for there cannot be any doubt that ordinary amino-acids, when linked up, form neutral amino-compounds as far as the links are concerned; or, as Fischer puts it, amino-acids become «amid-like anhydrides» or «polypeptids», which, according to the number of amino-acids they contain, are called di-, tri-, tetra-peptids, and so on.

As direct oxidation of arginin does not yield oxaluric acid, but guanidin-butyric or guanidin + succinic acid (Kutscher) or urea and ornithin, when treated with barium hydrate (Schultze), or arginase (Kossel and Dakin), Seemann reasons that the arginin group must be attached at its guanidin-end to other amino-acids,

[1] Burian, Ber. d. Deutsch. chem. Ges. 37, 708 (1904).

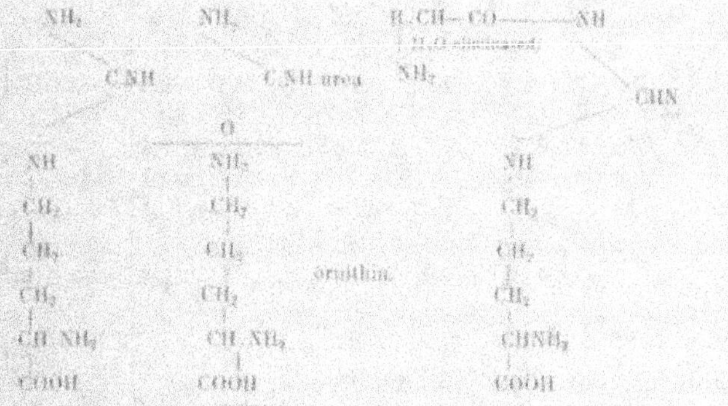

$$\text{NH}_2 \qquad\qquad \text{NH}_2 \qquad\qquad \text{R.CH---CO-------NH}$$
$$\text{C.NH} \qquad\qquad \text{C.NH urea} \qquad \text{NH}_2 \qquad\qquad\qquad \text{CHN}$$
$$\overset{\text{O}}{\text{—————}}$$

$$
\begin{array}{ccc}
\text{NH} & \text{NH}_2 & \text{NH} \\
\text{CH}_2 & \text{CH}_2 & \text{CH}_2 \\
\text{CH}_2 & \text{CH}_2 & \text{CH}_2 \\
\text{CH}_2 & \text{CH}_2 & \text{CH}_2 \\
\text{CH.NH}_2 & \text{CH.NH}_2 & \text{CHNH}_2 \\
\text{COOH} & \text{COOH} & \text{COOH}
\end{array}
$$

Arginin | arginase or ferram hydrate — ornithin   Arginin + another S amino-acid radical.

As examples of the way in which ring-compounds and sulphur is linked, we may take some of the polypeptids which Emil Fischer has obtained. Pyrrolidin carboxylic acid or Prolin (see p. 206) unites with alanin or amino-propionic acid (see p. 204) to form prolyl-alanin :

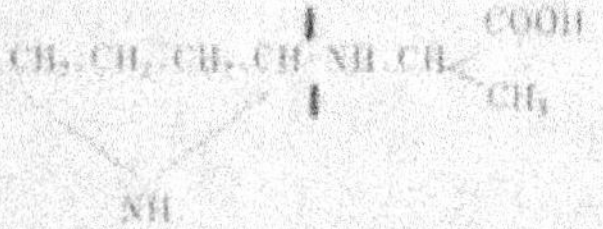

$$\text{CH}_2\text{.CH}_2\text{.CH}_2\text{.CH.NH.CH} \overset{\text{COOH}}{\underset{\text{CH}_3}{<}}$$

$$\text{NH}$$

Prolin—remainder.   Alanin—remainder.

and phenyl-alanin (see p. 206) may analogously be linked up with diverse amino-acids. Diglycyl-phenyl-alanin has *e. g.*, the constitution :

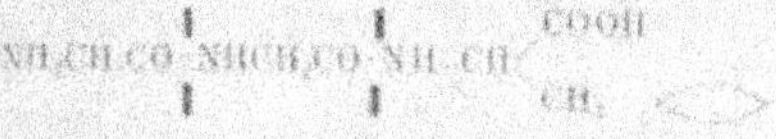

$$\text{NH}_2\text{CH.CO.NH.CH}_2\text{.CO.NH.CH} \overset{\text{COOH}}{\underset{\text{CH}_2}{<}}$$

Cystin, the constitutional formula of which is given on p. 207, Fischer has linked up, amongst other amino-acids, with glycocoll. Thus diglycyl-cystin has the formula :

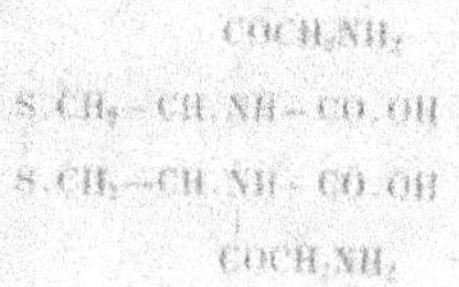

$$\text{COCH}_2\text{NH}_2$$
$$\text{S.CH}_2\text{—CH.NH—CO.OH}$$
$$\text{S.CH}_2\text{—CH.NH—CO.OH}$$
$$\text{COCH}_2\text{NH}_2$$

Iron is contained in most, if not in all, nucleo-proteids, and if we except the iron present in the haemoglobin, the main bulk of the remaining iron concerned in metabolism, is contained in the nucleo-proteids; nothing is known as to how the iron is linked up, but we know that it is present in a non-ionic or «masked» state, and that therefore it cannot give directly the Prussian blue reaction, or the ammonium sulphide- or haematoxylin-tests.

According to Ascoli iron does not fix on to the albumin at all, but to the nucleic acid or to the para- or pseudo-nuclein of the nucleo-albumin. Plasminic acid, which Kossel and Ascoli prepared from yeast, and which contains 27 per cent. of phosphorus, Ascoli believes to be a metaphosphoric acid, or the salt of such an acid with an organic base. Its most important property is that it renders iron «masked». If one add to a solution of metaphosphoric acid as much ferric chloride as can be kept in solution by the excess of acid, and if one then add ammonia to neutralisation and precipitate with alcohol and ether, a substance is obtained which gives the following reactions. It is soluble in water, hydrochloric acid, and ammonia; its iron does not react to small amounts of ammonium sulphide, and not immediately to larger amounts, and it does not give up its iron to hydrochloric-acid-alcohol except under certain conditions. Plasmin behaves exactly as does this metaphosphoric acid; it too contains iron, and also in a non-ionic form, as its presence cannot be demonstrated by either the Prussian blue reaction or by other direct tests.

When examining the products of partially digested silkfibrin, Fischer obtained a glycocoll-alanin compound, which arises by the union of one molecule of glycocoll with one molecule of alanin, there being given off two molecules of water. This glycocoll- or glycin-alanin-anhydride, was the first di-keto-piperazin discovered in a derivative of protoplasm.

$$
\begin{array}{ccc}
\ \ CH_2 \quad NH & & CH_2 \!-\! NH \\[-2pt]
H_2C\!\big\langle \qquad\quad \big\rangle CH_2 & \qquad O\!=\!C\big\langle \qquad\quad \big\rangle C\!=\!O \\[-2pt]
\ \ NH \quad CH_2 & & NH \!-\! CH_2 \\
\text{Piperazin} & & \text{Diketopiperazin or} \\
& & \text{Diglycocoll-anhydride}
\end{array}
$$

$$
\begin{array}{c}
CH_2 \!-\! NH \\[-2pt]
O\!=\!C\big\langle \qquad\quad \big\rangle C\!=\!O \\[-2pt]
NH \qquad CH \\
 | \\
 CH_3 \\
\text{Glycocoll-alanin-anhydride}
\end{array}
$$

Fischer has synthetized not only this glycocoll-alanin-anhydride, but two other di-keto-piperazins, namely

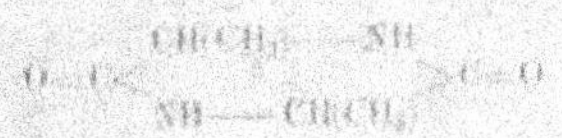

$$O=C\!\!<\!\!\begin{array}{c} CH\cdot CH_3 - NH \\ NH - CH\cdot CH_3 \end{array}\!\!>\!\!C=O \qquad O=C\!\!<\!\!\begin{array}{c} \overset{C_4H_9}{CH} - NH \\ NH - \underset{C_4H_9}{CH} \end{array}\!\!>\!\!C=O$$

Di-alanin-anhydride 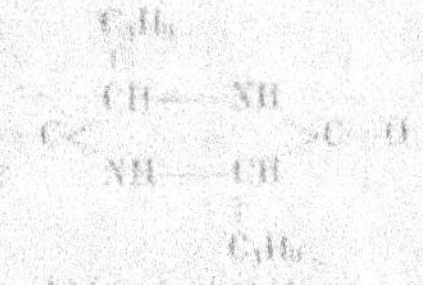   Di-leucin-anhydride or Leucin-imide

The occurrence of anhydrides of amino-acids in protoplasm appears to be beyond doubt.

On passing to bigger complexes we meet at once with great difficulties. Kossel pointed out in 1901 [1] that a systematic investigation into the quality and quantity of amino-acid constituents is the first essential, and to this we must all agree. He further proposed the theory that certain comparatively simple complexes, rich in diamino-acids, the so-called protamins obtained from ripe spermatozoa, might be considered as the nuclei round which all the others, chiefly mono-amino-acids are grouped. This view is, however, debatable. Emil Fischer [2] says «Kossel's proposal to assume a «protamin nucleus» in all albuminous compounds, and to make it the stepping-stone for a chemical system is going too far, and in this I concur for physiological reasons, partly because of the very work which Kossel and his pupils have done. After Bang [3] had pointed out that in immature spermatozoa histone takes the place of protamin, Kossel [4] showed that in some fishes, for example the salmon, the body-muscle is converted into protamin, while in other fishes, for example the cod, the muscle becomes only changed into histone. It follows therefore that protamin is a derivative of albumin, and that it cannot be considered from the physiological point of view as a nucleus of the albumin molecule, except we assume with Kossel that the conversion of skeletal muscle into protamin is the equivalent of removing the monoamino-acid «impurities» by means of a physiological process taking place in the testicles.

[1] A. Kossel, Bericht d. deutsch. chem. Ges. 34, 3211 (1901).
[2] Emil Fischer, Ber. d. deutsch. chem. Ges. 39, 530 (1906).
[3] Bang. Zeitsch. f. physiol. Chem. 27, 463 (1899).
[4] A. Kossel, Biochemisches Centralblatt 2, reprint, p. 10.

I shall show later that my researches into the functions of the nucleus allowed me in 1896 to draw another conclusion, namely that the nucleus is the agent by which mono-amino-acids are built up into bigger complexes. Kossel, to a certain extent, has also arrived at this conception, for he pointed out in 1905 [1] that the alloxur- or purin-bases, and further also a pyrimidin-derivative, which on hydrolysis gives rise to cytosin (or uracil) and thymin (see above) are not only rich in nitrogen, but also possess the C and N arranged alternately:

and that this chemical peculiarity was characteristic of that part of protoplasm which is concerned with the processes of propagation and the formation of new substances.

The Protamins above referred to, as shown by the following table, are characterized by the presence of a high percentage of di-amino-acids, which renders them strongly basic:

TABLE SHOWING THE COMPOSITION OF THE PROTAMINS

	Scombrin	Salmin	Clupein	Sturin	Cyclopterin	α-Cyprinin	β-Cyprinin
Alanin (α-amino-propionic acid)	+	0	+	+	?	?	?
Serin (oxy-alanin)	0	+	+	0	?	?	?
Amino-valerianic acid	0	+	+	0	?	+	?
Leucin (iso-butyl α-amino-acetic acid)	0	0	0	+	?	?	?
Diamino-valerianic acid (ornithin)	+	+	+	+	+	+	+
Diamino-caproic acid (lysin)	0	0	0	+	0	+	+
Histidin (imido-azol-alanin)	0	0	0	+	0	0	0
α-Pyrolidin-carboxylic acid	+	+	+	+	0	?	?
Tyrosin (oxy-phenyl-alanin)	0	0	0	0	+	0	+
Urea	+	+	+	+	+	+	+
Tryptophan (indol-amino-propionic acid)	0	0	0	0	?	0	0
Ammonia	0	0	0	0	?	?	?

[1] A. Kossel, Zeitschr. f. physiol. Chem. 44, 347 (1905).

The composition of protamins has been cleared up by Kossel's school in a very thorough manner. As will be seen from Kossel's figure on p. 218, it is possible to account for practically the whole of the nitrogen of the protamin salmin, while that of the albumin edestin of the Para-nut (Bertholletia) can only be accounted for to the extent of 58 per cent.

In this Figure the vertical line in the middle indicates in percentage figures the amount of nitrogen of those dissociation-products which could be isolated, the nitrogen-content of edestin was taken to be 18.64 per cent. (Abderhalden); the length of the horizontal lines indicates the ratio of the carbon to the nitrogen, except in the ornithin of the salmin and the leucin of the edestin in which cases the lines have been shortened.

In connection with the grouping of various radicals in the protoplasmic molecule attention must be drawn to the anti- and the hemi-groups of Kühne and Pick.

Anti-group.	*Hemi-group.*
Represented by gelatine	by casein
resists trypsin	is readily digested
not readily oxidized	readily oxidized
composed of hetero- and	of prot-albumose
deutero-albumose	
contains glycocoll, prolin and	tryptophane and
phenyl alanin.	tyrosin.

So far I have given a very short review of the purely chemical aspect of protoplasm, and shall now proceed to the discussion of the physical and physico-chemical aspects. In my first book, in which the Theory of Histology has been treated, I advanced certain views which since that time have also been brought forward by pupils of Ostwald and Nernst. In the first instance it is absolutely necessary to have a clear conception of what we mean with the terms «solution,» «electrolyte,» «hydrolyte,» and «colloid» (¹).

SOLUTION. — A substance, on coming into contact with a fluid, is said to pass into solution when its molecules separate from one another and diffusing into the fluid, mixt with the molecules of the latter. The resulting mixture, consisting of the

(¹) The following account is a reprint out of my *Chemistry of Proteids.*

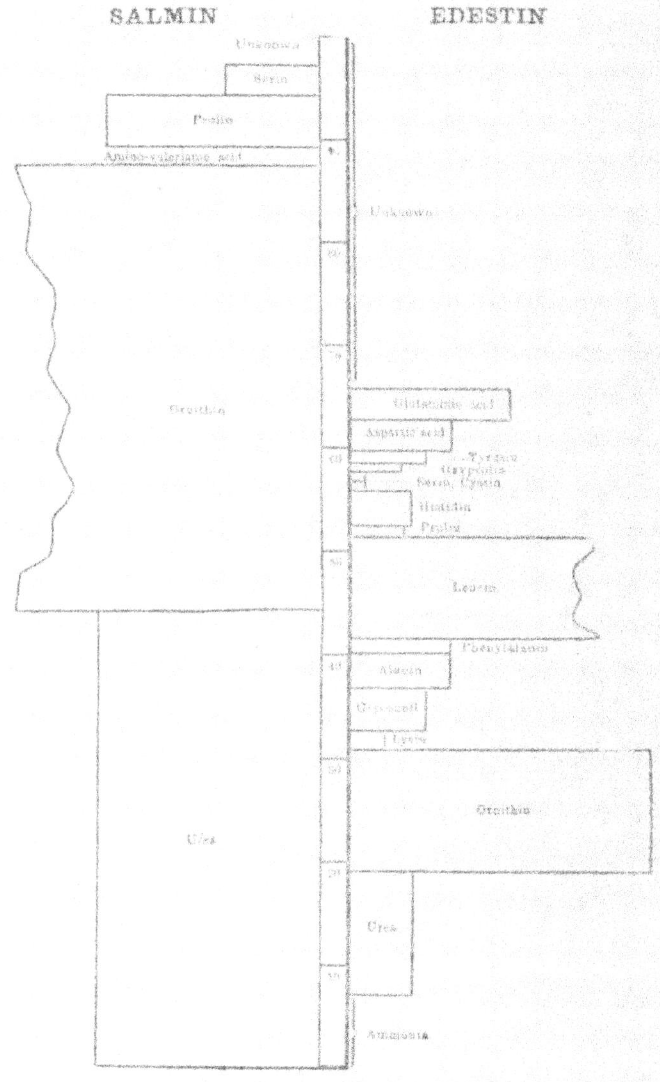
Distribution of Nitrogen in
SALMIN
EDESTIN
Unknown
Serin
Prolin
Amino-valerianic acid
Unknown
Ornithin
Glutaminic acid
Aspartic acid
Tyrosin
tryptophan
Serin, Lysin
Histidin
Prolin
Leucin
Phenylalanin
Alanin
Glycocoll
Lysin
Ornithin
Urea
Urea
Ammonia

molecules of the solvent and the solute (1), may form so homogeneous a system as not to interfere in any way with the transmission of light, or, to use a technical term, the mixture may be 'optically void,' i.e., contain no visible particles. On the other hand, the solute may consist of particles of such size as to interfere more or less with the transmission of light, when we speak of 'colloidal' solutions (see below) or of suspensions. All solutions are therefore mixtures of liquids or liquids and solids.

A substance in solution, as van't Hoff has shown, is in every way comparable to a gas. There is, however, one difference, for in the case of an ordinary gas the amount contained in the fluid is proportional to the amount of the same gas outside the fluid, or, in other words, the gaseous tension in the fluid is proportional to the partial pressure exerted by the gas outside the fluid. In the case of dissolved solids, however, the solid cannot leave the fluid, because the very fact of a substance dissolving at all depends on definite electro-chemical interactions. Brühl (2) has shown that the power of acting as a solvent depends on the latter possessing some atom which is potentially plurivalent; for example, oxygen in water is divalent, but capable of becoming tetravalent; the nitrogen of ammonia is trivalent but with a tendency to become pentavalent, and so on. To this must be added the conception that the body passing into solution may undergo an analogous change. In the light of Brühl's conception, and taking also into consideration that even pure water is partially dissociated, and possesses a high dielectric constant (3), following possibilities suggest themselves:—

1. The substance and the solvent, by mutually diffusing into one another, form mixtures without the solute undergoing electrical dissociation. This happens, for example, if sugar or mercuric cyanide dissolve in water, and also happens as the preliminary step in all cases where electrolytes dissolve; but in the case of electrolytes the primary «passing into solution» is followed by a secondary chemical dissociation as described below.

I believe, when diffusion takes place, that the solvent has one electrical charge, while the solute has the opposite charge.

---

(1) A solute is any substance which has passed into solution.

(2) J. W. Brühl, Zeitsch. f. physik. Chem. 10 1 (1892).

(3) A dielectricon is a substance without any electrical charge of its own, but capable of having an electrical charge induced in it.

The mixture being a binary system, it is impossible for an electrical current to pass through it, as this would mean moving both the solvent and the solute (¹).

2. The substance undergoes in the solvent electrolyte dissociation, as in the case of electrolytes of salts containing radicals capable of giving rise to strong positive ions or kat-ions, and to strong negative ions or an-ions. Thus in the case of common salt, sodium becomes $+$, while chlorine becomes $-$:

$$NaCl + xH_2O \rightleftharpoons Na\bullet + Cl' + H_2O$$

In this case an electrical current passes through the mixture of solvent and solute, because we are dealing with a ternary system consisting of a medium, the solvent, in which both negative and positive ions, derived from the solute, are freely movable.

3. The substance, being composed of a potential, strong kat-ion, and a potential, feeble an-ion, or *vice-versâ*, undergoes hydrolysis, which means that the weaker ion of the salt is replaced by a stronger ion derived from the solvent. If the solvent is water, and the weaker ion of the solute is electro-positive, its place is taken by the acid hydrogen-ion of water; if the weaker ion of the solute is electro-negative, then it is replaced by the alkaline hydroxyl-ion of water. Thus corrosive sublimate and water, or sodium carbonate and water, behave as follows:

$$NaCl + xH_2O \rightleftharpoons (NaOH) + 2H\bullet + Cl'$$
$$Na_2CO_3 + xH_2O \rightleftharpoons (H_2CO_3) + Na\bullet + OH'$$

4. The substance, being composed of two feeble radicals, forms with the solvent a hydrate which is only capable of undergoing complete dissociation if along with this substance another salt is present, by the dissociation of which either acid hydrogen- or alkaline hydroxyl-ions are liberated. See below, and also footnote² on p. 222.

ELECTROLYTE. — An electrolyte is defined by Arrhenius (³) as a substance which imparts to water, which itself is a non-conductor, the power of allowing an electric current to pass through it,

¹ Mann, *Physiological Histology*, 1902, p. 45. See also in his *Chemistry of Proteids*, pp. 26 and 27, under Ionizer.

³ Arrhenius, *Zeit f. physik. Chem.* 1, 631 (1887).

in virtue of the substance being in a state of electrical dissociation or ionisation, their being formed, while no current is passing, two sets of ions, the one having an electro-negative, the other an electro-positive charge.

HYDROLYTE. — If only one the components of a salt becomes an ion, while the other component transfers its positive charge to a hydrogen atom of the water, and thereby converts the later into the acid hydrogen-ion, $H^{\cdot}$, or its negative charge to the hydroxyl group, OH, of water, and thereby changes the latter into the alkaline hydroxyl-ion, OH', then the salt is said to undergo hydrolytic dissociation, and substances behaving in this manner may be termed hydrolytes. Examples of electrolytes and hydrolytes have been given under Nos. 2 and 3 in the previous paragraph on «solution».

COLLOID. This term was introduced by Thomas Graham [1] in 1861 for certain substances which differ from «crystalloids» in diffusing very slowly in water, in being unable to pass through animal bladders and vegetable parchment, and in not crystallising readily. Graham states: crystalloids and colloids «are like different worlds of matter», while I hold that all colloids are electrolytes, as explained on p. 225.

It is necessary to distinguish between insoluble, semi-soluble, and soluble states of colloids. A soluble colloid is one in which all the component particles carry definite electro-positive or electro-negative charges, as will be shown later, while an insoluble «colloid» is iso-electric, i.e. carries no electrical charges, and as long as a colloid remains in this insoluble state it exhibits none of the characteristics usually attributed to colloids and enumerated below. According to the nature of the particular colloid we are working with, the conversion of the insoluble into the soluble state is either comparatively easy or very difficult, and the more a colloid is rendered truly iso-electric, the more difficult is, other things being equal, to reconvert it into the soluble form. This reconversion in the case of albumins is often quite impossible, because when the iso-electric point is approached, the different groups of amino-acids in the albumin-molecule re-arrange themselves intra-molecularly to compensate for the removal of the electrically charged ions by means of which they were kept in

---

[1] Thomas Graham, *Phil. Trans.* 151, 183 and 373 (1861)

solution. In addition to this change, amino-acids may also be converted from real acids and bases, into pseudo-acids and into pseudo-bases [1].

Summing up our present knowledge, colloids, when «in solution», have the following characteristics:—

1. They polarise transmitted light.

2. Possessing a low osmotic pressure, they raise the boiling-point or affect the freezing-point of water only very slightly.

3. They are not coagulated irreversibly by a rise of temperature, provided electrolytes are absent and provided their chemical constitution does not become permanently altered.

4. They move either with or against an electrical stream which is being passed through them, and they are therefore either electro-positive or electro-negative, but they offer a great resistance to the flow of the electrical current, owing to their increased bulk and diminished surface.

5. They undergo hydrolytic dissociation, as in the case of arsenic trisulphide.

6. They are rendered more colloidal and are readily made insoluble by electrolytes, the potent ion of which [2] has an electrical sign the opposite to that carried by themselves, and they are made less colloidal by the addition of ions of the same sign.

7. Colloids of opposite electrical sign precipitate one another if they are in equivalent amounts, but if either of the two colloids is added in excess, then the colloidal precipitate, which was formed in the first instance, may re-dissolve.

8. One colloid in solution does not penetrate another colloid which forms a rigid system, or, in other words, colloids do not pass through animal or vegetable membranes.

9. As a rule they do not crystallise readily.

In support of my view that colloids are electrolytes the following facts may be mentioned.

Picton in 1892 divided arsenic-sulphide, As_2S_3, solutions,

---

[1] For a historical account of investigations into the nature of colloids up to the year 1905, see his *Physiology and Histology*, Clarendon Press 1905, pp. 1850, while for the more-recent work consult my *Chemistry of Proteids*.

[2] The potency of an ion is determined by the degree to which its electro-affinity is satisfied by the other ion with which it is linked together. If both ions have strong electro-affinities, as in the case of potassium chloride, then neither ion can exert its influence readily; but if one of the ions is weak, as, for example, the CO_3 radical in potassium carbonate, Na_2CO_3, and the Hg-radical in corrosive sublimate, then the stronger ion causes the hydrolysis of water, or may act on other substances of the opposite electrical sign which are dissolved in the water along with itself.

according to their physical state, into four classes, which he called α, β, γ and δ. The α-solution is termed a pseudo-solution, because under a magnification of 1000 diameters the fluid is seen to contain crowds of minute suspended particles in rapid Brownian movement. The β-solution, forming the transition to the γ-variety, is composed of particles so small as to be microscopically invisible. The γ-solution differs from the α and β ones in diffusing and exerting osmotic pressure, but it cannot be filtered through a porcelain filter without the solid separating out, while the δ-solution contains sulphide particles of so small a size as to pass readily through the filter.

Now Picton's α-solution is comparable to what is ordinarily called a colloid, an his δ-solution to what is usually termed an electrolyte. The difference between a colloid and an electrolyte is, therefore, in one respect, purely one of size, or a quantitative one; the difference becomes qualitative only in respect to the unit of electrical charge carried by each individual particle. Polarisation-phenomena therefore do not allow us to distinguish between electrolytes and colloids.

The first observer to point out that «inert» substances may decompose neutral salts in the presence of water, and that they may join either with the acid or basic radical set free, was v. Bemmelen, who investigated such porous substances as animal charcoal, silicic acid, and coagulated colloids. The fact that colloids may decompose such a «neutral» salt as barium chloride and induce its hydrolysis shows that colloids must be chemically active, i. e. that they must be electrolytes or hydrolytes.

We further know that ions travel with or against an electrical current and so do colloids (see above) under the general characteristics of colloids. They further undergo hydrolysis and combine with different metals in equivalent amounts (Whitney and Ober).

(0 per cent As$_2$S$_3$)	Chloride Solutions 25 ccm.	Amount of Salt added expressed in Grammes.	Free Chlorine remaining in Solution calculated as Acid.
100 ccm.	K	2.00	0.0038
100 ccm.	Ba	0.1094	0.0029
100 ccm.	Sr	0.1071	0.0012
100 ccm.	Ca	0.0706	0.0010

This table is exceedingly interesting, because it shows not only a marked difference between the monovalent potassium and the divalent barium, strontium and calcium, confirming Hans Schultze's observation that the relative coagulative power of mono-, di-, and trivalent metals varies greatly, but also shows, according to my opinion, that within the divalent metals the power of precipitating colloids increases with the diminishing electro-affinity of the metals [1].

When a colloidal solution becomes semi-soluble, or, in other words, more colloidal, when, for example, Picton's δ-arsenic-sulphide solution is changed into γ, then β, and ultimately into the α-variety, the following changes occur: — In a freshly prepared noncolloidal arsenic sulphide solution, As_2S_3 is dissociated into $[As(OH)]^{+++}$ and $3[HS]'$ and this dissociation is also met with in colloidal solutions, as has been shown by Freundlich. When the colloidal solution becomes less colloidal there occurs, according to my theory, a diminution in the amount of electrical dissociation; and this diminution is accompanied by a gradual increase in the size of colloidal particles. Picton and Linder were the first to notice that the size of the colloidal particles increases when the point of coagulation is neared, and that there is a reaction other than mechanical between solvent and solid, even in those cases of colloidal solution.

The change from an «electrolytic» into a «colloidal» solution I explain as follows: — «If to a solution containing a definite number of electro-positive (colloid + H)·-ions there is added an alkali containing the same number of electro-negative hydroxyl-ions, then the H· of the colloid and the OH of the alkali unite to form electrically neutral water, and the colloid, having lost its electrical charge, is precipitated; if however not a sufficient number of OH-ions are added to bind all the hydrogen-atoms, then the colloid aggregates re-arrange themselves into larger aggregates».

The observation that iso-electric, heat-coagulated albumin moves neither towards the anode nor towards the kathode, while after the addition of a trace of acid it moves towards the kathode, and after the addition of an alkali towards the anode, I explained in 1902 thus: — «As the proteid acquires the charge of

---

[1] Abegg and Herz, *Chemisches Praktikum*, Vandenhoeck and Ruprecht, Göttingen, 1900 [illegible], sixth edition, Macmillan, give the following table of electro-affinities:—

Kations arranged in descending order of their electro-affinities:—
K, Na, Li, Ba, Sr, Ca, Mg, Al, Mn, Zn, Cd, Fe, Co, Ni, Pb, H, Cu, Ag, Hg, Pt, Au.

Anions arranged in descending order of electro-affinities:—
Cl, NO_3, ClO_3, Cl, S_2O_3, Br, I, FO, CO_3, ClO, SO_3, SH, H_2BO_3, OH, CN, O, S.

the positive hydrogen-ion of acids, and the negative charge of the hydroxyl-ions of alkalies, we may assume the hydrogen- or hydroxyl-ions to unite with aggregates of proteid-molecules, and thus to form new ions consisting of the (colloid $+$ H)- or (colloid $+$ OH)'. The an-ion of the acid which was added (for example, the negative chlorine- or acetic-ions) or the kat-ion of the alkali (for example, the positive sodium-ions) become the companion-ions to the (colloid $+$ H)- or the (colloid $+$ OH)'- ions».

To the same conclusion as I expressed in 1902 in my *Physiological Histology*, namely, that colloids are electrolytes, have subsequently come Billitzer, working under Nernst, and Freundlich, working in Ostwald's laboratory.

Billitzer [1] arrived in 1903 at the conclusion that colloids may be regarded as ions, for he found it impossible to explain the movement of colloidal particles in an electrical field on v. Helmholtz's hypothesis [2] that a separation of the positive and the negative charge in electrolytes is brought about by the formation of a double electrical layer, which was so constituted that on two sides of a plane immeasurably thin (?) there were developed equivalent but opposite amounts of electricity.

Freundlich [3] explains the behaviour of colloids on the assumption that the surfaces of colloidal particles are semipermeable, which means that they allow of the ready passage of ions of the opposite electrical sign to that carried by themselves, i.e. of either kat-ions or of the an-ions, while the other ions which cannot enter the colloidal particles remain in the solvent. This explanation amounts to the same as that given by the author, namely, that the (colloid $+$ the entered ion) is an ion. Very interesting in this connection is an observation made by A. Fischer [4], who noticed that the basic dyes are absorbed at once by the acid nucleo-proteids, while with acid stains there is a delay, in about the proportion that methyl green will have stained already intensely, when acid fuchsin only just shows the faintest indication of staining. In the course of ten minutes, however, this difference disappears in material which was fixed in indifferent re-

[1] Jaq. Billitzer, *Ann. d. Physik*, 11, [illegible] und [illegible] (1903).
[2] H. v. Helmholtz, *Pogg. Ann.* 16[illegible], [illegible] (185[illegible]).
[3] See Lord Kelvin, *Nature*, 31st March and 14th May, 189[illegible].
[4] Herbert Freundlich, *Zeit. f. physik. Chem.* 44. (190[illegible]).
[5] A. Fischer, *Fixirung, Färbung und Bau des Protoplasmas*, 189[illegible], p. [illegible].

agents». Reversely «the acid dyes diffusing through the sections stain at first only the cytoplasm, and several seconds later the nuclei, which ultimately are also stained as intensely as the cytoplasm». Fischer failed to understand the importance of his own observations, for he uses his facts to prove the absence of any real difference in the absorptive powers of nucleins with regard to acid and basic dyes; while to me [1], Fischer's observations have this significance: each particle, either kat-ion or an-ion, has an aversion for ions of its own kind or those of the same electrical sign; thus the positive kat-ion $H^{\bullet}$ will not only repel other $H^{\bullet}$-ions, but also, for example, those of potassium, $K^{\bullet}$. On the other hand, positive kat-ions will readily unite with negative an-ions.

The view that colloids are electrolytes is further supported by the fact that colloids of opposite electrical sign precipitate one another, as has long been known to histologists. Romanowsky [2] in 1891 combined equi-molecular proportions of the basic methylene-blue and the acid eosin, and thus obtained the water-insoluble eosinate of methylene-blue [3]. Quite recently the same phenomenon has been studied by Biltz [4], who calls these unions «adsorption compounds».

After giving various further examples of the fact that hydrosols of opposite electrical sign mutually precipitate one another if they are mixed in equivalent amounts, he shows that mixtures of hydrosols possessing the same electrical sign — such as the purple of Cassius, which is a hydrosol of stannic acid and gold — are thrown down together by electrolytes having the opposite electrical load. He also found that the precipitating action of mixtures of electrolytes and colloids is an additive effect, and that in many cases an action which seems to be brought about by an electrolyte is caused at least partly by the presence of colloids. In this connection he draws attention to the work of Spring [5], who showed that solutions of the salts of plurivalent metals (such as aluminium chloride or ferric chloride) are not optically void, and therefore must contain colloidal hydroxides; and also to the work

[1] Mann, Physiological Histology, 1902, p. [illegible].
[2] Romanowsky, Zur Frage d. Parasitol. u. s. Therap. d. Malaria, St. Petersburg, 1891.
[3] Other instances are given in «Physiological Histology», pp. 441-461.
[4] W. Biltz, Mutual Interactions of Colloidal Substances, Ber. d. deutsch. chem. Gesell., 1905 (1904).
[5] Spring, Bull. de l'Ac. Roy. de Belg., 1900, p. [illegible].

of Mylius (¹), who accounts for metaphosphoric acid coagulating albumin, while orthophosphoric acid does not, by showing that metaphosphoric acid contains polymolecular particles, i.e. that it is in fact a "colloidal" solution. Mylius further shows that all acids which precipitate ordinary white of egg, after it has been diluted, contain complex molecules.

Biltz objects to a chemical explanation of colloidal solutions, and considers Bredig's view to be correct, namely, that the cause of the relatively great stability of pure colloidal solutions is the electrical difference of potential between the colloid and the solvent. I have to point out that according to all laws of physical chemistry the first essential for chemical interaction is the establishment of an electrical load, or, in other words, that only those substances which carry an electrical load are capable of acting upon one another "chemically". To say, as does Biltz, that we are dealing with adsorption-phenomena when a colloid is precipitated, is not giving an explanation at all, but amounts simply to stating the premise over again in a roundabout manner. If the cause of the adsorption is the ionic difference of potential between two substances, then adsorption means simply a chemical union.

The inter-relation of suspensions and colloids in viscid media, the behaviour of colloids upon one another, and how under certain circumstances one colloid may prevent the precipitation of a second colloid, is fully discussed by Arthur Müller (²).

In this connection the precipitation of colloidal solutions by the addition of (neutral) salts must be mentioned. Even if we assume that the added neutral salt does not interfere in any chemical manner with the colloid we are experimenting with, it is evident, if my view is correct—namely, that electroaffinities in equivalent intensities but of opposite sign attached to two radicals lead to these two radicals forming insoluble compounds—that salts which are soluble and capable of electrical dissociation must for this very reason be composed of ions which differ from one another as regards their electro-affinities. If, however, either the kation or the anion is stronger, then the unsatisfied balance of electro-affinity represents available energy which, when brought into contact with colloids, will lead to the precipitation of the

---

(¹) F. Mylius, *Ber. d. deutsch. chem. Ges.* **36**, 775 (1903). (The reader's attention is especially directed to this important paper.)

(²) Arthur Müller, *Ber. d. deutsch. chem. Ges.* **37**, (1904).

latter, provided that the colloid has an electrical sign which is
the opposite to that carried by stronger ion of the neutral salt.

If by adding water we dilute a solution of globulin made
with 1 per cent. of sodium chloride, i.e. with a neutral salt, the
globulin becomes precipitated, because the sodium of the NaCl
has a greater dissociation-tension or electro-affinity than has the
chlorine. As ions of opposite sign can only be present in equivalent amounts, it follows that the greater tendency of sodium to
form ions in water is checked by the smaller dissociation-tension
of the chlorine. It follows, therefore, that if we add a second radical, such as globulin, capable of becoming an electro-negative
ion, that the sodium may develop its full dissociation-tension
because of the formation of the compound:

$$[Na]' \begin{cases} CH_3 + \text{non-ionic } Cl \\ Globulin \end{cases}'.$$

Whenever by dilution with water the globulin is removed mecha-
nically from the sphere of action of the sodium, it ceases to be an
electro-negative ion and will commence to separate out, the
amount of separation depending on the amount of electrical change still carried by the larger aggregates.

Another explanation which is also possible, owing to the
amphoteric nature of albuminous compounds, is that the globulin
forms a complex ion with either the sodium kat-ion or with the
chlorine an-ion, according to the formulae

$$[Na' +]Cl + globulin]' \text{ or } [Na + globulin]' + [Cl]'$$

You may ask what right have we to consider protoplasm in
the same light as a salt? It was pointed out above that we may
isolate from protoplasm by its hydrolysis a number of fatty and
aromatic amino-acids, and therefore it is necessary to study
shortly what power these substances have of forming salt-like
combinations.

Strecker seems to have been the first to advance the view
that amino-acids fix metals by their COOH radical, while they
bind acids by the NH_2 group, and the same conclusion has been
arrived at by Bredig, Winkelblech, and Walker, who have studied
amino-acids in the light of physical chemistry. Bredig uses the
term amphoteric electrolytes for any substance «which may split
off, or unite with, H' and OH' ions, or, in other words, any substance which can play the part of an acid towards a base or that

of a base towards an acid. According to this definition, water is an amphoteric electrolyte because its hydrogen-atom H and its hydroxyl-radical OH may be converted into the chemically active ions $H^{\cdot}$ and OH' whenever water comes into contact whith certain salts, as will be shown more fully later. Alcohols $(C_nH_{2n+1}.HO)$ are also amphoteric electrolytes. Thus $(C_nH_{2n+1}.OH)$ can unite with sodium according to the equation $(C_nH_{2n+1}.O)-H+Na=C_nH_{2n+1}.ONa+H$, when the alcohol remainder $(C_nH_{2n+1}.O)'$ plays the part of an acid, the feeble kat-ion $H^{\cdot}$ being replaced by the strong kat-ion sodium, $Na^{\cdot}$. On the other hand, the hydroxyl-group OH may be replaced by a stronger an-ionic radical, such as a chlorine-ion; thus $C_nH_{2n+1}.OH'+H^{\cdot}Cl'=C_nH_{2n+1}.Cl+H_2O$. This behaviour of alcohols depends on the presence of the OH radical, and it will readily be seen that other compounds which contain this OH radical will behave analogously. Such OH compounds are, for example, serin and all phenols, $<\;\;\;>OH$. Alcohols differ, however, from ordinary hydroxyl compounds, as they only form alcohol-salts in the absence of water. These alcohol-salts on coming into contact with water dissociate hydrolytically, because water is hydrolysed by alcohol-salts.

The simultaneous presence of acid and of basic radicals in one and the same molecule as occurring in all amino-acids must of necessity lead to a weakening of the acid or basic characters of the molecule towards other individual molecules, and must also set up within the amphoteric molecule a tendency towards «internal salt-formation», by which expression we mean that the acid and the basic radicals of an amphoteric electrolyte will tend to mutually satisfy one another. Whenever this tendency becomes an accomplished fact, then the previously open-chain compound is converted into a «ringcompound». Thus

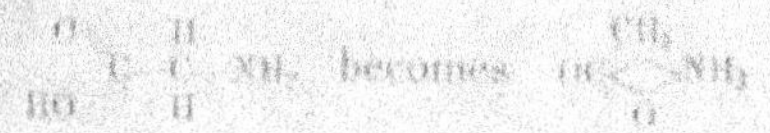

$$
\begin{array}{ccc}
O & H \\
\diagdown & | \\
C\;\;\;C-NH_2 & \text{becomes} & H_2C\diagup^{CH_2}_{\diagdown}NH_2 \\
\diagup & | & O \\
HO & H \\
\end{array}
$$

Chemically active glycocoll becomes chemically inactive glycocoll.

While glycocoll is in this inactive state it forms a true pseudo-acid-pseudo-basic compound; in other words, it cannot play the part of an-ion or that of kat-ion till the ring-like compound is re-converted into an open-chain. This change can only be brought about by subjecting the pseudo-acid-pseudo-basic molecule to the influence of ions. If active or inactive glycocoll is brought into contact with a strong acid, such as hydrochloric acid, then glycocoll-hydrochloride is formed:

$$\begin{matrix} O & & H & & & & O & & H & \\ & C & - & C-NH_2 + HCl = & & & & C & - & C-NH_3Cl \\ HO & & H & & & & HO & & H & \end{matrix}$$

while with sodium hydrate it forms sodium glycocollate and water:

$$\begin{matrix} O & & H & & & & O & & H & \\ & C & - & C-NH_2 + NaOH = & & & & C & - & C-NH_2 + H_2O \\ HO & & H & & & & NaO & & H & \end{matrix}$$

The proximity to or the remoteness from one another of the acid and basic radicals in the amphoteric amino-acid determines the ease with which an internal salt is made and unmade. As most of the normally occurring mono-amino-acids are α-compounds in which the basic NH_2-group is as close to the acid COOH-group as possible, it follows that the length of the primary chain does not much interfere with the internal salt-formation as long as only one NH_2 radical and one COOH radical is present:

$$\begin{matrix} CH_2 & \qquad\qquad & CH.CH_2.CH.CH_2.CH_3 \\ OC\langle\rangle NH_3 & \qquad\qquad & OC\langle\rangle NH_3 \\ O & \qquad\qquad & O \end{matrix}$$

Glycocoll. Leucin.

It is different, however, when two NH_2 and one COOH groups are present, or two COOH-groups and one NH_2 as in the case of the mono-amino-di-carboxylic and di-amino-mono-carboxylic acids.

The last point to be considered is the relative strength of the acid and the basic radicals in the amphoteric amino-acids. If the carboxyl-group COOH is replaced by the much more strongly acid sulphonic radical SO_3, then the basic character of the NH_2-group may be diminished to such an extent as practically not to make itself felt at all. This holds good, for example, in the case of sulphanilic acid, $C_6H_4(NH_3)(SO_2O)$. On the other hand, the basic character of the NH_2-group may be strengthened by the introduction of alkyl-radicals (methyl, CH_3; ethyl, C_2H_5) till it is 10 to 20 times stronger than ammonia (Winkelblech). The acid character of the COOH radical may hereby be overcome so completely as to prevent the latter from acting as an acid radical, at least at the ordinary room-temperature. Thus betain develops acid characters only at zero-temperature (Davidson). Glycocoll, sarcosin, and betain are in descending order less and less acid:

$$CO{<}{\overset{CH_2}{\underset{O}{>}}}NH_2 \qquad OC{<}{\overset{CH_2}{\underset{O}{>}}}NH.CH_3 \qquad OC{<}{\overset{CH_2}{\underset{O}{>}}}NH.CH_3.$$

Glycocoll   Sarcosin   Betain

The great inhibiting effect of the amino-group NH_2 on the carboxyl-group COOH is well seen by comparing acetic acid with amino-acetic acid or glycocoll. Thus $\frac{1}{25}$ normal acetic acid, dissociating only to the extent of 2 per cent. is 500,000 times more strongly acid than is amino-acetic acid, while according to Winkelblech the ratios of the acidity to the basicity of certain amino-acids are as follows:

	Acidity to basicity		Acidity to basicity
Aspartic acid	53 millions to 1	Asparagin	3000:1
a-amino-benzoic acid	4 millions to 1	Alanin	250:1
p	2.6 millions to 1	Glycocoll	120:1
m	1.5 millions to 1	Leucin	115:1
		Sarcosin	72:1

The most remarkable property of amino-acids is their strong hydrolysis, which means that the salts which amino-acids form with other acids or bases are very readily broken up by the ions of water. If a strong base is linked to a strong acid—if, for example, equivalent amounts of hydrochloric acid and of caustic soda are dissolved in water — then the acid hydrogen-ion of the HCl unites with the alkaline hydroxyl-ion of the NaOH to form neutral water, while the sodium- and the chlorine-ions form a neutral salt. In this case the negative chlorine-ions and the positive sodium-ions possess a great electro-affinity for one another, and therefore they do not unite with either the feeble, acid hydrogen-ions or the feeble, alkaline hydroxyl-ions of the water. But if, instead of two such strong radicals as sodium and chlorine, there be present one feeble radical, e. g. an amino-acid, in combination with a strong acid or a strong base, then the strong radical will not join up with the amino-acid, which is a more feeble radical than are the ions of water, but will combine with one of the ions of the water.

Generally speaking, any amphoteric electrolyte H.R.OH will

form, according to Walker, the ions H, OH, HR, and ROH, while the non-ionised portion must be either in the state of a hydrate $H\cdot R\cdot OH$ or that of an anhydride R. Therefore an equilibrium in the solution depends on the factors

$$\ddot{H} \quad OH \quad ROH \quad \dot{OH} \quad HROH \quad R$$

In working with amino-acids and with albumins it is necessary to constantly keep the salt-forming power of these substances before our mind's-eye. Glycocoll, being the simplest amino-acid, is therefore taken as a type.

Normal Glycocoll, $NH_2.CH_2.COOH$.—Winkelblech assumes that a watery solution of glycocoll contains 99.967 per cent. of hydryated but non-dissociated molecules

$$\begin{array}{ll} \text{Normal glycocoll.} & \text{Hydrated glycocoll.} \end{array}$$

while the minimal remainder is made up of a few ions and of non-hydrated glycocoll molecules. He explains the neutral reaction of a watery solution of glycocoll as being due to the want of dissociation of the hydrated amino-acid. Although then the presence of glycocoll leads to a union of the water-ions with the amino-acid, there is no hydrolytic dissociation of the newly-formed compounds. A hydrated amino-acid does not dissociate, because both the acid and basic radicals are very feeble.

Walker and I believe that the glycocoll molecules in watery solutions either form internal salts or that they unite in pairs, in such a way that the acid radical of one molecule links on to the basic radical of a second molecule:

Whatever change an amino-acid undergoes, whether it form a ring-like compound on becoming an internal salt, or whether it form double molecules, or whether it become hydrated, or whether it unite with acids, the originally trivalent nitrogen always becomes pentavalent.

Glycocoll Hydrochloride, $ClH.N.CH_2.COOH$ by hydrolysis, sets free neutral glycocoll $H.N.CH_2.COOH$ and hydrochloric acid, which then dissociates into the ions $H + Cl'$. The solution reacts strongly acid, owing to the hydrogen-ions, and it conducts the electric current mostly as hydrochloric acid, and to a very slight extent as the hydrochloride of glycocoll.

Glycocollate of Sodium, $H.N.CH_2.COONa$, by hydrolysis to neutral glycocoll and sodium hydrate are set free. The latter dissociates electrolytically into OH' and Na' ions. The solution has a strongly alkaline reaction, owing to the hydroxyl-ions, and it conducts the current mostly as sodium hydrate, and to a very slight extent as sodium glycocollate.

In connection with the union of amino-acids with carbondioxide Siegfried has made the following observation, which is of the greatest physiological importance:—

On saturating a mixture consisting of equal volumes of equinormal solutions of glycocoll and barium-hydroxide, an alkaline solution is obtained which remains clear when CO_2 is passed through it, and this continues to be the case till for each volume of glycocoll nearly two volumes of equivalent baryta water have been added. The solution so obtained gives off barium carbonate slowly on standing and quickly on boiling. Analogous results are obtained on substituting for glycocoll: i-alanin, l-leucin, sarcosin, phenyl-glycocoll, aspartic acid, glutaminic acid or asparagin, and on replacing barium-hydroxide by calcium or sodium hydroxide, and finally on substituting for CO_2 sodium carbonate.

Analyses of the compounds which glycocoll, i-alanin, l-leucin, sarcosin, and phenyl-glycocoll form with calcium-hydroxide and CO_2 have shown that these amino-acids must contain the radical

$$R-N\begin{matrix}H\\ \vert\\ COOH\end{matrix}\qquad R-N\begin{matrix}H\\ \diagdown COO\end{matrix}\qquad CH_2-N\begin{matrix}H\\ \diagdown COO\end{matrix}$$
$$COOH\qquad\qquad COO-Ca\qquad\qquad COO-Ca$$

Carbamino-acid radical.   lime-salt of salt.   calcium carbamino-acetate or calcium glycocoll-carbonate.

that is, the normal lime salts of the hitherto unknown dibasic carbamino acids of the glycocoll series. These compounds are therefore formed by the amphoteric amino-acids, simply adding CO_2, which thereby becomes de-ionised.

Quite analogous to the amino-acids behave the peptones, crystalline serum-albumin and dialysed horse serum. Siegfried points out that the anion of CO_2 in the blood appears in a new light, especially in connection with the hypothesis of Setschenow as to the conversion of serum-albumin into carbo-albumin by the action of CO_2, and also in connection with the carbo-haemoglobin of Bohr.

The double nature of amino-acids, *i.e.* to act either as acids or as bases, is interfered with as soon as one of NH_2 or COOH radicals is bound up. Curtius and Göbel have shown that glycin-ester, $H_2N.CH_2.COOC_2H_5$, and E. Fischer that other amino-acid esters are strong bases (as already mentioned in connection with sarcosin and betain); Schiff, on the other hand, found methylene-compounds to be acids, as the amino-radical is joined to formaldehyde, thus alanin is approximately neutral, while methylene-alanin is strongly acid:—

$$
\begin{array}{ll}
CH_3 & CH_3 \\
| & | \\
CH.NH_2 & CH.N=CH_2 \\
| & | \\
COOH & COOH \\
\text{Alanin} & \text{methylene-alanin}
\end{array}
$$

The presence of a second NH_2 or COOH group does not alter the general character of an amino-acid, but the basic character predominates in lysin, and the acid character in glutaminic acid, but notwithstanding this the latter can act as a base, for it forms chlorides.

Albumins behave in exactly the same way as do the amino-acids. According to Sjöqvist, Cohnheim, Cohnheim and Krieger, Erb, Bugarszky and Liebermann, and von Rohrer, albumins react as bases towards acids, being in some cases even more basic than the amino-acids. According to von Rohrer albumins are about 500 times more basic than is distilled water, and according to Sjöqvist about 71.2 more feeble than is anilin. With acids they form salts which undergo great hydrolysis.

Different albumins differ not only in their capacity for binding acids, but give different curves, when these are so constructed as to show that dissociation depends not only on the concentration but also on the excess of the acid. If a weaker acid be taken instead of hydrochloric acid, then the dissociation becomes even more marked.

Albumins behave quite analogously when they combine with bases. Bugarszky and Liebermann and Spiro and Pemsel have shown that sodium albuminate exhibits marked and varying hydrolysis. One essential difference exists, however, between albumins and the simple amino-acids: the albumins are pluri-acid bases and pluri-basic acids.

The behaviour of albumins towards salts will have to engage our attention next. Spring was the first to point out the importance of the mobility of ions, for on comparing solutions having the same conductivity (chlorides of K, Na, Rb, Li, Cs, NH_4) he found that they produced flocculation in the order of the mobility of their ions, except in the case of lithium chloride, which takes much less time to coagulate than does the potash salt, because lithium chloride undergoes hydrolysis and thereby gives rise to the formation of hydrogen-ions, which possess the greatest mobility, and this has been confirmed by Posternak.

Other interesting points discovered by Posternak were that the same acid radical produces in different salts different effects:—

HCl	NH_4Cl	KCl	NaCl
0·388	0·385	0·389	0·395

and that the same acid which in dilute strengths favours solution, causes precipitation when it is concentrated. This fact is attributed to a change in the electrical conductivity, thus

Strength of HCl	Molecular concentration	Conductivity
1/1000	0·0270	0·85
1·475/1000	0·185	0·84

In the first case the quotient $\dfrac{\text{dissociated molecules}}{\text{non-dissociated molecules}} = 19$, while in the second case it is 6.

Ordinary albumins being electro-negative are coagulated, according to Hofmeister and Pauli, by kat-ions in the following order:—

$$Li > Na > K > NH_4 > Mg$$

while the electro-negative an-ions tend to prevent coagulation in this order:

$$H > SO_4 > PO_4 > citrate > acetate > Cl > NO_3 > Br > I > CNS$$

Posternak has now observed the very interesting fact that if the reserve-material of the seeds of Picea dissolved in 1:1000

HCl be taken, that the order of the above salts is inverted, the electro-positive albumin is now precipitated by an-ions in this order:

$$CNS'>I'>Br'>NO_3'>Cl'> \text{acetate}$$

while the coagulation-inhibiting kat-ions follow in this order:

$$Mg''>NH_4'>K'>Na'$$

This phenomenon is interesting in connection with the phenomena exhibited by heat-coagulated albumin, which may behave either as a kat-ion or as an an-ion. Pauli has also drawn attention to the fact that the above order, in which salts precipitate electro-negative albumins, is the same as that in which they prevent the imbibition of water by gelatine-plates and in which they increase the melting point of gelatine.

Pauli has carefully investigated the effect which is produced on egg-white by the addition of the neutral salts of the alkalies and of magnesium. In the first instance he confirms Schäfer's observation that two salts in combination will do what one salt by itself is unable to do, for if potassium or sodium chloride and sodium acetate be used in such strengths as not to cause coagulation, they will on being mixed give rise to coagulation, and $KCl + NaC_2H_3O_2$ will produce a greater effect than if $NaCl + NaC_2H_3O_2$ are used. In the former case the kat-ion is different in the two salts while in the latter case they are the same. The dibasic magnesium sulphate+ the monobasic sodium chloride also augment mutually their coagulating efficiency.

If the coagulating values of a series of kat-ions are indicated by $f, f', f'', \ldots$ and the inhibiting values of a number of an-ions by $h, h', h'' \ldots$, then by combining electrolytes the three following states are possible:

$$\sum f, f', f'', \ldots \gtreqless \sum h, h', h'', \ldots$$

which means that it is possible to add to a solution of a coagulating electrolyte other electrolytes which either increase or diminish or leave unaltered the coagulating power of the first electrolyte.

In the following table Pauli has arranged the kat-ions in ascending order from left to right, magnesium being the feeblest and lithium the strongest kat-ion, while the anions are so arranged that the one with the fullest inhibiting power, namely, fluorine, comes first, while the strongest inhibitor, namely, thiocyanate, comes last.

Kations → Anions ↓	Mg	NH₄	K	Na	Li
Fluoride	[illegible]	[illegible]	[illegible]	[illegible]	[illegible]
Sulphate	[illegible]	[illegible]	[illegible]	[illegible]	[illegible]
Phosphate	[illegible]	[illegible]	[illegible]	[illegible]	[illegible]
Citrate	[illegible]	[illegible]	[illegible]	[illegible]	[illegible]
Tartrate	[illegible]	[illegible]	[illegible]	[illegible]	[illegible]
Acetate	[illegible]	[illegible]	[illegible]	[illegible]	[illegible]
Chloride	[illegible]	[illegible]	[illegible]	[illegible]	[illegible]
Nitrate	[illegible]	[illegible]	[illegible]	[illegible]	[illegible]
Chlorate	[illegible]	[illegible]	[illegible]	[illegible]	[illegible]
Bromide	[illegible]	[illegible]	[illegible]	[illegible]	[illegible]
Iodide	[illegible]	[illegible]	[illegible]	[illegible]	[illegible]
Thiocyanate	[illegible]	[illegible]	[illegible]	[illegible]	[illegible]

It will be seen from the table that the feeble precipitating power of magnesium and ammonium is already interfered with by the acetates and chlorides, while potassium is not affected by nitrates, and so on.

The criticism which I have to make Pauli's very important investigations on the salting out of albumins, which are fully detailed elsewhere [1], are that he has not taken into account that the addition of a solid soluble salt to the solution of a second salt must render the salt already in solution more concentrated, because it has to abstract water before it can pass into solution itself. Pauli has further assumed throughout that the salt only act upon one another, and not also on the albumin. If we consider what effects, especially the halogen salts, have in preventing, for example, the setting of gelatine, we must bear in mind that an analogous change may very well be produced in egg white, and that for this reason in the above table the iodides and thyocyanates have apparently so strong an inhibiting action on all kat-ions. The formation of double salts has also not been taken into account, nor has sufficient attention been paid to the amphoteric character of the albumin. That, finally, so called

---

[1] Mann, *Chemistry of Proteids*, chap. 8.

"neutral" salts are in reality not neutral, but are composed of
ions in which either the negative or the positive electro-affinity preponderates has already been explained.

The Structure of Protoplasm.

Contemplating organised nature what strikes me most is its
great stableness as compared with the unstableness of inorganised
matter. This view may at first seem paradoxical, but is never-
theless true. If we bring $NaCl$, KNO_3 and H_2O together, even
assuming that the water remains passive, we shall have $NaCl$,
KNO_3, $NaNO_3$, KCl and the ions Na, K, Cl, NO_3, which
means that many of the original $NaCl$ and KNO_3 molecules have
lost their individuality. It is different with protoplasm, for as
long as it is living it possesses the power of attracting or shutting
out other units according to the special characteristics which it
has acquired by evolution. The fundamental characteristic of
protoplasm is its colloidal nature, which means that it is composed of very large aggregates each of which has only a unit
charge of either $+$ or $-$ electricity. Diagrammatically an ordinary electrolyte and a colloidal electrolyte may be represented in
this way.

$$\left[X_3\right]^{+}\ \text{or} \qquad\qquad \left[X_{100000}\right]^{+}\ \text{or}$$

ordinary electrolyte   colloidal electrolyte

What leads to the formation of colloidal matter?

There is one factor which we may assume to be constant,
namely, our solvent water. When water comes into contact with
different salts, we find that the radicals which go to form the
salt, possess the power of becoming ionised to different de-
grees.

The greater the power of a certain radical to become either
a kat-ion or an an-ion the greater will also be its influence on
other radicals, because its chemical power is in direct ratio to
its capacity of becoming ionised. The less its power of forming ions the more will it tend to unite with other units similar
to or identical with itself, because the least difference of potential must always be developed in a community of identical
units.

We thus have on the one hand such chemically exceedingly
active substances as the halogen and oxy-acid salts of the alkalis

[e.g. KCl KNO₃, K₂SO₄] and on the other hand the chemically inactive paraffins [CH₄, C₂H₆]. While the former because of their great ionic power in the presence of water will always interact with other active units and thus lose their individuality, paraffins on the other hand will under the same circumstances remain inactive. It is to me exceedingly interesting to see how our most primitive ancestors, the paraffins, by evolution gave rise to alcohols, aldehydes and acids, and thereby gradually acquired the power of interacting with the environment.

$$
\begin{array}{ccc}
\quad H \quad H & \quad H \quad\; OH & \quad NH_2 \;\; OH \\
H-C-C-H & H-C=C & H-C-C \\
\quad H \quad H & \quad H \quad\; O & \quad H \quad\;\; O \\
\text{ethane} & \text{acetic acid} & \text{glycocoll}
\end{array}
$$

While an ordinary mineral acid such as hydrochloric acid in semi-normal strengths is dissociated into ions to the extent of 100 per cent., acetic acid is dissociated 3 per cent., and amino-acetic acid or glycocoll forms only a few ions. Thus we have an inert compound, the paraffin, become a chemically active compound, namely, acetic acid, and the latter changed into a chemically less active substance, namely, glycocoll. There is however, one great difference between acetic acid and glycocoll, for the former can only interact with kat-ions, such as sodium, while the latter interacts with both kat-ions and an-ions being amphoteric in nature. It is this very property which also leads to the formation of internal salts, namely, to the pseudo-acid-pseudo-basic compounds. Internal salt formation satisfies the affinities of the compound in question for negative and positive radicals, and thereby safeguards it to a great extent against an inimical environment containing free acid or basic groups, as I pointed out in my *Physiological Histology* in 1902, p. 27. This view has been confirmed in a remarkable way by the researches of Wakelin Barratt [1], who found that Paramaecia may unite with small quantities of acid and larger quantities of alkalies without losing their neutral reaction or power of surviving.

Attention has already been drawn to the fact that a whole

---

[1] J. O. Wakelin Barratt, *Die Wirkung r. Säuren u. Basen auf lebende Paramaecien; Zeitsch. f. allgem. Physiol.* 4, 1904 (1904) and 1906; *The Reaktion des Protopl. in ihrem Verhältnis zur Chemotaxis*, p. 87.

series of fatty and aromatic acids exists in protoplasm, and as each of these possesses only feeble acid or basic characters owing to its amphoteric nature, the acids readily unite with one another and form thereby large colloidal aggregates, which in a chemical sense are slow to act, and thereby preserve their identity.

It must not, however, be assumed because protoplasm appears in many instances in the living condition homogeneous that therefore it is structureless, nor should we mistake appearances which have been produced by re-agents for normal structures

The chief conclusion I arrived at, in 1902, in my *Physiological Histology*, as far as fixing is concerned, was that histologists should beware of all fixing re-agents which are electrolytes, such as the salts of the heavy metals and acids, for all of these establish differences of potential and thereby lead to a more or less pronounced separation or dissolution of colloidal matter, according as to whether the more active ion has either the opposite or the same charge as that carried by the colloidal aggregates. I am convinced that many of the appearances which have been described as normal protoplasmic constituents are artefacts due to the action of electrolytes, but if we do not use electrolytes for fixing purposes, but employ non-electrolytes such as osmium tetroxide (OsO_4) or formaldehyde (OCH_2) dissolved in isotonic "normal" salt solutions, we will still find definite differentiations of the protoplasm. As non-electrolytes act by forming additive compounds, without setting up differences of potential, we have every right to suppose that structures which we may see after the use of aldehydes and osmium tetroxide have existed under living conditions.

Amongst the most readily recognized appearances in protoplasm, are the zymogen granules of gland cells. Granuleformation is in every respect identical with the formation of an emulsion; as in the case of milk (till the specific gravity factor makes itself felt) we have a balance between the size of the fat globules and the fatty acids and alkalies present, so in the cellplasm. If we assume a cell-plasm to have a definite acid and basic capacity, and the granules which are excreted by the nucleus to be either basic or acid in character (or by a subsequent change to become acid or basic), then the size of the granules and also their number will be determined by the amount of acidity or basicity of the cell-plasm. It has been pointed out that neutralisation of a number of charges on individual small units, will bring these units together into bigger aggregates, each of which will have its own charge as long as an ion having the opposite charge is present in the solvent, and this also holds good for the zymogen granules. To me a discharge of zymogen-granules by the cell means simply that by a chemical stimulus the difference of potential between the cell-plasm and the cell-granules becomes disturbed, in consequence of which the granule-phase becomes separated from the plasm-phase; as further all zymogen-granules in the cell-plasm are in an inactive state and in a rabbit remain so even after twenty-two days inanition, while the cell-phase is greatly reduced, we may say that the latter is the more changeable of the two phases, which again means that by an appropriate stimulus, such as the entrance of electrolytes into the cell, the cell-plasm will be made to become more colloidal, in consequence of which it will shrink and thereby force the granules to the surface of the cell.

The zymogen-granules I chose as a type of transient structure, for they are formed day after day only to be used up again in the general economy of the animal or plant, and under this heading come also reserve materials such as starch, glycogen, fatty compounds, &c.

As a type of a structure which is constant under certain definite conditions, we may take the fibrils of nerve-cells. We know that all nerve-phenomena are accompanied by definite changes in potential and we also know that such changes can only be due to chemical alteration in the plasma of which the various cell-processes are composed. It is exceedingly instructive that given one nerve-cell or a chain of nerve-cells they remain fibrillar only as long as they are and can be made use of. As soon as afferent impressions or stimuli cease to act on a nerve-cell and its processes, there occurs a disappearance of the fibrillar structure, showing that the fibrils are but the paths along which normally impulses are sent and also that stimulation is the cause of nerve-fibrils being formed. We have thus in the nerve-cell a mechanism so constituted that irritation (stimulation) leads to coagulation along definite tracts, which allow change set up at one end to travel till it reaches the other end.

Of recent years a great deal of attention has been paid to

intra-cellular channels, as found in nerve-cells and various gland-cells (crescents of Gianuzzi, parietal-cells of the stomach, liver-cells, &c.). It may be that all these passages are excretory channels, or that some may serve for the absorption of food material. There is *a priori* nothing against the permanence of such intra-protoplasmic ducts, especially if we have to do with excretory tubes, for if we commence with a non-differentiated plasma, capable of reacting to electrolytes, it will follow, if the secreta be at all chemically active, that they must induce a coagulation of the plasma which surrounds them. Whether the cytoplasm so coagulated will remain coagulated, till the next time excreta are to be got rid of, or will become again homogeneous, is determined by the amount of coagulation the cell-plasm has undergone, and by the presence or absence of electrolytes capable of undoing the coagulation produced by the secreta or excreta. Very good examples of such intra-cellular tracts produced by nuclear substances diffusing into the cell-plasm will be found in the papers by Goldschmidt, who follows R. Hertwig in calling the structures in question, Chromidial-apparatus. It is quite impossible to enter into all the various differentiations which have been described in connection with protoplasm, and therefore I shall limit myself, as far as Bütschli's statements are concerned, in saying that in many instances there is undoubtedly a honey-comb-like structure, which seems to have been devised to bring about a ready diffusion of food material and of gases.

In this connection it may be pointed out that in all animals and in most plants the stability of the cytoplasm depends on the presence of an ample supply of oxygen. It is not necessary to assume, as is generally done, that the oxygen serves only for purposes of oxidation, that it is always used up; for just as haemoglobin in the presence of oxygen takes up the latter and becomes oxyhaemoglobin, so do I believe that many compounds, especially in the nucleus, are kept constantly in an oxidised state, and that the oxygen-bond forms a link in the chain of chemical compounds to which I shall refer later.

Into the question of the centrosome and the part it plays during mitosis, it is necessary to go somewhat more fully. After

[1] R. Goldschmidt, *Zoolog. Jahrbuch* (Zoology), 21, Heft 1, 1905, and *Arch. f. Protisten-kunde*, 5, 1905 [illegible].

Sachs had explained division of the cell as depending on centres of attraction dividing the nucleus between them. Fol in 1873 [1] described the fibrils which pass outwards from what is now known as the centrosphere, and compared the appearances to the picture presented by iron-filings which arrange themselves round the two poles of a magnet. The same conception has been developed by Giard [2], who explains the formation of the spindle as due to physico-chemical phenomena and the establishment of electrical or electro-magnetical poles in the nucleus; by Ziegler, who made a magnetic model [3]; by Gallardo [4], who made an electro-static model by using a suspension of quinine-sulphate in oil of turpentine, and showed «that the introduction of a third terminal put to earth produced a deviation of some of the fibres from the belly of the spindle to itself—the figure being, in fact, a striaster, such as sometimes occurs in dividing cells [5]»; by Hartog [6], who speaks of the cytoplasmic figure of the dividing-cell being a strain-figure, under the action of a dual force, analogous to magnetism, and still more to statical electricity; he calls the force at play «mitokinetic force». Hartog, on the strength of his magnetic models [7], finds that the spindle-fibres, astral rays, the outer limiting membrane of the cytoplasm, the nuclear wall, and the free chromosomes along the cell-spindle, must all possess a high permeability to mitokinetism as compared with the other structures of the cell. «A spindle figure can only be obtained in a field with the two unlike poles of a dual force ...; as the diffusion, osmosis, and surface-tension phenomenon are of similar character at the two poles of a cell, they cannot be the forces involved in the spindle».

I shall revert to this later.

Darbishire [8] says: «A consideration of the ontogeny and phylogeny of the centrosome seems to point to the conclusion that amphiasters, spindles, and fibres have no actual existence,

[1] Fol, Die erste Entwicklung des Gerrostenier; Jenaische Zeitschrift, vol. 7.

[2] Giard, Bull. Sc. 7, 258 (1879).

[3] Ziegler, Untersuchungen u. d. Zelltheilung; Verh. Deutsch. Zool. Ges. (1897).

[4] Gallardo, Essai d'interprétation des figures karyokinétiques; Ann. Mus. Buenos Aires (1896), and Interpretacion dinamica de la division celular (1909).

[5] Quoted from Marcus Hartog's paper, Proc. Roy. Soc. 76, 357 (1905).

[6] M. Hartog, Compt. rend., June 20th, 1904, and Proc. Roy. Soc. 76, 548 (1905).

[7] Made with glycerine, gelatine or balsam (which two later are allowed to set), and with magnetic oxide of iron (Fe_3O_4).

[8] A. D. Darbishire, The Centrosome, Trans. Oxf. Univ. Junior Scient. Club, 1905.

but are the track of the influence which the centrosome or its homologue exercises on the chromosomes, owing to the arrangement of the constituents of protoplasm along the lines of that influence, like iron-filings in a magnetic field... The word influence is used because it is sufficiently vague to prevent the reader from thinking that one had any conception of what it is. Darbishire agrees with Boveri in the views expressed by the latter in his book «On the Centrosome» that «the binary division of the cell is brought about by the binary division of the centrosomes, and also that the abnormal, multiple spindles seen in cases of polyspermy (Henneguy) are due to the abnormal number of centrosomes present. Hertwig's view, that the multipolarity of figures is caused by a superabundance of chromatic material, Rabl's conception that centrosomes are pulled out passively by a bipolarity of the cell, or Heidenhain's notion that centrosomes go passively to predestined places in the cell, are also not tenable. At the end of his paper Darbishire gives my views, which I shall state later.

Lillie (*) has likewise applied magnetic forces to explain the factors by which chromatic filaments and chromosomes become arranged in definite patterns during mitosis. By stringing small cubical pieces of cork at distances of about six millimetres along a delicate silk filament, and piercing the corks with small, similarly oriented, magnetised needles, floating this contrivance on water, and subjecting it to the influence of a magnet, he obtained the same appearances as are seen during the mono-spirem stages of karyokinesis, while the aster-stage could readily be demonstrated by stringing the magnets along a number of flexible wires capable of being bent into any desired shape.

During the last four years (†) I have taught that the centrosomes play the part of electrolytes by coagulating the cell-plasm or nuclear sap, as the case may be. As coagulation of a colloidal substance means that the colloidal particles aggregate to form bigger units, coagulation is equivalent to a contraction of the colloidal matter. If the colloidal particles possess adhesiveness, coagulation will produce an elastic system, arranged either in the form of a foam, or a net, or filaments, and the greater

---

(*) Ralph S. Lillie, _Biological Bull._ 8, 193 (1905).
(†) See end of Darbishire's paper.

the amount of coagulation, the greater will also be the contraction of the coagulated material. When a change is produced in colloids by the action of electrolytes having an electrical load opposite to that carried by the colloid which we are enabled to see with the help of the microscope, we speak of structure; if the change is of such a nature as not to be resolved by the microscope, we say the substance is homogeneous. By coagulating a colloid we may produce a system doing an enormous amount of work, provided there are fixed points to which the coagulating mass can attach itself. It is very instructive to take two similar vessels, containing an equal amount of globulin solution made by extracting ground lentils with 5 per cent NaCl, to add an equal amount of acetic acid sufficient to cause coagulation, and finally, to leave one vessel undisturbed while the other is shaken for one minute. In the former the coagulated material will separate out quickly, while in the second vessel, owing to the original system having been broken down, there are no fixed points to serve as attachments of the coagulating material, and in consequence of this the coagulated globulin separates out very slowly, owing to the original points from which the coagulation started having been disturbed; instead of having one contracting system there are now many systems.

In a cell about to divide the increased activity of the centrosome is an index of electrolytic changes taking place in it. Increased chemical activity always means that by the influence of some other chemically more active radical or ion there is induced in, or has been transferred to, the original inactive or sluggish matter the power of diffusion, which expresses itself in a lowering of the surface tension. In consequence of the latter a centrosome will divide and may do so completely, or the two daughter-centrosomes may for a time be still adhering to one another by a delicate bridge. The increased activity, called forth by electrolytes, by imparting the same electrical charge to the two centrosomes, will force them apart, and the centrosomes in their turn by liberating material which combines with the surrounding colloidal matter give rise to the formation of the spindle and the rays proceeding from the centrosphere. Continued action of the centrosomes on the cytoplasm or *vice versa* must lead to a contraction of the original fibrils formed in connection with the centrosome because of the increased coagulation, and must lead to a separation of the chromatin segments, and their migration towards the centrosomes if the latter are fixed points.

We have thus to explain the various changes set up in cytoplasm during glandular secretion, during mitosis and so on, on purely physico-chemical grounds. The different means by which coagulation may be set up I have fully discussed in my books on the *Theory of Histology* and the *Chemistry of Proteids*, and it will suffice now if I enumerate the headings: (1) Setting of colloidal solutions by lowering of the temperature; (2) Conglutination or aggregation by mechanical means owing to dissolved colloid passing spontaneously out of solution and forming delicate surface pellicles exhibiting many of the characteristic properties of solid matter, as thereby the total energy of surface tension becomes diminished [1]; (3) Coagulation due to alterations in the electrical tension between the colloid and its solvent; (4) Salting out of albuminous substances owing to an increase in the concentration of salts; (5) Precipitation of colloids due to a withdrawal of hydrogen-radicals of the CO·O—H and the hydroxyl-radicals of the oxy-acids and phenol-compounds; (6) Precipitation due to the removal of salts as in the case of globulins; (7) The formation of irreversible salts owing to metals, such as calcium or mercury having low dissociation-energies; (8) The formation of additive-compounds: the amino-acids uniting for example with aldehydes; (9) The «spontaneous» coagulation of albumins due to factors which are not yet fully recognised; (10) Coagulation by means of heat.

The osmotic properties of protoplasm have been so fully studied by Overton that his papers ought to be carefully read by everyone [2], and I have only to say that I fully agree with the conceptions put forward by him.

To me the protoplasmic structure means simply an equilibrium for the time being between colloidal aggregates which differ from one another in their constitution (and which are prevented from becoming inert or dead material by the presence of inorganic and organic electrolytes). Two important papers by Pauli [3] and Hofmeister [4] have also appeared dealing with protoplasm from the physico-chemical and the chemical points

---

[1] W. Ramsden, Proc. Roy. Soc. **72**, 156 (1903).

[2] E. Overton, *Ueber d. allg. osmotischen Eigenschaften d. Zelle, &c.; Vierteljahrsschrift d. Naturf. Ges. Zürich*, **40**, (1895) und **44**, 88 (1899); und *Zeitschr. f. physik. Chem.* **22**, 189 (1897).

[3] Pauli, *Der colloidale Zustand und die Vorgänge in der lebendigen Substanz; Braunschweig, Vieweg*, 1902.

[4] Hofmeister, *Die chemische Organisation der Zelle; Braunschweig, Vieweg*, 1901.

of view, and I have to content myself by drawing attention to them, with the exception of quoting one passage from Hofmeister: «Even now, we may say, that the contemplation of the cell as a machine working with chemical and physico-chemical means leads nowhere to problems which could compel us to assume other than known forces, and, as far as we can see, there is no reason for that resignation, which either expresses itself in an «ignorabimus» or in vitalistic deductions».

Definition of Protoplasm.

At the beginning of this paper Hugo von Mohl's reason for speaking of protoplasm was given. He conceived it to be the mother substance of the nucleus and the cell-envelopes. This conception is, however, no longer tenable. In my paper «What is Life?» I pointed out in 1898 (¹) that «organic individuals possess the power of creating around themselves a new environment, the cytoplasm, which has the following functions: (1) To elaborate possible inorganic or organic food substances and thereby to make them directly assimilable by the nucleus (chloroplasts and zymogen granules). (2) To protect the nucleus from deleterious influences outside the organic individual (as proved by the removal of the whole or greater part of the cytoplasm, invariably leading to the death of the nucleus). (3) To either attract food to the cell or to move the cell towards the food by means of the centrosomes which are to be regarded as special locomotor organs (viz. centrosomes in white blood corpuscles [M. Heidenhain], the basal globules at the base of cilia) (v. Lenhossék). (4) To prevent all inter-communication with the outer world by the formation of cysts (amœba) or callus on sieve plates (plants), whenever deleterious agencies are at work».

«Organic individuals, within physiological limits, are independent of chance, as the combination of compounds peculiar to each individual leads to the formation of a new environment consisting of complex carbon compounds, which in their turn by acting on the world at large so modify the latter as to make it directly assimilable by the nucleus. The nucleus in its turn forms its organic environment or cell-plasm by which it is kept in existence».

(¹) Mann, *Trans. Oxford University Junior Scient. Club*, 1899.

This conception was based on the researches of my pupil Lily Huie, who for the first time showed by definite experiments [1] that the nucleus is the organ for forming cytoplasm.

A typical gland-cell of the insectivorous plant Drosera rotundifolia contains in its resting condition a vacuolated cell-plasm with zymogen-granules, and a nucleus with large nucleolus and very scanty nuclear basophil chromatin. A similar cell, when examined 20 to 30 hours after feeding with egg-white, shows that the cell-plasm has mostly disappeared; that the nucleolus is also reduced to a mere shadow, while the basophil nuclear chromatin is enormously increased, having divided into 3 distinct chromatin segments. The same appearance may be obtained within one hour if the cell be fed on peptone. Two to three days after feeding the nucleus is engaged in re-building the cytoplasm, while seven days after feeding the cell-plasm has been completely reformed and the nucleus has assumed again the appearance it shows during the resting condition.

In conclusion let me give an abstract taken from my book on the *Chemistry of Proteids*.

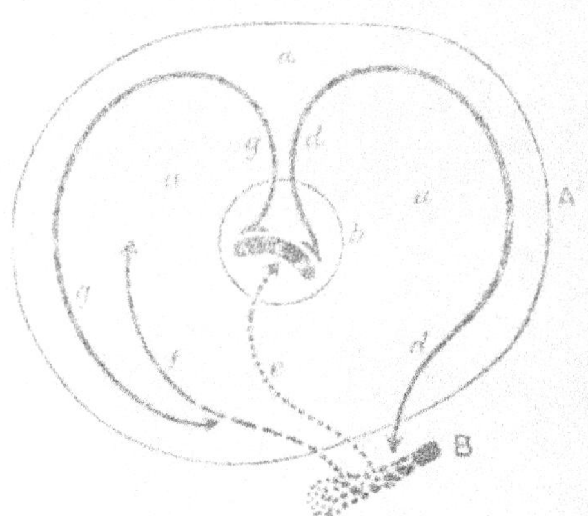

"We have to distinguish between the origin of organic compounds and that of life. To be able to make marsh-gas, alcohols, aldehydes, acids, amino-acids, peptids, peptones, and albumin, however great an achievement in itself, is not the same as making

[1] Huie, *Quart. Journ. Micr. Sc.* 39, pp. 387 and 42, 203 (1899).

life. To many people a living cell consists of «protoplasm», a substance they imagine to be one exceedingly complex body. They do not realise that in a cell we have a not very large number of comparatively simple compounds which only collectively form the protoplasm. What constitutes life, is the presence of a number of such «organic» compounds, capable of mutually re-acting upon one another, and thereby giving rise to new compounds, which cannot re-act chemically with the mother-substances from which they are derived, but which by inter-acting with new radicals give rise to a cycle of events.

«In the above diagram I have endeavoured to make my meaning clear. From the nucleus two arrows pass outwards: the one on the right represents the formation of "extra-cellular" zymogen granules, which have the function of ionising extraneous chemical compounds in such a way as to make them available to the cell-individual. These enzymes change, for example, albumin into albumoses, peptones and amino-acids. The arrow on the left of the figure represents «intra-cellular» zymogens, the function of which is a constructive or de-ionising one; they bring about an aggregation of those amino-acids and peptone-like bodies which have been liberated from proteid-food by the extra-cellular enzymes. The aggregates so formed constitute the main bulk of the cell-plasm, and they are subsequently partly transformed by the activity of the nucleus into the extra-cellular and intra-cellular zymogens already alluded to. The cycle of events just described is what we call life. Cessation of life, or death, will be produced either by the inability to procure food, which is necessary to counterbalance the wear and tear necessitated by the conversion of one chemical compound into another one, and this amounts to death by starvation, or secondly, by the inability of the nucleus to digest the food, and so make it available to the individual cell. In addition to these two kinds of physiological death, we have another form due to violence, as, for example, by the application of excessive heat or cold or inorganic (corrosive sublimate, &c.) or organic (bacteria) poisons.

«What must be the ultimate aim of chemical biology is to establish the sequence of events in the cycle from simple to more complex substances and the disintegration of the latter for the purpose of liberating energy and of so acting on other chemical compounds as to make those available to each individual cell.

«If we want to proceed systematically and not by guesswork

we have to pursue histological research based on a sound knowledge of chemistry and physics, and thus we shall be able to
understand and to modify the events in the life-cycle, for we will
be able to accelerate and to slow down nuclear and cytoplasmic
activities. The importance of such research in connection with
cancer and all fevers cannot be over-estimated.»

As von Mohl's conception of the physiological function of the
nucleus is no longer tenable, let us discontinue the use of the
word «proto-plasm» and substitute for it the term «plasm».

Comptes rendus des séances

Présidence: M. Mattoso Santos

Sont présents: MM. Albrecht (Francfort s/M.), Benda (Berlin), Feyo e Castro (Lisbonne), Kanon (Kioto), Mlle. Loyez (Paris), Mann (Oxford), Mattoso Santos (Lisbonne), Parra (Mexico), Pinto de Magalhães (Lisbonne), Ramón y Cajal (Madrid), Romiti (Pisa), Silva Tavares (S. Fiel), Celestino da Costa (Lisbonne), M. Athias (Lisbonne).

Election du Bureau définitif:

M. Romiti propose que le Bureau provisoire reste définitif, ce qui est accepté par l'assemblée.

Le Président remercie et prononce l'allocution suivante:

Mesdames, Messieurs, chers collègues: Γνῶθι σε αὐτόν, si cette maxime résumait pour Thalès la suprême aspiration du savoir humain, tant de siècles après, nous devons encore répéter avec le philosophe de Milet, quoique dans un sens moins métaphysique, «Connais-toi toi-même.»

Et c'est par notre belle science qu'il faut commencer; c'est elle qui nous apprend comment se composent les machines, où se produit cette énergie si complexe dans la variabilité de ses manifestations morphologiques, physiologiques, psychiques, qu'on appelle la vie.

Certainement les conceptions d'un anthropomorphisme outré, qui pendant des siècles ont dérouté la science, se sont depuis longtemps effondrées. On n'étudie plus l'homme comme un microcosme, pour rapporter sur les êtres qui l'entourent tout ce que l'on y trouve; on rebrousse chemin: on part de ceux-ci pour arriver à celui-là. L'homme c'est toujours le but — connais-toi toi-même; mais, sous la continuelle poussée du travail scientifique, on a substitué à d'aussi vagues que fantastiques abstractions, l'analyse, maintes fois trop détaillée des faits, peut-être, mais, par contre, permettant d'appuyer sur des fondations solides et durables l'œuvre scientifique.

Des découvertes menèrent à de nouvelles recherches, d'où sortirent de nouvelles découvertes. Ce long et persistant travail d'analyse entassa une masse énorme de faits qu'il fallut classer.

De là des divisions et des subdivisions successives, des groupements qui s'arrogent parfois une indépendance qui commence à devenir gênante, quand on veut se placer à un point de vue plus élevé que le seul classement systématique, quoique nécessaire, des connaissances acquises.

Voilà pourquoi de tous les côtés se fait sentir le besoin d'un travail de rapprochement et de concentration.

De l'histologie à l'anatomie, passant par l'embryologie, on tient à faire l'histoire de l'apparition, du développement, des différenciations et des transformations des molécules vivantes.

On ne se contente plus de connaître la forme, la structure et les rapports de position des parties qui composent un être vivant, on s'enquiert de l'origine de ces parties, d'où et comment elles sont venues.

De la monère à l'homme, on demande quel est l'enchaînement de tous les êtres vivants; on se procure dans la phylogénèse ce qui dans l'ontogénèse a été abrégé ou sauté; on fouille dans la paléontologie à la recherche des anneaux qui manquent aux chaînes morphologiques.

De leur côté, les sciences morales et sociales, nous les voyons mettre largement à contribution l'ensemble des sciences anatomiques pour la résolution de leurs problèmes.

Mais que de lacunes à combler, que de vides à remplir!

Et cependant, combien de matériaux avez-vous déjà ajoutés, chers collègues, à ceux qu'ont amoncelés vos devanciers! Et vous voilà encore à l'œuvre, et vous venez aujourd'hui continuer votre besogne dans notre ville, dans notre Lisbonne, flattée de voir siéger dans son enceinte le XV Congrès international de médecine, fière de vous recevoir.

Ces réunions sont pleines de charme. Elles rapprochent les membres de la grande famille scientifique, elles donnent de la cohésion aux efforts individuels, elles orientent notre tâche; elles nous rassemblent par un commun amour sous un même drapeau — celui de la science.

Soyez les bienvenus.

Avant de terminer, veuillez me permettre, Mesdames et Messieurs, de reporter un instant mes souvenirs vers celui qui, en ce moment, devrait vous souhaiter la bienvenue, vers le prof. Serrano, qu'une mort inattendue nous a enlevé.

Dès la constitution de la section d'anatomie de ce Congrès, un nom fut proposé pour en assumer la direction, celui du prof. Serrano. Nous ne pouvions tous qu'applaudir à un semblable choix. Il a consacré toute sa vie à l'étude de l'anatomie et se montra, jusqu'à la dernière heure, soucieux de la grandeur et du progrès de la science qu'il a tant aimée et à laquelle il a apporté le concours de son esprit éclairé et méthodique.

Son traité d'ostéologie humaine est là pour attester ses facultés de travail et d'examen, sa judicieuse critique et son grand savoir.

Appelé à lui succéder, je ne saurais invoquer en ma faveur auprès de vous que le grand désir de bien servir la science.

M. MATTOSO SANTOS propose ensuite les noms suivants pour la présidence d'honneur: MM. les prof. Anderson (Galway), Benda (Berlin), Eternod (Genève), Kamon (Kioto), Loewenthal (Lausanne), Mann (Oxford), Mitrophanow (Varsovie), Musgrave (St. Andrews), Paes Leme (Rio de Janeiro), Parra (Mexico), Ramón y Cajal (Madrid), Regaud (Lyon), Romiti (Pise), Stieda (Königsberg), Swale Vincent (Winnipeg), Waldeyer (Berlin), Warfvinge (Stockholm).

Présidence de M. ROMITI

M. ROMITI: Je remercie de tout mon cœur M. le président et le Bureau du Congrès de l'honneur de m'avoir compris parmi les présidents d'honneur de la section d'anatomie, et je suis bien honoré de pouvoir commencer les travaux de la section en donnant la parole à M. Cajal (de Madrid) pour faire sa communication.

Histogénèse des nerfs

Par M. RAMÓN Y CAJAL, Madrid

Il y a quelques années, à la suite des recherches de His, des nôtres, de celles de Retzius, Lenhossék, Kölliker, Harrison, etc., dominait presque sans conteste dans la science neurogénique la

doctrine monogéniste ou du développement continu des cylindres-axes des nerfs. En se basant sur les révélations concordan-
tes de la méthode de Golgi et des procédés ordinaires de coloration, ces auteurs soutinrent l'opinion que les dendrites et les expansions fonctionnelles des neurones tiraient leur origine de la
métamorphose et de l'accroissement du protoplasme d'un seul
élément nerveux embryonnaire, le *neuroblaste* de His; ils affir-
maient, en outre, que les cellules de Schwann apparaissant tardivement dans l'intérieur des cordons nerveux ne sont pas des neuroblastes périphériques émigrés, mais des éléments mésodermiques incapables de jouer aucun rôle dans la création des cylindres-axes, se bornant exclusivement à les protéger en élaborant
une gaine adventice. Cependant, en ce qui concerne l'origine de
ces éléments accessoires, il y avait des savants qui, tout en
admettant sans réserve la théorie de la continuité, acceptaient
aussi la nature ectodermique des cellules de revêtement (Lenhossék, Harrison, etc.)

Presque simultanément à l'apparition de la doctrine monogéniste commença aussi à se répandre une autre hypothèse à laquelle, malgré la faiblesse de ses preuves, se rangent actuellement un grand nombre d'histologistes. C'est la *théorie cellulaire*,
imaginée il y a longtemps par Balfour, Beard et Dohrn, puis re-
jetée par les embryologistes les plus autorisés et maintenant,
avec une profonde conviction, par des savants aussi compétents
que Bethe, Capobianco et Fragnito, Joris, Berta, O. Schultze,
Kohn, etc.

D'après cette conception les axons moteurs embryonnaires
seraient composés de chaînes de neuroblastes, c'est-à-dire, par
des corpuscules allongés et soudés par leurs bouts. C'est dans
l'intérieur du protoplasme de ces chapelets que se produiraient,
en vertu d'un processus de différenciation, les cylindres-axes;
tandis que, une fois le développement de la substance conductri-
ce achevé, les noyaux des chaînes cellulaires resteraient en place
pour devenir des corpuscules de Schwann (*lemnoblastes* de Lenhossék).

Cette hypothèse soulève de très graves objections quand on
veut l'appliquer à l'histogénèse de la moelle et autres centres nerveux; c'est ainsi que la plupart de ses adeptes s'en servent exclusivement pour éclairer le mécanisme de la formation des nerfs
périphériques.

Cependant, en dépit de toutes les difficultés, il y a aussi des

savants tels que Fragnito, Berta, Pighini, etc. qui admettent la
conception caténaire pour se rendre compte de l'apparition des
dendrites et des voies nerveuses centrales. A en croire ces auteurs, la cellule nerveuse adulte résulterait de la fusion et de la
transformation d'une colonie de neuroblastes, dont les noyaux fi-
niraient par être réabsorbés.

Enfin, on trouve encore les savants qui, se rangeant en principe à l'hypothèse caténaire, admettent, pour expliquer l'accroissement des neurones et la formation des prolongements protoplasmiques, l'intervention d'une sorte de blastème intercellulaire
continu, lequel se condenserait progressivement autour des neuroblastes de la substance grise (Sedgwick, Bethe, Joris, etc.).

Une telle discordance de solutions touchant un sujet aussi
important que celui de l'origine des nerfs et des prolongements
dendritiques, tient tout simplement à l'emploi de méthodes imparfaites absolument incapables de colorer sélectivement le protoplasme nerveux embryonnaire. De plus, par une aberration de
critérium très étonnante, ces auteurs ont laissé de côté, sans jus-
tification aucune, le seul moyen technique susceptible de nous
fournir des images nettes et décisives à l'égard des premières
phases de l'évolution embryologique: le procédé du chromate d'argent. Il est vrai que ce procédé est très délicat et qu'il faut, pour
y réussir, de la patience et de la persévérance; mais la valeur
d'un moyen technique ne se mesure pas par la commodité de
son application, mais par sa puissance analytique et la netteté
de ses révélations.

Étant donné cet état d'incertitude et d'anarchie d'idées, il
nous a paru qu'il y aurait quelque intérêt à étudier une autre
fois et scrupuleusement la question, à l'aide d'un nouveau procédé d'imprégnation déjà employé dans ce sujet par nous d'abord,
et puis par Berta et Fragnito. Nous voulons dire le procédé du nitrate d'argent réduit (formolé avec fixation préalable dans l'alcool), lequel colore assez énergiquement, depuis le 3e jour de
l'incubation chez le poulet, les neuroblastes et leurs expansions
dendritiques et cylindraxiles.

Déclarons d'abord que les recherches récentes que nous
avons entreprises chez les embryons d'oiseaux et de mammifères,
à l'aide de ce moyen analytique (ainsi qu'avec les procédés ordinaires), confirment pleinement la doctrine classique fondée sur
les révélations de la méthode de Golgi. En réservant pour un autre travail plus étendu la description détaillée avec figures des

résultats obtenus, nous nous bornerons ici à exposer sommairement les conclusions les plus importantes.

1. Dans les stades les plus précoces (peu avant le commencement du 3º jour de l'incubation chez le poulet) les neuroblastes se montrent dans nos préparations tels que His, nous et Lenhossék les avions décrits et figurés, c'est-à-dire sous la forme d'un corps pyriforme presque entièrement rempli par le noyau et pourvu d'un seul prolongement dirigé vers la périphérie: l'expansion primordiale ou cylindre-axe. C'est dans l'endroit du protoplasme donnant naissance à cet appendice et dans l'intérieur de l'axon même que s'initie la différenciation neuro-fibrillaire. C'est seulement plus tard, du 3º au 4º jour de l'incubation, qu'apparaîtra le réseau neuro-fibrillaire, très mince et fort pâle d'abord, du côté convexe ou interne du neuroblaste.

2. Il y a aussi, comme nous l'avions reconnu depuis longtemps, des neuroblastes très embryonnaires portant dans leur côté épendymaire un appendice radial. Cependant nous croyons que cette forme bipolaire se présentant souvent dans des neuroblastes très peu développés n'est pas aussi précoce que la mono-polaire.

3. Le bout terminal de l'axon embryonnaire, qui siège encore dans l'épaisseur de la moelle épinière, présente un renflement conique à base périphérique correspondant incontestablement au cône d'accroissement décrit, il y a longtemps, par nous, Lenhossék et Retzius dans les préparations de la méthode de Golgi. Néanmoins, en comparant les renflements terminaux imprégnés par les deux procédés, on observe des différences qui nous révèlent que les cônes d'accroissement sont des organes complexes se composant principalement de deux facteurs: charpente neurofibrillaire terminée brusquement dans l'épaisseur dudit renflement (parfois en forme de pointe de pinceau ou de brosse); et substance protoplasmique incolorable par le nitrate d'argent, mais facilement révélable par le procédé de Golgi; cette matière cytoplasmique coiffe le faisceau neurofibrillaire en projetant des appendices ou des lamelles irradiées.

4. L'examen des embryons de poulet plus avancés (du 5º au 10º jour) et même des fœtus de mammifère démontre que les axons en voie d'accroissement siégeant dans la substance blanche ou dans les tissus extra-nerveux offrent un renflement terminal qui devient progressivement olivaire et qui ressemble notablement aux massues ou boutons libres que nous avons trouvés récemment dans les nerfs adultes en voie de régénération. Un grand

nombre de ces boutons se rencontrent chez le chat et le lapin (fœtus très avancés) dans les systèmes de la substance blanche très tardivement différenciés (substance blanche cérébelleuse, pédoncules cérébelleux, tubercule acoustique, etc.).

5. La poursuite des fibres nerveuses de la racine antérieure à travers le mésoderme dès le 3° jour de l'incubation démontre péremptoirement la continuité des axons avec le corps du neuroblaste moteur de la moelle, ainsi que leur parfaite indépendance des corpuscules adventices ou intercalaires. Cette démonstration est d'autant plus aisée que les cylindres-axes en question prennent une teinte rouge ou une couleur café noir transparente se détachant très clairement du fond jaune constitué par les tissus mésodermiques.

6. De prime abord, et ainsi que l'ont fait remarquer un grand nombre d'histologistes, notamment His et Kölliker, l'intérieur des racines motrices et sensitives est dépourvu ou presque dépourvu de noyaux. Chez les oiseaux, ceux-ci commencent à pulluler entre les faisceaux de fibres nerveuses embryonnaires après que les racines ont gagné la périphérie et sont arrivées à destination (du 4° au 7° jour de l'incubation ; chez les mammifères le processus d'infiltration des nerfs par les *lemmoblastes* ou corpuscules de Schwann s'effectue plus tardivement ; ainsi, il n'est pas encore initié dans les nerfs bulbaires des embryons de lapin de 25 millimètres. D'ailleurs, cette infiltration est plus avancée dans les branches nerveuses périphériques que dans les gros cordons, particularité qui ne parle pas en faveur d'une origine médullaire ou ganglionnaire des cellules de revêtement.

7. On peut en dire autant des bifurcations de trajet et des arborisations périphériques terminales des axons moteurs ou sensitifs ; ces branches isolées, en voie de croissance active à travers les tissus mésodermiques, ne possèdent d'abord aucun noyau satellite marchant d'une façon absolument indépendante par les interstices des cellules connectives ou musculaires embryonnaires.

8. Les dendrites des neuroblastes apparaissent dans les neurones moteurs pendant le 4° jour de l'incubation, et très souvent dans le segment initial de l'axon. Dans les jours suivants elles s'accroissent progressivement, se dichotomisant à plusieurs reprises, et se colorent très intensivement par le dépôt métallique. Il est superflu d'affirmer que, de même que les axons, ces prolongements cellulaires ne se créent pas par fusion de chaines neuroblastiques, ni par condensation d'un blastème indifférent, mais

par la projection continue du protoplasme somatique. Dès le commencement de leur formation, les expansions protoplasmiques renferment un squelette neuro-fibrillaire fasciculé en continuation avec le réseau du soma et les filaments conducteurs de l'axon.

9. Ainsi que plusieurs embryologistes l'ont reconnu, toutes les voies situées dans la substance blanche de la moelle, le bulbe rachidien, le cerveau moyen, etc., se composent d'abord de cylindres-axes nus et indépendants, en continuation avec les neuroblastes d'association. L'apparition de corpuscules nucléaires intercalaires, c'est-à-dire de cellules neurogliques, s'effectue très tardivement, et ceux-ci ne peuvent, par conséquent, collaborer au processus de croissance et de ramification des fibres nerveuses centrales.

10. Jamais il ne nous a été donné de surprendre durant les premières phases évolutives des neurones, ni plus tard lorsque les dendrites ont fait leur apparition, des anastomoses intercellulaires. A mon avis, les unions en chaîne ou en *syncytium* colonial signalées par Fragnito, Berta, Joris et d'autres tiennent à une apparence de fusion résultant du fait de l'accumulation dans les mêmes espaces interépithéliaux de plusieurs neurones embryonnaires, lesquels se serrent et s'accolent très intimement. Mais pareil aspect, que naturellement n'offrent pas les neurones isolés ou écartés des pléiades cellulaires, s'évanouit du moment que la charpente neuroglique et les arborisations nerveuses terminales se développant et s'interposant entre les corpuscules nerveux, écartent les somas et les dendrites, décelant enfin leur parfaite individualité.

De tous ces faits d'observation s'ensuit la conclusion générale que nous n'avons aucune raison pour réviser ni corriger la conception monogénétique de His, laquelle, après avoir résisté vigoureusement à l'épreuve des nouvelles méthodes neurofibrillaires, nous semble une doctrine scientifique définitive et désormais inébranlable.

DISCUSSION

M. HELD: Je suis content que les nouvelles observations de M. Ramón y Cajal viennent confirmer la théorie et les expériences de la continuité génétique des cylindraxes qui, au moins pour les fibres motrices, est une nécessité au point de vue pathologique.

M. SILVA TAVARES: Je demande à M. Ramón y Cajal d'abord si les méthodes de Schultz colorent uniformément tous les éléments nerveux, inclusivement les neurogliques; deuxièmement, comment expliquer les divergences d'opinion à propos de la forme et nature des éléments nerveux, et les faits paraissent si clairs, comme les rapporte l'éminent histologiste espagnol.

M. MARCK ÁTHIAS: Je félicite vivement M. le Prof. Cajal des brillants travaux faits avec ses nouvelles méthodes, travaux qui apportent un appui d'une énorme valeur à la théorie du neurone telle qu'elle a été exposée par M. Waldeyer. Je prie seulement M. Cajal de bien vouloir me dire ce qu'il pense au sujet de l'origine des cellules que l'on trouve éparses au milieu du mésoderme et qui, d'après les partisans de la théorie caténaire, seraient des neuroblastes ayant probablement émigré du tube neural.

M. ROMITI: Je demande à M. Cajal comment on peut expliquer les résultats obtenus par Pertonaito (de Parme) au moyen de la méthode de Golgi, e comment les mettre d'accord avec ce qu'il vient de communiquer.

M. GUSTAV MANN: The facts that fibrils make their appearance comparatively late, that there is a marked increase in the fibrillation according to the amount of work a nerve cell does and that the fibrillation of nerve cells and axis cylinders disappears very soon if one prevent the stimulation of nerve cells, have led me to the conclusion that the nerve fibrils are the result of the stimulation of the nerve cells by electrolytes. The gradual growth of axiscylinders at the periphery must be explained by assuming that certain molecules resulting from the action of electrolytes on a previously homogeneous plasm leads to these molecules arrange themselves along definite strands because the least difference of potential or with other words the greatest amount of surface tension is always developed if molecules of the same kind are brought together and therefore the resulting fibrils are in a state of the greatest possible stability.

M. CAJAL répond à M. Benda: Les réseaux de neurones sensitifs périphériques, décrits récemment par O. Schultze dans les larves de salamandre et de triton, comportent une interprétation en harmonie avec la conception honogénique de He...

Mes recherches faites à l'aide de la méthode du nitrate d'argent démontrent que les cordons protoplasmiques, prétendus pleins et anastomotiques de Schultze, sont des faisceaux de très fines fibrilles dépourvues de myéline et entourées de cellules de revêtement prises par mécompte pour des neuroblastes émigrés.

Au niveau des points nodaux du réseau nerveux dudit auteur se trouvent constamment des divisions des axons embryonnaires dont la ténuité extrême, la proximité, la disposition fasciculée, etc., ont été la cause de plusieurs erreurs.

En outre, ces plexus compliqués, ayant l'apparence de réseaux grossiers dans les préparations communes, ont été aussi observés par moi dans les muscles des larves de batraciens et même dans ceux des embryons de mammifères.

Réponse à M. Tavares: Les divergences d'opinion dans de pareilles questions tiennent à des causes multiples.

Laissant de côté certaines influences psychologiques, je crois que la cause principale du manque d'accord entre les savants est l'imperfection des méthodes employées, méthodes non sélectives, lesquelles sont incapables de colorer sélectivement le protoplasme nerveux en le séparant optiquement de celui formant les cellules neurogliques et les corpuscules de Schwann embryonnaires. Il est vrai que ce pouvoir sélectif manquant aux procédés communs, nous le trouvons dans la méthode de Golgi employée dans l'argument par nous, Lenhossék, Retzius, etc., mais malheureusement l'application de ce mode d'analyse aux premières phases de l'évolution des neurones est très difficile; ainsi la plupart des auteurs modernes se sont servis des colorations ordinaires. De plus, dans ce domaine, les révélations du chromate d'argent, n'étant pas contrôlées comme celles obtenues dans les centres nerveux adultes par la méthode d'Ehrlich, ont été prises avec une excessive méfiance.

D'ailleurs, nous ne devons pas oublier que, quand les procédés ordinaires ou réductifs ont été employés par des savants d'une grande expérience et sagacité, tels que MM. Kölliker, His, Lenhossék, Harrison, etc., on a obtenu des résultats absolument concordants avec ceux fournis par le chromate d'argent.

À mon avis, les idées actuelles de l'école de Bethe sur l'histogenèse des nerfs ne sont pas le fruit immédiat de l'observation, mais l'effet de la généralisation, au domaine du développement des nerfs, des hypothèses très hasardeuses sur les connexions des cellules nerveuses adultes; je fais allusion à l'existence supposée des réseaux inter et péri-cellulaires.

Réponse à M. Athias: La question de la nature et de l'origine des cellules de Schwann des nerfs embryonnaires est très difficile. Les polygénistes admettent une origine ecto-dermique, opinion à laquelle se rangent aussi quelques partisans de la doctrine de la continuité (Lenhossék, par exemple). Mais il faut l'avouer, à l'état actuel de la science il est impossible de résoudre ce problème, parce que les moyens analytiques dont nous disposons ne permettent pas de différencier, dans les premières phases de l'évolution ontogénique, les cellules connectives ordinaires de celles-mésodermiques ou ecto-dermiques) mélangées à ces dernières et destinées à devenir des corpuscules de Schwann.

Cependant, en faveur d'une origine mésodermique parlent d'abord la similitude de ces cellules adventices avec les éléments conjonctifs ordinaires, ainsi que le fait que dans les nerfs en voie de régénération l'axon jeune, d'abord nu, semble attirer successivement au moyen peut-être d'un processus chimiotactique) les éléments mésodermiques embryonnaires de la cicatrice.

Ajoutons que d'après nos observations les cellules de Schwann de la portion plus développée des fibres régénérées n'offrent jamais de phénomènes de multiplication.

Réponse à M. Bonnier: Dans les préparations de Perroncito faites avec la méthode de nitrate d'argent, outre des faits bien établis et concordant avec ceux décrits par nous, se révèlent probablement des dispositions bizarres dont la signification n'est pas facilement déterminable; telle est par exemple l'existence de boutons non terminaux donnant origine à des branches ou des plexus nerveux fort compliqués. N'ayant pu examiner ces préparations, tout ce que je suis en mesure d'affirmer à cet égard, c'est que dans des coupes très nombreuses colorées d'après habile méthode, j'ai trouvé constamment les axons en voie de croissance se terminant librement au moyen de boutons absolument libres.

En ce qui concerne le problème de la régénération des nerfs, nous sommes d'accord, M. Perroncito et moi, au moins dans les points essentiels.

À mon avis les faits absolument décisifs en faveur de la doctrine de Waller sont:

a) Existence de continuité entre les fibres nouvelles de la cicatrice et celles du bout central.

b) Présence, dans l'extrémité libre des fibres marchant à travers la cicatrice, et le bout périphérique de boutons terminaux libres constamment orientés vers la périphérie.

c) Enfin le fait que toutes les divisions des fibres jeunes abordant le segment périphérique, en siégeant dans l'intérieur de celui-ci, ont les branches dirigées en sens centrifuge.

Ces faits, il faut l'avouer, ne sont pas bien nouveaux, car ils ont été en grande partie découverts par Waller, Ranvier, Vaulair et Struebe, faits qui, suivant le mode critique de certains savants, ont été simplement écartés ou oubliés pour être trop incommodes à la conception polygénique ou hypothèse caténaire.

La composition des corpuscules rouges du sang

Par M. Eugen Albrecht, Francfort s/M.

A. — La couche superficielle des globules rouges du sang des vertébrés est formée par une substance lipoïde qui, chez les mammifères, consiste exclusivement, ou presque exclusivement, en une lécithine se fondant et se détachant en forme de gouttelettes, etc., à 49.55° C. Cette température varie selon les différentes espèces, mais est constante pour chacune. La lécithine superficielle des globules rouges des mammifères ne se teint pas par les substances qui sont attirées fortement par les lipoïdes (Overton) ordinaires; mais la lécithine extraite du sang par les méthodes usuelles ne se teint pas non plus. Par l'extraction avec l'alcool à 63° on obtient une seconde substance lipoïde sous forme de petits grains se colorant fortement avec le Neutralrot et qui paraît être en relation intime d'une part avec l'hémoglobine, d'autre part avec la lécithine de la surface.

Les preuves principales données pour la nature lipoïde de la couche superficielle des érythrocytes sont:

1. sa liquéfaction et les déformations des globules rouges produites par la chaleur (Albrecht);

2. sa dissolution, souvent après formation de protubérances myéliniques par l'éther, le chloroforme, la benzine, etc. (Albrecht, Köppe);

3. sa dissolution (saponification) souvent avec formation de figures myéliniques par le KOH, NH (Albrecht).

B. — Tandis que chez les mammifères la quantité de la lécithine superficielle est relativement considérable, elle est relativement petite chez les batraciens (Albrecht et Hedinger et M. Plehn); tandis que la formation de l'épaississement marginal des disques des mammifères est due à elle tendance à des formations «myéliniques», Albrecht, Weidenreich), la formation du *Randreifen* de Meves (qui n'est qu'une partie différenciée et épaissie de la membrane continue, Weidenreich) est due principalement à une autre substance lipoïde combinée avec la lécithine se fondant à de beaucoup plus hauts degrés, donnant de très belles figures myéliniques avant sa dissolution par KOH, NH₃, par le toluol, le chloroforme, etc. (Albrecht et Hedinger et M. Plehn).

C. — La couche lipoïde superficielle suffit aux exigences physiologiques suivantes:

1. elle cause une forme des globules rouges à surface très grande, de sorte que l'échange des gaz entre l'hémoglobine et le plasma ambiant ait lieu le plus facilement, le plus vite et le plus également possible.

2. Les épaississements marginaux donnent à ces formes de disques une très grande stabilité; de l'autre côté, la nature demi-solide de l'enveloppe permet aux globules rouges de subir des déformations mécaniques très considérables sans qu'ils perdent la faculté de restitution formale. En se fermant rapidement après toute lésion soit superficielle soit plus profonde du globule rouge, elle en conserve longtemps la forme; et elle conserve aussi aux fragments des érythrocytes (soit déchirés par force mécanique, soit divisés sous l'influence de la chaleur) au moins une partie de leur valeur physiologique (méracytes de Giglio-Tos, microcytes, poïkilocytes, etc.).

3. Les couches superficielles servent de membranes semiperméables aux érythrocytes, ce qui explique la faculté de ceux-ci de réagir différemment envers les différentes substances dissoutes dans leur ambiant (Hamburger, Köppe). Jusqu'à une certaine dilution des sels du fluide de suspension, les membranes s'imbibent seulement de l'eau qui pénètre dans l'intérieur et gonfle les globules, sans être dissoutes elles-mêmes (Hamburger, Overton, Albrecht, Weidenreich); à de plus hauts degrés de dilution elles sont peu à peu saponifiées et dissoutes à cause de l'ionisation progressive de l'alcali du médium (Albrecht et Hedinger).

4. Comme toutes les substances graisseuses (Exner, Hofbauer et d'autres), celles de la surface des érythrocytes possèdent une attraction spéciale pour l'oxygène; de sorte qu'il paraît très vraisemblable qu'elles l'accumulent en «solution solide» (in fester Lösung) et le fassent passer ensuite à l'hémoglobine du globule rouge (Albrecht). En tous cas, cette qualité facilite beaucoup le passage de l'oxygène par la paroi de l'érythrocyte.

5. De même, les surfaces lipoïdes des érythrocytes amassent en elles toutes les substances dont le «Teilungscoefficient» pour les lipoïdes surpasse celui pour l'eau, comme l'éther, le chloroforme, l'alcool, etc.; d'un côté elles servent donc de porteurs de ces

substances au système nerveux, et ailleurs, de l'autre côté elles
sont cause de l'action directe et intense de ces substances sur les
érythrocytes.

6. Il a été possible de démontrer d'une façon évidente que toutes les déformations bien connues des globules soit par les différences de concentration du milieu, soit par la chaleur, par les
agglutinines ou par les ambocepteurs des hémolysines sont conséquence des altérations de la paroi lipoïde d'un contenu liquide
des globules rouges (Albrecht, Albrecht et Hedinger, Weidenreich).

D. — L'intérieur de l'érythrocyte ne contient pas d'éléments
structurés (Albrecht, Weidenreich); c'est un fluide plus ou moins
homogène où l'hémoglobine se trouve en solution. Pour qu'elle
sorte du globule rouge (hémolyse) il est nécessaire que, hors de la
destruction partielle ou, pour la plupart, totale de la membrane
lipoïde, il s'établisse une altération des parties superficielles du
contenu (deuxième couche corticale, peut-être formée par une léci-
tho-cholestérine? changement des corps albuminoïdes ou lipo-pro-
téides de la surface?)

Après la perte de la couche lipoïde superficielle le globule
rouge peut maintenir, souvent longtemps, la forme sphérique qui
en résulte (Albrecht).

E. — Le noyau des érythroblastes des mammifères contribue
très probablement à la production de la lécithine superficielle
(décomposition myélinique de la chromatine comme chez les cellules nucléées nécrotisées (Albrecht)); en outre il contribuera à la
formation de l'hémoglobine (Fe); peut-être donne-t-il naissance
aussi à une ou plusieurs substances qui, elles aussi, se combi-
nent facilement avec l'oxygène et servent d'oxygénophores comme la couche lipoïde superficielle. C'est rendu vraisemblable par
le fait qu'à l'action des alcalis sur le noyau des amphibies on
voit déjà avant la dissolution de la membrane monter de grandes
masses de vésicules gazeuses de la surface du noyau à celle de la
cellule où elles disparaissent (Albrecht et M. Plehn et Hedinger).
Le reste basichromatique condensé du noyau des mammifères est
détruit par expulsion au plasme et dissolution.

F. — Ainsi, tout ce qui est connu d'essentiel sur la structure physique et chimique des érythrocytes, les caractérise comme de petits corps oxygénophores (et gazophores en général),
dont chaque partie montre un extrême degré d'adaptation et de
perfection spécifiques.

Contribution à l'étude de la structure des fuseaux neuro-musculaires

Par M. F. A. GEMELLI

J'ai pu, à l'aide d'une modification de la réaction de Golgi [1], déceler l'existence, dans les plaques motrices, d'une structure caractéristique [2]. A l'aide de la même méthode, j'ai pu voir des faits semblables dans les fuseaux neuro-musculaires, que je vais vous présenter.

Avec ma méthode sont mises en évidence, dans le prolongement cylindraxile qui aboutit aux fuseaux, de nombreuses neurofibrilles, lesquelles, le plus souvent, courent parallèles entre elles; rarement elles se croisent, et jamais elles ne s'anastomosent. Une fois arrivées dans les ramifications du cylindraxe, à l'intérieur des fuseaux, elles se divisent, s'anastomosent plusieurs fois, le plus souvent entre elles, au point de former dans l'intérieur des terminaisons de la plaque un réticulum qui, par sa nature et son aspect, doit être considéré nerveux. Ce réticulum est extrêmement fin.

J'ai constaté aussi une particularité que je juge d'un grand intérêt en ces temps où l'on discute si fort sur les connexions intimes du système nerveux.

Outre la fibre médullaire qui forme les diramations terminales typiques bien connues, un second système de fibrilles nerveuses, d'une extrême finesse, pénètre dans les fuseaux. Elles se propagent au dedans de la gaine de Henlé de la fibre médullaire qui va former la terminaison typique de la plaque et, sitôt parvenues à la lanterne de celle-ci, elles se divisent le plus souvent en plusieurs rameaux.

J'ai réussi également à voir les terminaisons des fibrilles susmentionnées; un grand nombre d'entre elles viennent se mettre en contact avec l'arborisation terminale de la fibre médullaire et se prolongent directement dans l'intérieur de celle-ci, avec le réticulum que j'ai décrit plus haut.

Ces faits, que je crois très importants, viennent compléter mes travaux sur les plaques motrices, ainsi que les travaux de Dogiel et de Kolmei sur la structure réticulaire de certaines ter-

[1] Anatomischer Anzeiger, B. XXVII, octobre 1905; Rivista di Scienze Biologiche e naturali, tom. 1905.

[2] La Névraxe, Louvain, V. 7, F. 1, 1905; C. R. de la Société de Biologie, 21 octobre 1905.

minaisons nerveuses. Je crois aussi que la continuité, décrite par moi, dans le réticulum et les fibrilles secondaires fournit une preuve en faveur des idées de Apáthy.

SÉANCE DU 21 AVRIL

10 h. du matin

Présidence : M. RAMÓN Y CAJAL

Sont présents : MM. Albrecht, Bouin, Cajal, Celestino da Costa, Mlle Denn (Chicago), M. Ramon, Mlle Lewes, MM. Athias, Mattoso Santos, Pacheco (Coïmbre), Paes Leme, Parra, Pinto de Magalhães, Silva Tavares, etc.

M. MATTOSO SANTOS communique à l'assemblée que M. Bouin a dû rentrer précipitamment en Italie et présente ses compliments aux membres de la section d'anatomie.

Définition, structure et composition du protoplasme

Rapport par M. G. MANN, Oxford (v. p. 202)

DISCUSSION

M. ALBRECHT : 1) — Je crois qu'ici il ne nous sera pas possible de discuter la partie chimique et physico-chimique de la communication qui vient d'être présentée. C'est pourquoi je fais observer seulement qu'il m'a été très intéressant d'entendre que M. Mann a prononcé déjà avant Hállitzer la pensée que les colloïdes sont des électrolytes. Pauly a prouvé, du reste, que les protéides purs ne sont pas électriques du tout.

2) — Quant aux hypothèses de structure cellulaire que notre éminent collègue nous a exposées, je crois que la plupart n'ont pas encore de base suffisante dans mes observations sur la cellule tissu et c'est pourquoi ses conclusions, déduites principalement de la théorie électrochimique des colloïdes, ne me paraissent pas acceptables.

Surtout je n'admets pas encore prouvée l'idée que dans la cellule vivante et par les sels circulants des coagulations analogues à celle produite par le HgCl, jouent un rôle dans la formation des structures intracellulaires.

Je ne saurais non plus accepter la pensée que les fibrilles nerveuses naissent d'une coagulation effectuée par le stimulus (décomposition électrolytique) et n'existent pas sans cette irritation. Cette manière de voir ne nous expliquerait pas : a) la pluralité des fibrilles dans chaque prolongement de la cellule nerveuse; b) leurs directions déterminées et leur isolement; c) leur formation ayant la fonction analogue à celle des stries musculaires, etc.

L'explication donnée de la contraction des fibrilles de la radiation mitotique par coagulation ne me paraît pas suffisante non plus; d'abord elle nous fait voir prendre peut-être une petite rétraction des Spindelfasern, mais pas leur contraction parfaite et disparition suivante; ensuite Conklin, Bütschli et moi, nous avons vu qu'il y a des mouvements de liquide le long de ces «fibrilles», et il n'est point prouvé qu'elles soient solides.

On ne pourra pas maintenir non plus l'opinion que ce soit le noyau qui «forme» le cytoplasme. Il y a une «inter-action» continuelle entre le noyau et le cytoplasme, un échange de matériaux des deux côtés — j'en parlerai dans ma communication suivante —; mais on ne pourra pas conclure de la que cette affirmation que le cytoplasme soit une fonction spécifique du noyau. Au contraire; s'il y a quelque chose prouvée dans cette question, c'est que le cytoplasme doit «former», nourrir le noyau, substituer ce qu'il a perdu par le métabolisme fonctionnel, puisque le cytoplasme doit puiser des capillaires, etc., les matériaux dont le noyau a besoin pour sa reconstitution.

Sur la structure du protoplasme

Par M. Eugen Albrecht (Francfort s. M.)

L'époque de l'histologie et cytologie purement descriptive est passée. Sur la base qu'elle nous a fournie il s'élève déjà un édifice assez considérable, qui croît de jour en jour: c'est celui de la microchimie et de la microphysique physiologiques, inauguré principalement par les travaux de Traube, Berthold, Bütschli, de Vries, Quincke, et continué par un assez grand nombre de collaborateurs s'augmentant toujours.

Ce sont principalement les études physico-chimiques modernes dont l'application systématique à l'étude de la cellule nous permet de tracer au moins en général les lignes fondamentales d'une nouvelle conception du plasme, extrêmement fertile en explications relativement simples de phénomènes vitaux paraissant très complexes et donnant incessamment de nouvelles directions heuristiques de théorie et de méthode.

Seulement, il ne faut jamais oublier que tout ce que les nouvelles recherches physiques et chimiques nous offrent de suggestions doit être vérifié par l'étude de la cellule même et autant que possible, par l'étude de la cellule *vivante*.

Ce que je crois pouvoir établir comme base assurée de notre connaissance des structures les plus importantes du protoplasme non différencié, ce sont les constatations suivantes:

1) Le protoplasme se trouve en général à l'état liquide. La preuve principale en est donnée par la dissolution en forme de gouttelettes (*tropfige Entmischung*, Albrecht) qui, en est présentée dans le cytoplasme vivant, ou peut être produite déjà par l'action de la solution de sel physiologique.

2) Selon la concentration relative des cristalloïdes, des colloïdes, de l'eau, ce liquide cellulaire peut apparaître sous diverses phases (Hardy); comme émulsion de gouttelettes (Berthold, Albrecht), comme structure écumeuse (Schaumstructur, Bütschli) aux espaces plus ou moins larges; parfois peut-être de véritables structures de réticulum passagères peuvent-elles se former (Hardy, Pauly, Haber), bien que pour la cellule vivante cela ne paraisse prouvé nulle part.

3) Il est très invraisemblable qu'il y ait des cellules ou des états de cellule parfaitement homogènes. Probablement il y a toujours cette différenciation en cytochyme et cytenchyme, soit sous forme de médium de suspension et éléments suspendus, soit sous forme de parois relativement stables (Schaumwände) et contenu de ces chambres intracellulaires moins viscide. La densité du cytenchyme des émulsions peut varier très considérablement, de gouttelettes soutenant évidemment beaucoup d'eau (grande partie des ainsi-dits vacuoles y appartient) a certains «grains» de sécrétion très viscides, aux fibrilles solides comme celles du muscle strié, ou aux cristaux intra-cellulaires. Il doit être remarqué que la «Wabenstructur» des préparations fixées n'est très souvent que le produit de l'altération artificielle de la phase d'émulsion de la cellule vivante.

4) Pour faire comprendre la possibilité d'une naissance de parois fluides, de gouttelettes intracellulaires dans le mélange de colloïdes et de crystalloïdes en solution que représente le cytoplasme, il suffirait donc de recourir aux différences des concentrations relatives de ces ingrédients que nous venons de dénommer, mais l'étude de la cellule vivante montre que cette manière de voir ne serait pas juste. A la vérité c'est une catégorie généralement négligée de substances cellulaires à laquelle il faut attribuer la plus haute importance dans la formation de ces parois, etc., intracellulaires. Ce sont les *lipoïdes* de la cellule dont j'ai pu démontrer la présence, souvent en quantité surprenante, dans toutes les cellules investiguées. Ce sont elles qui, en se saponifiant, en s'étendant en forme de lamelles fines ou, au contraire, en élevant, en forme de graisses génuines, la tension de surface des parties du fluide qu'elles renferment, font naître une variété très grande de formations intracellulaires. A cause de la facilité avec laquelle elles peuvent être rendues visibles sous des formes myéliniques (par le KOH, etc.), j'ai proposé pour toutes ces substances le nom de *substances myélinogènes*. Elles se trouvent dans le nucléole comme dans la

surface du noyau et maintiennent la séparation entre le nucléole et le suc nucléaire comme entre le noyau et le cytoplasme; elles sont répandues partout dans le cytoplasme sous forme de petits grains à forte réfraction et attirant pour la plupart très vivement le «Neutralrot» et les autres réactifs colorant les lipoïdes d'Overton. Ces derniers granules que j'ai appelés *liposomes* se régénèrent probablement continuellement et surtout dans les cellules sécrétoires par l'afflux de chromatine plus ou moins décomposée et de myéline provenant du noyau.

La formation des «Chromidien» de Hertwig et de Goldschmidt est probablement due à une augmentation considérable de ce transport nucleo-cytoplasmique dans les cellules à action chimique très énergique.

5. Le type de formations de gouttes intracellulaires qui se réalise le plus fréquemment est le suivant: couche superficielle de substance lipoïde (myélinogène), souvent fortement colorable; deuxième partie superficielle riche en substances albuminoïdes; reste du suc contenu riche en eau et cristalloïdes, avec peu de substance albuminoïde, souvent probablement parfaitement sans colloïdes.

Il est évident que par des différences chimiques de chacune de ces trois couches bien de différences vitales cellulaires comme intracellulaires soit passagères soit constantes peuvent être produites; et il est sûr que la recherche de ces différences nous résoudra beaucoup des énigmes de ces prédilections et aversions singulières des cellules pour certaines substances qui ont toujours été prises pour une des plus fortes preuves du vitalisme. Ainsi, par exemple, Gurwitsch a démontré que pour la sécrétion rénale il y a trois sortes de vésicules ou de gouttes intracellulaires différentes (dont l'une à surface lipoïde) qui servent probablement de condensateurs et de transporteurs des substances que la cellule prend du plasme pour les sécréter. De cette manière aussi il se rétablit naturellement toujours la différence de concentration («das Konzentrationsgefälle») nécessaire pour que les matières spéciales attirées par les diverses cellules y entrent toujours de nouveau, quand même il n'y en ait qu'une petite quantité dans le sang capillaire. (Je ne parle pas ici des autres moyens dont la cellule se sert pour le même effet, comme la condensation du sucre en forme de glycogène, etc.). C'est dans ces petites gouttelettes à paroi lipoïde aussi où nous devons probablement chercher les prisons des ferments divers de la cellule vivante comme Hofmeister les a postulées.

Le *noyau* de la cellule (excepté à l'état de division mitotique) appartient au type de gouttes cellulaires indiqué; surface myélinogène, couche chromatique, suc nucléaire plus ou moins riche en cristalloïdes et en colloïdes.

Le nucléole, le plus souvent compacte, peut, lui aussi, apparaître quelquefois sous la même forme («vacuoles nucléolaires», etc.).

6) La conservation de la *forme externe* de ces liquides cellulaires est garantie pour les cellules fixes et pour beaucoup de cellules mobiles par les parois solides des cellules. Ces parois, elles aussi, sont probablement toujours imprégnées de lipoïdes, comme je l'ai pu démontrer pour l'épithélium alvéolaire du poumon. Il en résultera pour les cellules fixes plus ou moins des avantages que j'ai énumérés pour les globules rouges du sang comme effet de leur paroi myélinique.

La question de la semiperméabilité des parois cellulaires des animaux présente pour le moment de très grandes difficultés.

L'hypothèse de la semiperméabilité nous expliquerait beaucoup des singularités dans les phénomènes de résorption et de sécrétion, etc. Mais les preuves y font défaut jusqu'à présent.

7) Les cellules nues à mouvement amiboïde possèdent une couche superficielle mince, huileuse, telle que la théorie l'exige. Pour les leucocytes c'est prouvé par les changements qu'ils subissent sous l'action de l'alcali ou de l'éther; ils se comportent comme des boules revêtues d'une substance graisseuse. Nous avons donc le droit d'expliquer leurs mouvements par les changements de leur tension de surface ainsi que Quincke, Bütschli, Verworn, Rhumbler, J. Bernstein, l'ont rendu vraisemblable.

8) La cellule animale représente donc, pour la plupart, et sauf les différenciations spécifiques, une petite chambre à paroi solide, imprégnée de lipoïdes et contenant un liquide composé de colloïdes, de cristalloïdes, d'eau. Ce dernier peut se composer ou bien d'un liquide contenant en émulsion plus ou moins de gouttes aux parois différenciées elles aussi, ou une quantité variable de petites chambres aux parois viscides renfermant un liquide différent.

Les parois intracellulaires des deux groupes contiennent probablement toujours des substances myélinogènes qui sont fournies en partie des liposomes persistants du cytoplasme.

Le noyau cellulaire appartient aux gouttes cellulaires à surface myélinogène et se trouve en interaction constante avec le cytoplasme.

Discussion

M. C. BENDA: Dans mon rapport je m'occupe de quelques-unes des questions traitées par M. Albrecht; en ce moment je conviens seulement en ce qu'il n'est pas permis d'appliquer le nom de «Chromidies» à ce que j'ai nommé «Mitochondries», que j'ai démontré être essentiellement organiques en poursuivant les conditions dans lesquelles elles se présentent dans les différentes phases de la vie cellulaire.

M. SILVA TAVARES: Je prie M. le prof. Albrecht de vouloir expliquer si les corpuscules qu'on voit dans les cellules, après l'immersion dans l'hydrate de potassium pendant des heures, sont vraiment des produits non artificiels, et quelles en sont les preuves.

M. ALBRECHT répond à M. Benda: Je n'ai pas nommé la mitochondria en parlant des chromidies, parce que je n'étais pas sûr de l'identité des formations décrites sous les deux dénominations. Si M. Benda les déclare identiques, je partage naturellement son avis que dorénavant le nom de mitochondria devra être employé pour ces formations.

Réponse à M. Tavares: Les liposomes peuvent être vus dans la cellule intacte, pourvu qu'on se serve de grossissements assez forts et de l'immersion à l'huile. Le KOH les rend seulement plus visibles en les agrandissant sous forme de corps myéliniques et en rendant plus transparent le reste du cytoplasme. Les investigations ont été faites surtout sur les cellules hépatiques et rénales du lapin, de la souris, etc.

Di una nuova terminazione nervosa della Epidermide Umana: «Sistema del Plnea Nervosa»

(Sur une nouvelle terminaison nerveuse de l'Épiderme humain — Système de l'épi nerveux)

Par M. MARIO ANDREA ROSSI (Mexico)

Le produzioni nervose della epidermide umana, scoverte sin qui e descritte dagli autori, come: fibre intraepiteliali — cellule di Langerhans —, menischi tattili e cellule nervose, non possono costituire un lusso inesplicabile di terminazioni isolate, senza un nesso sintetico, che ne faccia un sistema concreto, in rapporto con una sensazione della pelle.

Nell'anno 1890, interno dell'Istituto scientifico, diretto dal prof. Otto von Schrön, a Napoli, impresi a studiare il difficile problema, attraverso le incertezze del metodo Ranvier; portando nella tecnica il contributo di nuovi metodi e sottoponendo, il primo fra tutti, pezzi di cute, impregnati al tricloruro di oro, al processo dell'incolloidinamento ed alla lima del microtomo.

Quattro anni di amoroso lavoro: Settantasei prove tentate, su pelle fresca, con soli nove risultati apprezzabili e tre dimostrativi: la sicurezza palmare che vi ha, nella epidermide umana, un sistema nervoso terminale, il quale abbraccia, in un insieme armonico e logico, le quattro produzioni intraviste e descritte isolatamente, m'indussero a pubblicare, sulla *Riforma Medica*, dell'Agosto 1893, una monografia, intitolata: «Le terminazioni nervose di senso, della pelle dell'uomo», nella quale descrissi e dimostrai, con numerose tavole in cromolitografia, il nuovo sistema della Pinea Nervea.

Ulteriori studi, compiuti nella città di Messico, per compilare una relazione e preparare una grande dimostrazione microscopica, da sottoporre alla osservazione ed alla critica del primo Congresso medico nazionale, tenuto in Gennaio 1906, mi pongono in grado di presentar al Congresso medico internazionale di Lisbona le seguenti conclusioni, appoggiate sopra una preziosa collezione di preparati microscopici:

1.°—Vi ha nella pelle dell'uomo un sistema concreto epidermico di terminazioni nervose di senso, al quale si collegano le produzioni, descritte come: fibre intraepiteliali, cellule di Langerhans, menischi tattili e cellule nervose semplici.

2.°—A questo sistema, mai descritto prima del 1893, venne imposto il nome di «Pinea Nervea».

3.°—Il sistema nervoso pineale è costituito da:

A.—una fibra nervea midollata, la quale si diparte dalla rete sub-papillare, s'innalza nella epidermide, attraverso di uno zaffo epiteliale o di una papilla nervosa, e, dopo poco, si rigonfia in un «Bulbo Pineale».

B.—Dal bulbo pineale si diparte, in tutti i versi, una serie di fibrille amieliniche—fibrille primitive—le quali tosto si risolvono in espansioni lanceolari, a guisa di foglioline di albero: foglioline od «elementi pineali».

C.—La fogliolina pineale si continua, dal suo apice, in una corta fibrilla amidollare—fibrilla secondaria—che va a mettere capo in uno dei poli di un ganglio intrinseco della epidermide o cellula di Langerhans.

D.—Dagli altri poli della cellula nervosa multipolare, ganglio intrinseco o cellula di Langerhans, muovono, in tutte le direzioni, fibrille amieliniche, più sottili, o fibre intraepiteliali, che, biforcandosi, vanno a disperdersi, appuntite e senza rigonfiamenti bottonuti, tra le cellule mucose dello strato di Malpighi.

4.°—Il sistema pineale epidermico costituisce una vera arborescenza, che ha radici nella rete nervosa del derma e spande rami e foglie tra gli elementi dell'epitelio.

5.° — La interpretazione funzionale di cosiffatto organo, riesce così della massima facilità. Le fibre epiteliali, intrecciate, in rete fittissima, nello strato germinativo, raccolgono, dal mondo esterno, le impressioni sensitive, cui presiedono, e le trasmettono, per più vie, al ganglio o cellula multipolare di Langerhans. Qui vi più impressioni si raccolgono in una sola e forse sono rinforzate (rocchetto moltiplicatore); dirigendosi, per la fibrilla secondaria, verso la fogliolina pineale, di sconosciuta interferenza, e, per la fibrilla primitiva, verso il bulbo pineale, dove convergono tutte le impressioni, dipendenti dalla parte di cute, soggetta alle terminazioni arborescenti di ciascun sistema pineale.

Dal bulbo, le varie percezioni, raccoltesi e concretizzate in sensazione unica, sono indirizzate verso l'organo centrale.

6.° — Ai fisiologi il determinare con quale sensazione cutanea debba trovarsi in relazione la pinea nervea e se la sua prossimità al mondo esterno non giustifichi, sino ad un certo punto, l'ipotesi, che possa rappresentare la raccoglitrice e la trasmettitrice della doppia sensazione tattile, assai più dei corpuscoli Meissner-Wagner e della clava di Krause.

<hr>

SÉANCE DU 21 AVRIL

(à 1 heure)

Président: M. PAES LEME

Nomenclature histologique, cytologique et embryologique; bases d'une classification

Rapporté par M. NATHAN LOEWENTHAL, Lausanne (V, page 16),
et M. KARL BENDA, Berlin ().

DISCUSSION

M. AGABBITI (): Nous devons savoir gré à M. Benda de ce qu'il a osé se prononcer contre le fétichisme des chromosomes dominant dans la cytologie depuis si longtemps. À la vérité, il n'est ni moins vraisemblable que dans la cellule, dans le noyau vivant se décomposant, se restituant, la masse que l'on croit spécifique, portant des qualités héréditaires de la cellule, y reste intacte et inerte. Du reste, Guttewski qui, a démontré par des expériences d'hybridisation, d'une

____

() Sera publié à la fin du volume, si M. Benda nous l'envoie à temps, ainsi que nous le lui avons demandé lors de la clôture du Congrès.

façon très nette, l'importance du cytoplasme pour la transmission des qualités par l'hérédité.

2º Aux conclusions de M. Benda concernant la base d'une nomenclature des organes élémentaires de la cellule on ne pourra que consentir. Seulement il sera nécessaire de nous réserver le droit d'appeler organes cellulaires aussi ces formations constantes qui, comme bien des granulations cellulaires, la striation musculaire, les fibrilles nerveuses, ne peuvent pas être dérivées d'une formation visible existant dans le spermatozoïde ou dans les blastomères.

— Après avoir présenté son rapport, M. BENDA montre quelques préparations de *Mitochondries* colorées par ses méthodes ; ces préparations sont :

1º Mitose des blastomères de Triton. Fuseau achromatique, chromosomes et mitochondries.

2º Division de maturation, spermatocytes de Blaps (Coléoptère).—Mitochondries en bâtonnet, participant à la mitose, formant un fuseau autour du fuseau ordinaire.

3º Mitose des blastomères de Triton. Coloration à l'hématoxyline ferrique. Fuseau achromatique, chromosomes (métaphase) et vitellus.

4º Spermatocytes et spermatogonies de Bombinator en repos. Les mitochondries forment des accumulations autour de la sphère.

SÉANCE DU 23 AVRIL

(à 10 heures du matin)

Présidence : M. G. MANN.

Assistance: MM. Benda, Celestino da Costa, Mlle. Dunn, M. Kamon, Mlle. Loyez, MM. Mann, Athias, Mattoso Santos, Paus Leme, Parra, Pinto de Magalhães, Silva Tavares, Waldeyer.

Métamérisation embryonnaire, son importance au point de vue de l'anatomie comparée

Rapport par M. ROULE, Toulouse (v. page 301)

DISCUSSION

M. MATTOSO SANTOS : Je crois qu'il y a lieu de distinguer deux origines aux faits de métamérisation que l'on peut constater chez les vertébrés : une *ancestrale*, dont toutes les effets se présentent avec une allure spéciale, mais gardant cependant le cachet de leur origine ; une autre, *actuelle*.

La première se révèle surtout dans le mode de formation des *mérosomites* (segments primordiaux) et dans la différenciation de ceux-ci en *épimères* (myotomes), *mésomères* (néphrotomes) et *hypomères*. La provenance et l'évolution de ces segments décèlent des rapports entre les vertébrés et les annélides, qui nous induisent à admettre pour ceux-là une souche *zoonitaire*, quoique très éloignée, sans doute.

La seconde, représentée par la *vertébralisation* et les dispositions morphologiques corrélatives, est tout à fait propre aux vertébrés.

Entre la forme allongée, la vie pélagique active, la nature des mouvements de ces derniers animaux et leur façon métamérique, il faut sans doute reconnaître une liaison, mais tantôt d'effet, tantôt de cause.

Je considère donc qu'il y a chez les vertébrés des faits de métamérisation : les uns, indices, restes même, d'une ancienne structure métamérique très profonde, que de successives coalescences adaptives ont de plus en plus masquée, dont en effet on ne peut parfois constater la nature que par l'embryogenèse, — tandis que d'autres, relevant plus ou moins directement de ceux-là, ou, au moins, procédant de l'organisation acquise, apparaissent, s'affirment et deviennent dominants dans cet embranchement.

Dans l'embryologie des vertébrés il faut, à mon avis, tenir compte de ces deux ordres de faits.

Some points of convergence and divergence in the human and other animal types

Par M. RICHARD J. ANDERSON, Galway

The arrangement and shape of the skeletal parts in mammals, the similarity in attachment and action of muscle groups, if not individual muscles, find greatest «human» expression in those orders most nearly allied to man, that is in those in which specific characters are least marked. The forms of greatest divergence are those in which the number of digits is reduced. The vascular system shows varieties that one may naturally expect to see, having regard to the embryonic conditions. The history of development represents, or is a recapitulation of the history of types. One has naturally looked to the nervous system for answers to some difficult questions. A very large number of mammals have well convoluted brains, and the brain itself is of considerable weight in elephants, and many cetacea, owing probably to the great surface and muscular distribution tracts. The brain is relatively large in some monkeys and some birds, and even in the chicks during development; the size of the brain is larger in proportion to the size of the body. It will be remembered that Owen was quite in favour of a classification of mammalia according to the degree of convolution of the brain. The approach of the brain of the higher apes to man is evident enough especially in the case of the Oran-utan. The occipital lobe is well developed in man, so that those who distinguish man by his altruistic (i.e. his self-denying, self-sacrificing) faculties,

and find reason for locating these qualities in the occipital lobes
may find here some crumbs of comfort. The occipital lobes of
certain microcephalic individuals (pathological) have been examined by the late Professor Giacomini and others (e.g. Cunnin-
gham). One can easily see, by referring to the figures given
in Duckworth's Anthropology, that a striking resemblance is
presented in the parietal region of the microcephalous individual to the parietal region in gorilla, and in the posterior lobe
(occipital) one sees a resemblance to that of the Chimpanzee[1].

It is said that the condition in microcephali is due to an
arrest of development; this would quite «fall in» with our ideas
of progressive changes in the continuous type. It is well to know
that the Ursidae have brains that present a by no means distant resemblance to the human brain at, I think, about the six-
teenth week of intra-uterine life, but that bears are very much
altered in certain directions, so as to constitute a carnivor type
quite different to that of dogs and seals and cats everyone knows.
The plantigrade type shows clearly where one may look for resem-
blances. The structure of the hands and feet have led morphologists very early to form estimates of the morphological status
of individuals and classes. There is, however, the conditional
and functional value of the eye, as well as the ear and larynx,
which in time may lead to central nerve development. The
parietal lobe is regarded as expressing the intellectual type of
the individual or race. The lower part of the frontal should,
perhaps, be included. We have then the centres that are inter-
associated in the work of the hand (and arm) and the eye, head,
and laryngeal movements.

It would seem from the position of certain centres that the
upper part of the parietal lobe is the more intellectual, but this is
not held by several eminent morphologists, who attribute to the
lower parietal portion the highest functions, and cite the brain
descriptions of several eminent individuals as confirmatory.

It will be admitted that the hands and arms, legs and feet,
have much to do with the relation of the individual to outside
objects, also the eyes, ears and larynx in a pronounced and general, though less apparent way. Pose, feature, style of movement, are inter-associated with the expression of the emotions,

____

[1] Kükenthal — Weissbere

which in the course of time may become quite complete, in response to composite poses or features. The power to imitate is soon apparent in man, and whatever value pose or feature may have in evoking forms of emotion or thought, they certainly meet with some response in children that are still very young, although they may only be temporarily implanted and create merely a taste, for the nerve tracts do not all seem to be developed very early.

The susceptibility to training emphasizes the mammalian groups. In the Avian orders imitation plays an important part, even in their own social lives. The building of nests, imitation of movements, and of articulate sounds are associated with apparently the musculo-cutaneous sensory apparatus. The head musculature has an important function in indicating and registering the operations of the parts of the brain that have to do with emotions. It keeps pace with the development of the brain, «Sie steht im engsten Connex mit dem psychischen Leben». This musculature or these muscles are grouped around the eye, ear, mouth, and nose. They appear thus to be essentially bound up with these important sense organs. «Durch sie wird das menschliche Antlitz zum Spiegel der Seele» (Wiedersheim). The variations of the muscles of mankind have been for many years a curious and interesting study, and, in many instances, as is well known, the exact condition of muscles in the lower orders or classes of animals is represented in special individual muscle groups of a limb or part, in man. The attempt to accomplish some task by methods which animals employ may serve to influence the segregation of certain of these muscles, if the work be begun early. But, where the division or production of a muscle is part and parcel of the progressive development of the general musculature, one may naturally seek an explanation in the anatomical conditions which prevail in the earlier stages of development.

The expressions of the psychical actions by general pose or gesture must be associated with those of the face, viz., in rendering the working of the mind as given by the face muscles.

Training can do much to effect the muscle performances, and the psychic operations of animals, muscle anomalies, or indeed anomalies of any kind have not been studied in many animals owing to want of material and observers, rabbits and domestic animals are studied in our Biological Laboratories or in Veterinary Schools. It so happens, however, that anomalies are rare in rabbits, which is to be expected, perhaps in other animals also, not so in all as we learn from the records of Macalister and Testut. Anomalies of bones are of great value sometimes as one sees in what direction a bone has grown or increased, and the response to altered nutrition or change of force is registered. One can have no difficulty in following the grounds given by some anatomists for regarding anomalies as induced by altered forces in embryonic or early life. The change of force in early life may lead to arrest of development or to a sudden change of growth, and an organ may thus gain the form possessed by the same organ in another type. The high importance of the muscle system which lays the foundation of the structural knowledge the animal gains of the outer world seems the most important. Irregularities in the viscera as in vessels have been noted, but many of the latter are easily referable to developmental causes, or to the enlargement of collateral branches. The muscle anomalies may even be complemental and one muscle may develop more, because some other has developed less. Leaving these possibilities to one side, one expects to have certain changes in musculature due to the association of human beings with other animals which are for their activity admired and imitated. It is not possible for an adult man to adopt the plans of the monkey or the rhinoceros in getting fruit or obtaining roots, but his feeble attempts to use their methods may influence the young who seek to train themselves muscularly to the condition of that of their seniors, so that muscle poses and impressions may begin very early. It seems clear that one might train an animal within certain limits to do the work usually assigned to another. This training if done early and kept up may lead to change of pose and movement. The early association of the foal is never forgotten, so that one should not rear a young horse with a donkey. Its paces are not altered with ease in after years, and never with pleasure. The goat, however, is a favourite with most horses owing to its peaceful and restful habits when tame. If then one take the trouble to study the points which seem to influence most the young animal one finds that muscle pose seems the most potent factor.

In the case of human beings the inquiry has not been far enough carried in the very young, but the value of muscle sense increases as the dexterity of the limb is less in evidence (relativity, of course, to the value of the organs of special sense).

The anomalies, therefore, in feature or pose in the negro, taking the Caucasian in the average anatomical records, as the referred to condition, may arise from his tendency to imitate the objects in nature.

The examples given by various observers seem to bear out this. One sees the result of this tendency in several countries. But the appearance or reflection of animals in man is almost as striking as Dr Matheus, of Eckmann Chatrian, could have wished. I do not mean the change in the mouth or eye which Dr. Louis Robinson mentions as present in the horse trainer, or the Army Sergeant, but the horsey impression that the faces of some men get, who spend much time with, and admire, horses; this development is furthered by the observation of those animals during early youth. The features are often as equine, as was the voice of Gulliver after his sojourn in the land of the horse nation. There may be associated with this equine ejaculations, or a whinnying, or even a neighing tone in the voice. One must have noticed this in some military people. The influence of the dog and sheep, as well as of the fowl and ox, appeals to many, and there is little doubt that other animals would be equally effective if greater opportunities were given to them (the elephant played an important part in early civilization). How can one tell anything about these? I fancy by a careful study of the skeleton in men of different races.

A double jugal occurs more frequently in some races than in others (¹), and the *tuberositas malaris* is well developed in some groups. There may be an absence of the lachrymal bone which is sometimes found divided (or double), the *crista buccinatoria* is variously developed.

The superior maxilla gives evidence of an occasional articulation with the temporal, which is approached in some other mammals by the prolongation of the superior maxilla along the jugal, or the growth of jugal backwards. The squamous part of the temporal touches the frontal rarely in man, but the temporal by means of the zygoma does reach the frontal in the horse. It is found, however, that wormian bones that exist in man and primates may, by uniting with one or other of two bones, give rise to anomalies which would not attract attention if the wormian bones join a third to make this latter larger. Taking these facts into consideration, and remembering how easily bony deposits creep along tendons and membranes, it is clear that some anomalies probably arise from attempting to assume a particular pose. This may, indeed, interfere with the nutrition of the parts. Wormian bones may arise where the condition affects the skull. The muscle change may affect the muscle impression and thus the bones feel the result. The actions or pose of impressive people or animals affect the impressionable, so that they repeat these actions, &c., often unconsciously, just as the clown imitates the clever feats of the trapezist consciously but simply, for he follows the jump of the former, by jumping over his own hat. The imitations of the horse, dog, or domestic fowl which are often seen in the five-year old boy or girl, are more the result of the concurrent pleasure which accompanies the actions. The modification of pose and action in the horse, ox, dog, elephant, camel, &c., is due to training which is furthered by the register of the movement by the organs of sense. The process of moulding is materially curtailed. The state of training must be again acquired after a period of rest. This is easier in times subsequent to the first. A repetition becomes necessary in many cases in dogs. Pointers are said to be efficient after the first training, but this does not hold for «setters». Training does lead to developmental peculiarities which may be emphasized by in-breeding and selection, and so even without imitation quite decisive changes may take place; so also in birds, but imitation is common in this class. The varieties of dogs and bears that one sees do not arise necessarily from artificial or natural selection. The dog order may be polyphyletic, but it is not improbable that Arctocyon is the ancestor of the chief groups in our own land and North America. It is not strange that man should present anomalies sometimes which are represented by normal structures in reptilian groups. These for obvious reasons are more likely to resemble those found near the direct line. Specialization for running, jumping, flying, burrowing clearly widens the chasm. Where a specialized group appears as an offshoot of a less specialized type one might naturally expect similarities occasionally arise, hence one looks rather to the lizard or crocodile for illustrations of possible human anomalies. The lemuroid type is nearer the parent stem than other primates, and clearly nearer the main stem than many other mammals. Some morphologists wish to place the former on the level near edentates, which is not without reason. The coronoid process has considerable importance in some groups, but this process of the lower jaw is not large in monkeys, in which muscles make often from impressions on the body of the jaw itself. Darwin has quoted Francis Galton to show the effect of heredity in a movement of the arm and hand which led to a slight abrasion of the nose in a person who, whilst somnolent, raised his arm and allowed it to drop somewhat suddenly. The same movement continued through the son to the grandson. Darwin also gives, it will be remembered, an instance of shrugging of the shoulders being hereditary. He notes that Englishmen (Irishmen *a fortiore*) do not give expression to inability in this way. That a different interpretation of the latter phenomenon is possible, I have noted elsewhere. In warm, temperate Europe and in other hot or tropical places birds are numerous and fowl-keeping is common amongst the civilized. The influence of the pose in animals upon men is unmistakable, and the thrusting forward of the wings in birds, especially in scrapers and runners, is very pronounced. It is very likely that artists took their ideas of angels' wings from this elevation of the wings in birds, and so when the artistic expression was possible it gave the effect akin to the shrug which one often sees. If the pose express impossibility it is accidental, though, perhaps, not inappropriate, as it may suggest impossibilities in any individual not aerial, or future possibilities. Darwin, indeed, says that an Eastern raised his shoulders when asked by a Western to climb to an elevated position. The Augurs in ancient times attached much importance to the mode of flight of birds and the groupings and the individuals were regarded as having direct connection with the wishes or thoughts of the gods. In modern times everyone knows that, for some people, birds indicate adversity or prosperity. The wing pose in ostrich and fowl must be an instinctive attempt to do what their weight, etc., prevents them doing. The five (or more) fingered type is primitive, so that one easily sees that the artistic training became impossible in large groups of animals at a very early period from the disappearance of digits, but capacity for active and close training has increased and the persistance of

impressions, due to training, is in some very great. Mammals
outside the human type are not imitative; birds, at least a very
large number of species, are imitative. Now the parietal bones
seem to be developed symbiotically with the parietal lobe, this
is not quite so, as has been shown elsewhere, but one may see
that the large arched square parietal bones in man, and the primates generally, are quite different from the parietal bones of
other groups. They are in the former more nearly an expression
of brain development, and especially of parietal development.
The symbiotic connection of the brain and other tissues has been
long suspected. Professor Schiefferdecker, of Bonn, has gone far
to prove it. The parietals in birds are large, thin at first and
developed over the optic lobes with which they are symbiotic.
The bones get thick in barn door fowl, but remain thinnish in
several groups. The bones are square, and, where they have got
thick, the changes are in response to changes in musculature, and
relative brain recession, perhaps. The bones get thin in several
primates in response to pressure from within, and the absorption
of the bony material from the central parts of the bone in order
to supply some of that substance to the adjacent ridges. Turner
found a divided parietal which is not easily explained, unless
one assume that a second centre was made further out. The
inner pair may then have represented the primitive parietal (optic)
ossicles, whilst the lower may have represented the re- and post-
frontals of reptiles. Wormian bones are so very frequent, however, that one often seeks most advisably an explanation which
involves a question of nutrition.

Referring again to the examples of muscle change in man,
which are so numerous, and which have evidently some relation
to the imitative power of man, the blending of the frontal muscle,
with some others (pyramidals), was found in a Lulu woman.
This may have been due to causes different to progressive development, as gorillas have the same arrangement. So a New Cale-
donian had a musculus frontalis like a gorilla. Skin muscles
are better differenciated in Whites, less so in Yellow races, and
least so in Blacks (Chudzinski quoted by Duckworth).

Orbicularis palpebrarum Zygomaticus Major, and Platysma,
blended in Aboriginal Australians (Chudzinski, Turner, Macalister, etc.).

One must admit that the *flexor longus pollicus* and flexor in-
dicis are specialized products of the human race, on which nu-

merous factors have always been at work, and no explanation, in conformity with the theorie of imitation, can explain the existence

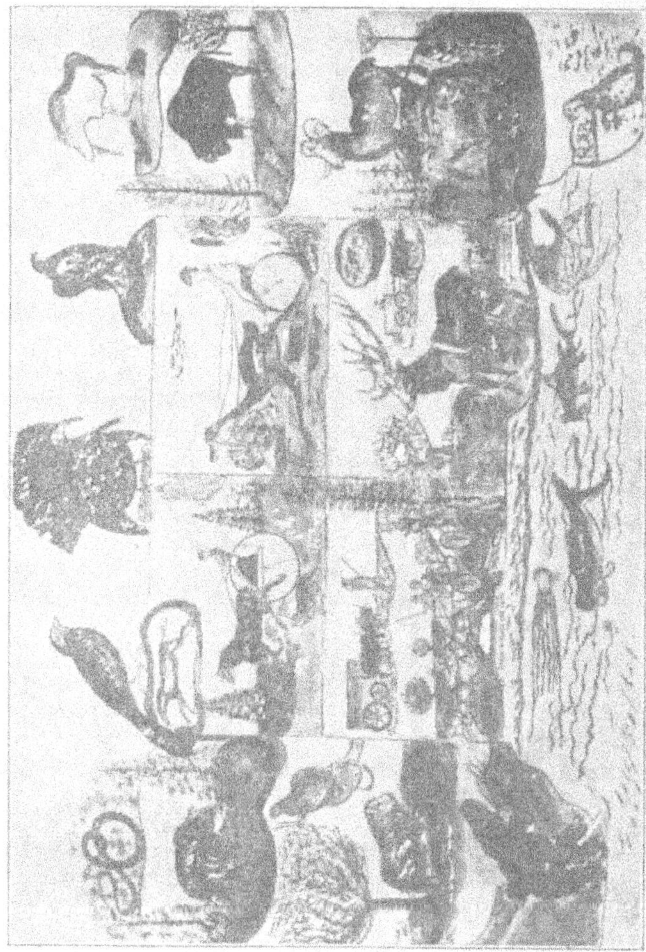

PLATE I.

of a united astragalus and scaphoid in man, which is only found in a few reptiles, and indicate embryonic modification of the centres akin to what obtains in Crocodiles. The Caucasian race has

been best studied. It is likely that one could get better material
for research in tropical climates. The researches of some well-
known anatomists bear out this. Though anomalies are not few
as judged by the immense work of Professor Gruber, yet human
anatomy is founded on average conditions in Caucasians, and
the individuals have been largely submitted to the same conditions of life. The men of the tropical field and forest have for
generations been subject to influences that trees and animals
engender when they develop in the highest and most aggressive
fashion. One must take each anomaly and endeavour to find
its proper position—embryological, mechanical, retrospective, pro-
spective or complemental. Is it likely to be produced in a child
in its most impressionable years? It will then be easier to find
out whether an anomaly is (or is possibly) referable to "mechanical" causes, as Kohlbrügge suggests. If a considerable number
of people different from the white race, which we have always
with us[1], be examined, one may get a clearer notion of the causes.
Professor Waldeyer has shown that the Gorilla has a much
less advanced spinal chord than homo, the size of the upper part
and even the lumber enlargement show the requirements for
skilled action. His investigations show that the Cuneus and Pre-
cuneus are very well developed in the negro, so is the Lobulus
precentralis, and the parieto-occipital sulcus is well developed on
the mesial cerebral surface. It seems not improbable that the
native of a tropical climate, or the child, who as well as his
forebears has been influenced by the animals, plants and scenery
of his country, might, by his actions, influence other types of the
genus Homo more efficiently than the original types of animals
would do. Powerful and forceful animals, or objects, deeply
impress the various types.

Most people will admit that the American people descended
as they are from Europeans who went there in the days of Co-
lumbus, and since then, have been influenced by the American
Indians in pose and feature. The troublesome times in the past
caused the impressions of the Redmen to be burned deeply into
the minds of Europeans. The immigrants seem to have strengthened the race, which in places has yielded to overtaxed energy.
There are so many factors at work that one is told that the race

---

[1] Insight points out that anatomical material is not of local origine in some cases.

is changing decade by decade, and the locality which has its own special value yields to the work of the incomers from the West. It has been endeavoured by means of simple sketches to show what leading agents are at work in certain parts of North America. The influence of steam and telegraph one cannot foreshadow. Four hundred years have permitted natural influences to have sufficient power for the moulding of the type. Contrary to what happens in the individual, the last years seems the most powerful, but the accumulated results of tradition, the cultivation of a vivid imagination, and the long isolation from old-style Europeans, have enabled the purely American influences to strike deep root. This convergence seems to be but a form of imitation. A type with characteristic form and feature is not easily effaced, and so we may expect a continuance of the type, locally at least, for many years (Plate I).

The influences that have served to mould the far-Eastern type might perhaps be best explained by those who have long experience of the different types or varieties of type to be found in land that see the sun so many hours before us Europeans. The habits of some would surely tend to develop depth of chest and breadth of head, if one can at all draw conclusions on the very imperfect data which one possesses, and it seems equally certain that the habits of some groups would tend to develop the long-headed type. Spherical shells contain, of course, more than shells of the same superficial content and some other shape, and if the body of an animal were perfectly free from external forces working at points on its contour, it seems that a circular cylindrical form would evolve itself. Once forces begin to act, not in an isolated manner, but continuously, or intermittently, from birth to maturity, strenuously or placidly, a response might be given by the muscle and skeletal parts. Putting this question to one side, it seems pretty certain that of outside objects, plants, and the scenery of the plain, influence the vast majority of the Eastern groups more mountains or animals. The former suggest slow development and steady than growth, and the latter activity, perhaps boisterous activity. The study of animals leads man to learn the expedients of animals and to become more resourceful. An influence which is partly, no doubt, purely biological, is sought from the traditions of the races which have had sages or heroes. One loses so much by lack of interest in animals (except man) that exclusiveness leads

to placidity Eastern architecture is apparently imitative or complementary, but the influence of this on children must be great.

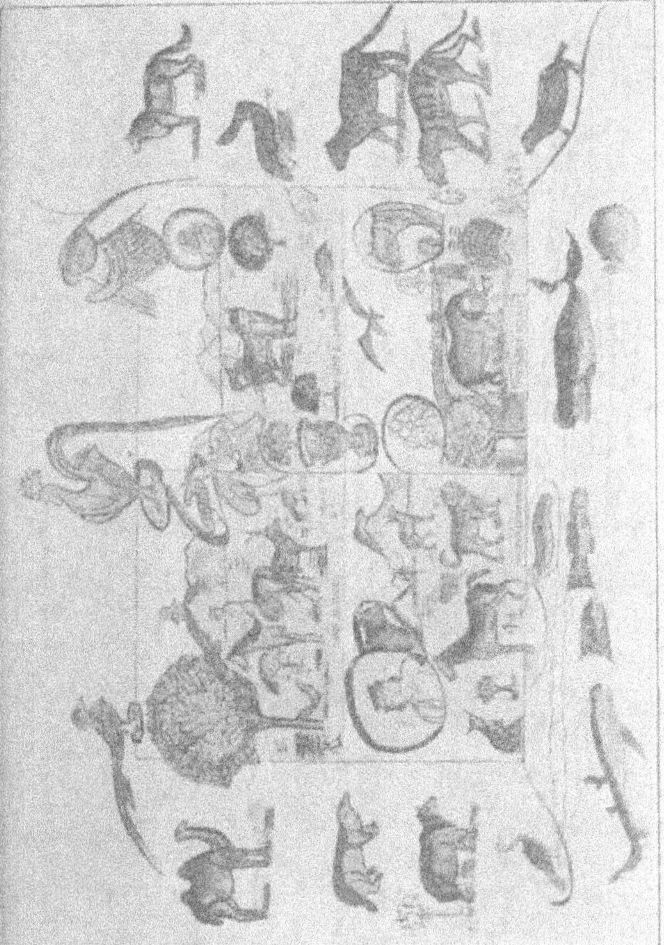

PLATE II.

Factors that influence man of the Eastern Holartic Region, Plants, Rivers, Human Beings in a placid non-aggressive serious state and Square Architectural Structures — Art.

The musculature seems from some records ([1]) to show a pro-
gress from tendon to muscle, and on to a division and increase

---

([1]) Stuart, Jal. A. & P., quoted by Duckworth.

in the number of tendons; this evidently shows that the energies of the nervous system are concerned with details, and new

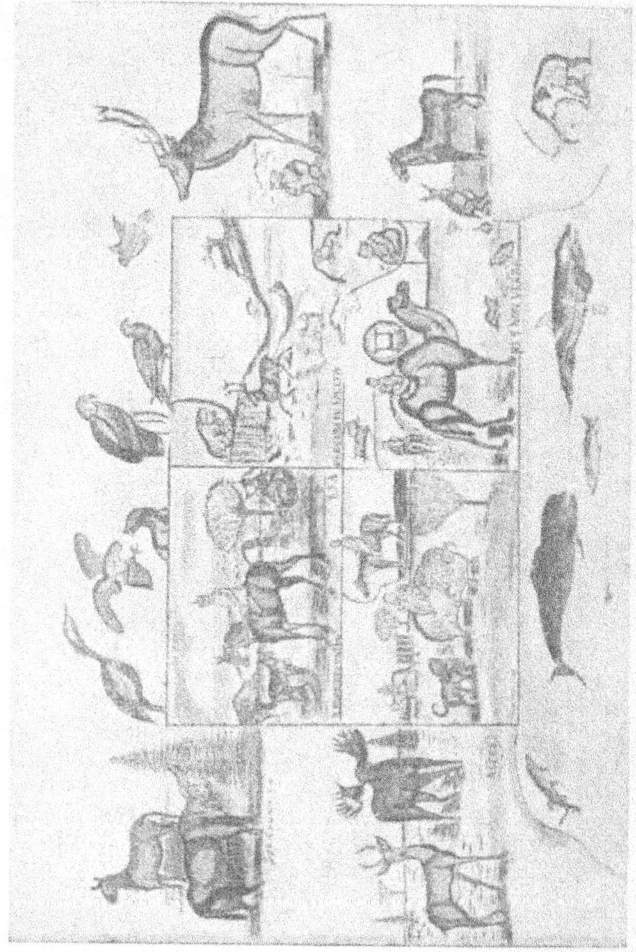

PLATE III. — URALIAN WATER SHED.

The Dwellers are interested chiefly in, and influenced mainly by Agricultural Work, Domestic Animals of the Field, Horses, Cattle, and Sheep, Forest and Flat Lands, Architecture in Towns, Pastoral Pursuits in the Country.

muscle or tendon slips are provided for dexterous expression of detail (Plate II).

Contrast the result of Flower's and Murie's dissection of

a Bojos woman, which shows the reverse tendency; and examples appear of structures that seem to have retained or acquired the Simian or the Canine type.

The admiration that birds and elevated creations are to have affected Eastern sports. Amusements, generally speaking, are believed to represent the chief simple, and impressional features of operations more serious and troublesome.

The types in other lands also have been susceptible of modification. One group forms the central Eurasian types, varying greatly in character. One cannot go into the question further than to say that there are the people of the plains and the forest; and those who are influenced by mountains and rivers. Horses seem to have had an immense influence on some populations (see Brehm). The ox and the sheep, camel and reindeer have their local effects. The forests are local. The architecture, churches and academy get hold of the contemplative. Architecture may stir up the strenuous or soothe the overstrung nerves. It seems natural to look to selection and environment as main factors in evolving the greyhound and the bulldog. The first is stretching out for «the beyond», and the other is concentrated on the personal accompaniments within the narrowest limits consistent with power (Plate III).

Landscape and colour, Mountain, River, Lake and Sea, have often gained attention. The effects of the steam machinery and motors have not had time yet to directly influence the types. The curtailment of the activities for reasons different from those given for the condition in the extreme East may give rise to kindred anatomical varieties (Plate IV).

The angular buildings suggest activity, whilst the curved lines of others suggest repose. Exuberant nervous developments find an expression in Horses (racing and training). The cult of architecture and the training of animals produce a certain change in groups which reproduce the same important factor in their time (Plate V and Plate VI). We notice, therefore, that the divergence is partly due to causes which were at work in separating the Bimana from the parent stem, and that in many respects this divergence is not so great as in various mammals and in birds, and that the structure of the central nervous system shows us that provisions are made for the increased skill of the hands and feet, the eye, ear and larynx. That the differences between different races of men are inconsiderable compared with the differences between man and the highest living primates has been long admitted. Cuvier and Meckel amongst the later anatomists dwelt on the anatomical characteristics as

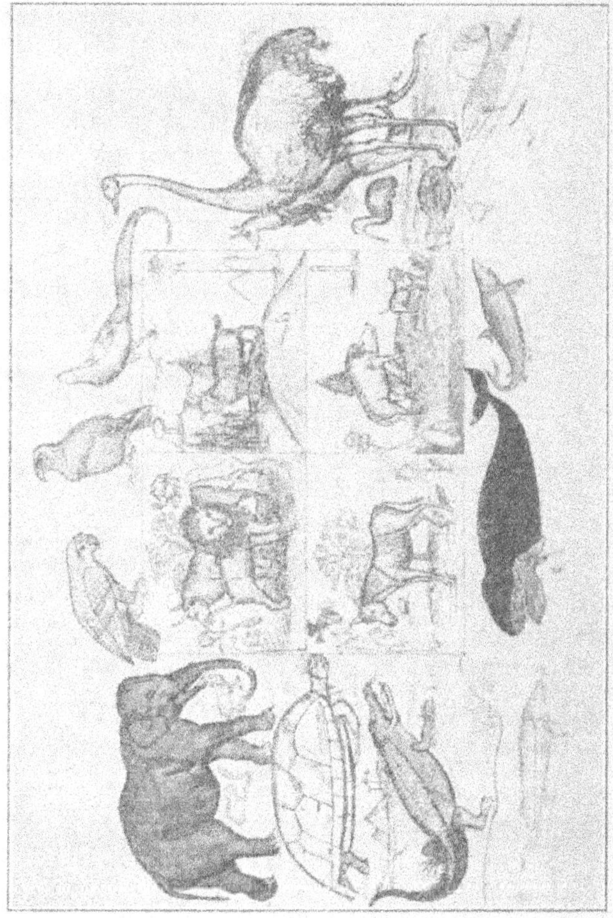

PLATE IV.

indicating more a modification advantageous to each case but unfitting the animal with the modified organ for movements that possibly exist with the unmodified organs. The statement of Cuvier that man can speak is objected to by Huxley who failed

to understand that Cuvier meant that man had the power to
develop speech which is closely associated with the power to
imitate the pose, feature, attitudes or voice of any living thing.
Waldeyer has shown that this is associated with enlargement

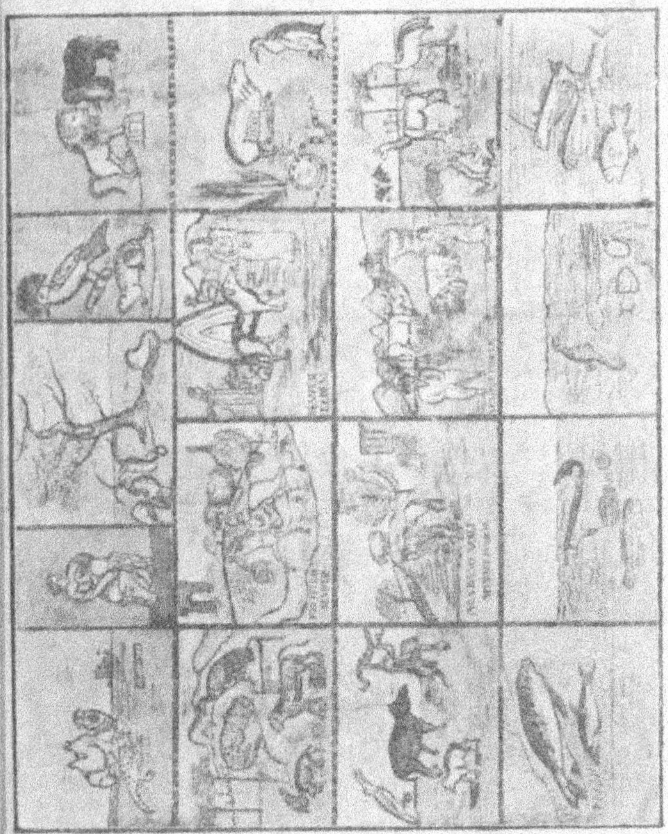

PLATE V

Factors that Turn Man against the Mob; Museum, Horse-show, Miniature Agriculture, Domestic Predatory Animals, Open and Shady Architecture. The Arts and Nature

of the spinal cord, as well as with a decided advance in brain
development not merely size but an increase in the number of
nerve fibres. The location of the centres of speech and dexterity
in the parietal and frontal lobes gives prominence to these parts.
The effects of training on animals has been to modify the organs. The hereditary traits are the most potent. The modifi-

cations in men are due probably to one of the causes given
by Macalister, in almost every case, but it seems that modi-

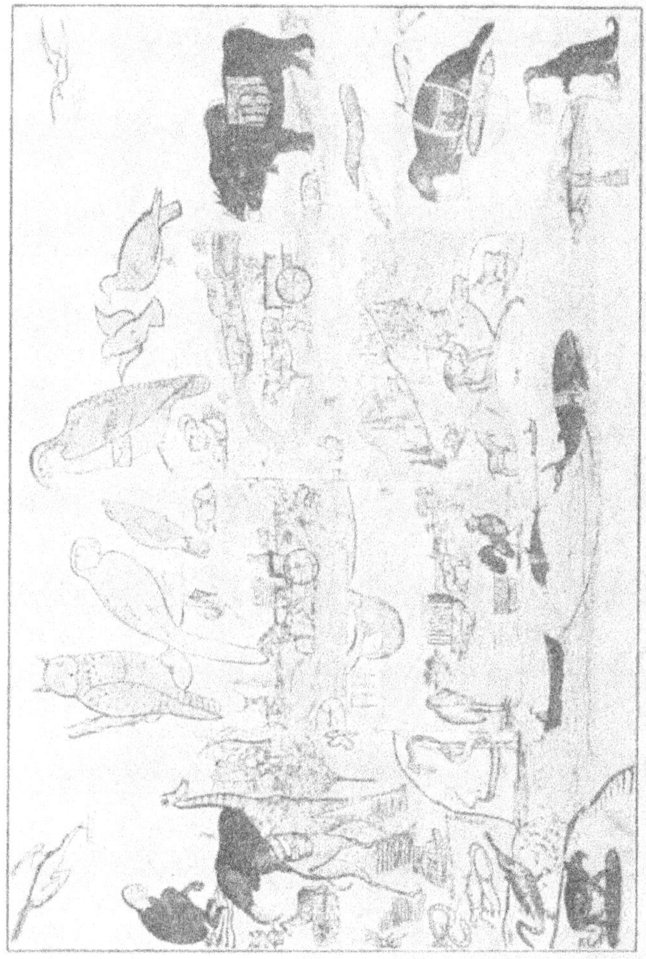

PLATE VI.

Scythian Groups, chiefly influenced by the graceful, harmonious coherent and predictive movements of Men and Animals.
The Arts, Trained Work, Architecture, Agriculture of the more extensive kind.

fications or freaks, apropo of nothing, may arise, which are
sometimes looked upon as a reminiscence of the past, or a pro-
phecy of future attainments. One cannot find out whether these

anomalies are transmissible. There is no proof that actual anatomical varieties are transmissible (Krause). The anomaly results from some ancestral peculiarity which is latent (Testut and others). They may, or some may result as the outcome of mechanical work (Kohlbrügge and others). Pathological changes apart, it is certain that food and early discipline in animals affect their competence. Human beings are influenced especially in early years, tastes are created, desires to move and act in certain ways. The featural result and pose may simulate hereditary traits. Mental tendencies and traits may arise which may appear to be hereditary. Divergences are the results of long continued influences that mould the individual; natural training and natural selection (with all its complicated varieties) are amongst these. Man, although he seems one of the least modified forms and exhibits features that connect him with a very distant past, he soon observed the advantages that many animals possess, in being specialized. He has learned to imitate many of these, and his voice is susceptible of treatment as well as his hands and feet. Convergences in muscle or skeletal parts have been aided by this. When unable to modify himself he succeeds by the work of his hands to construct models that express his feelings or his aspirations, and from these models or work of art he himself can again idealize the expression. The suggestions of Weismann remove some of the difficulties. Everyone knows the fact but not its range, that a slight embryonic change leads often to readjustment. (1.) It is certain, therefore, that man is not nearly related to any other primate. (2.) Anomalies are mostly retrospective or imitative that resemble those forms permanent in the higher primates. (3.) Crocodilia are probably nearest the ancestral strain, at least of the living reptiles. (4.) The nervous system at a very early age expresses in the sense organs the value of the material employed in the construction. The subsequent (relatively) or absolute disappearance of these may mean the provision of a valuable substance for consumption elsewhere (Lankester).

Some notes on the mandible and jugal in primates

Par M. RICHARD J. ANDERSON (Galway)

The Jugal and Mandible in Primates present sufficient interest from the nature of their connections and shape to render a survey of these bones not unacceptable.

Lemur (Macaco Varius?) (Fig. 1) presents for examination a wide zygoma. The arch of each is farthest out at the junction of the middle and posterior thirds of the orbit. The Jugal reaches

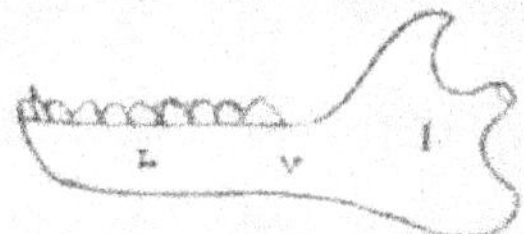

to the middle of the lower border of the orbit. The lower jaw is 7.5 cm long. The dentary one centimetre broad, and the ascending portion 3.8 cm from coronoid to lower border, and 2.5 cm from before back. The symphysis is receding and 1.25 cm in length. The Masseter surface is well-marked, the fossae on the angles which are prominent are marked.

A specimen which is named ruffed lemur (probably L. Macaco) jaw 6.2 cm × 1.2 cm, ascending ramus from coronoid to lower margin 2.9 cm by 1.8 cm broad, the zygoma is flatter and a deep fossa is situated below the coronoid process on the outside. There is a marked impression on the outer surface of the ascending part of the ramus, this reaches down to the angle and is continued over the surface of this for some distance, whilst in the preceding specimen which is older the impression does not reach beyond the base of the process, the inner surface, however, of the angle is excavated, and the lower border is here turned in. The impression on the outside does not reach so far down on the younger specimen but is deeper above.

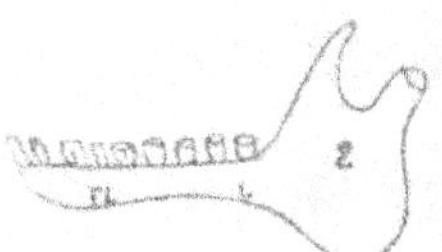

Galeopithecus (Fig. 2) has a very strong zygoma formed by a strong jugal which reaches quite over the arch and caps the small arch which is formed partly by the maxilla, the lower jaw is duply sculptured by the temporal and masseters. The fossa inside the angle is not conspicuous. The angle is large and round. The ascending part of the ramus is broad below 2.5 cm long and does not rise higher above the terminal part of the dental margin than it sinks below the lower border. The lower margin of the jaw is convex behind, concave in front. It bends down near the symphysis which is 0.6 cm long. The length of the Mandible is 5.2 cm, it tapers and is 0.68 cm broad in front.

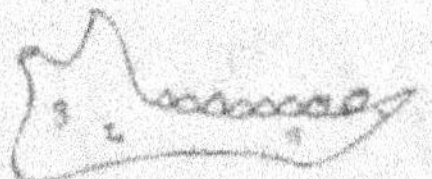

Loris gracilis (Fig. 3) has a wide jugal that reaches half over the zygomatic arch, is 1 cm broad from before back. The zygoma is strong. The coronory process is pointed and curved upwards and backwards. The mandible is 2.5 cm long and 0.8 cm broad. The ascending part is 1.5 cm from the tip of the coronoid process to the angle which extends downwards and backwards resembling in this respect some American monkeys. The outer surface is hollowed except at the angle. The posterior part of the coronoid process is concave.

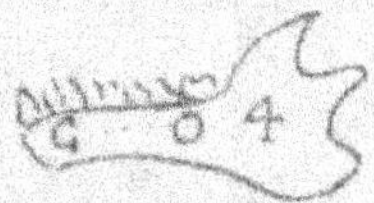

The jugal in Galago (Fig. 4), is very slender at its point of junction with the frontal, and stretches underneath the zygomatic process of the temporal, back to the fossa of articulation, but does not form a part of this. The arch is slender but prominent. The jaw is 4 cm long 0.4 broad in front and 2.2 cm from coronoid process to the lower border. The galagos have the mandible with its lower hind edge produced backwards.

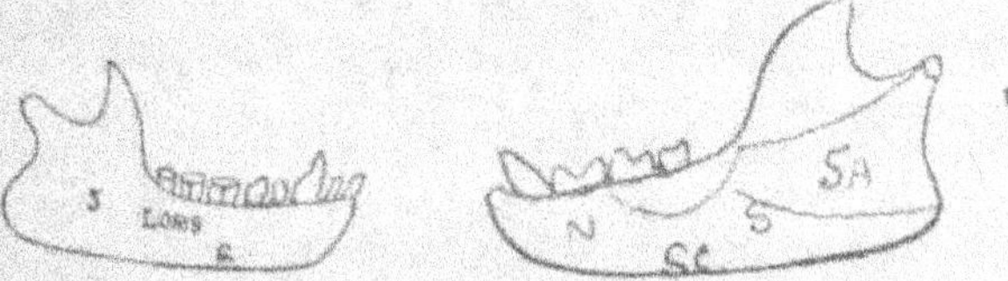

Lepolo lemur (Fig. 5) has a strong zygomatic arch formed by the maxilla capped by the jugal, which is very slender near its junction with the frontal. The length of the lower jaw is 3.7 cm and the breadth 0.7 cm in front. The ramus is 1.4 cm from the coronoid apex to lower border, the ascending portion is 1.25 cm broad, hollowed in the lower border with a very prominent angle. The outer surface is concave. The inner surface presents a deep fossa internal to the angle. The Temporal fossa is not conspicuous, the ridge above is feebly marked. The symphysis is oblique, strong and bony.

The mandible is short and deep in the Aye-aye (Cheiromys). The condyle as in Galeopithecus is short. The coronoid is «better-marked» (Owen) than the condyle.

The large rounded angle and the symphysis are both produced backwards, Owen notes, and the angle is broad and round. The coronoid process in Cheirogaleus «is very high» (Owen).

It will be seen that in several members of this group the ascending portion of the mandible is very large, and takes its character from the muscular attachments, which are very pronounced in Galeopithecus. This portion of the lower jaw must form a very important protection for the soft parts. The coronoid process which is large in all, curved and hooked in some, seems to have extended into the tendon of the temporal. The impression on the outer surface is often well marked, so that the muscles attached require deep impressions. The fossa internal to the angle is also very conspicuous.

The mandible is not so much spread in Cheirogaleus Melanotis as it is in Cheirogaleus milii (Forbes). The angle of lower jaw is pointed and hooked in Microcebus myoxinus. Here and in other cases the lower jaw extends its ossification into the tissues or tendons. The angle of the lower jaw in Microcebus furcifer is much produced backwards and downwards. The angle of the lower jaw is not produced downwards in the true Lemur (F.). Hapalemur has a very characteristic lower jaw that is massive in front and possesses «a very long symphysis», its angle also being very large. The angle is produced downwards, inwards, and backwards even more than in Indris (F.). The Indrisinae have the lower jaw provided with a large angle, which is produced backwards, the line of union of its two halves being long, and its lateral movements very limited. The line of union of the two halves of the lower jaw is shorter in Indris brevicaudatus than in Avahis, its angle is very large» (F.). Of fossil species, referred to by Forbes, Megaladapis has the two halves of the lower jaw ossified together.

«The angle of the mandible (in Microchaerus) being produced into a large hook-like flange» (Flower and Lydekker quoted by Forbes).

The chin in Omomys, another fossil Lemur, according to the same observer, is described as longer and less rounded than in Anaptomorphus (Eocene). Adapis from the Upper Eocene of France, England and North America, has the lower jaw «deep and stout».

Salient features of the lower jaw are brought out better in the Lemuridae than in any other group. The angle and coronoid process are so developed that the origin and uses of coronoid process, angle and ascending ramus are demonstrated. The muscles can be grouped so as to illustrate two «couples», as they are called by the mathematicians, for moving the ascending portion around an axis passing through the articulation. Where latent movement is allowed the same principal is to be observed. The extension of the processes is undoubted and the advantage of the bone as a support is clear enough. It is evident that the temporal muscle has gained more power for the «Couple» separating from the masseter. Hapale Jacobus. The jugal reaches the point of junction of the external border of the orbit with the superior border and articulates with the parietal, not with the temporal

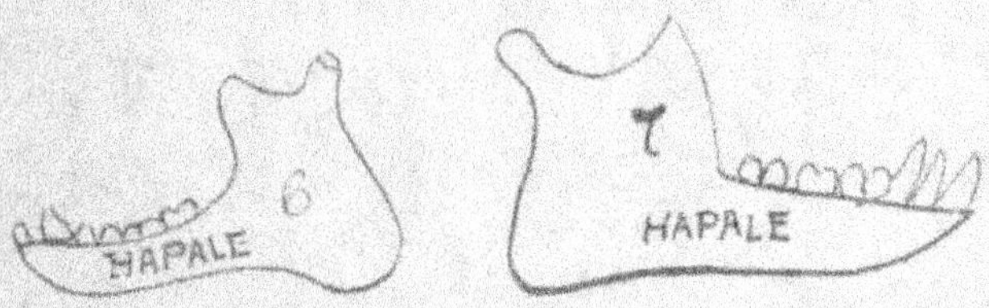

which articulates with the parietal by a short suture (Fig. 6 & 7). The zygomatic arch is 2 mm broad, and then one half is formed by the jugal. The mandible has a large ascending portion, an angle that projects back and down, a slender coronoid process and a condyle that reaches nearly as high, a quadrangular impression on the outside does not reach the angle which is much hollowed internally and the point inverted, the mandible is 3 cm long, 5 mm deep at the dentary part and 8 mm deep at the ascending part. The symphysis is 8 mm long and solid. It may be mentioned that the upper half of the ramus is more deeply impressed than in lower part.

Another specimen (Jacobus) gives a somewhat broader ascending portion of mandible 7 cm a little broader than the last, and the lenght of the entire jaw 27 mm, the height of the ramus is 17 cm. The impressions are distinct.

The jugal is perforated by a facial nerve in Platyrrhines.

In Brachyurus the jugal is touched by the parietal, and the lower jaw is dilated behind.

The jugal in Pithecia mariquonum reaches the parietal. There is a sphenoparietal suture. The ramus has an ascending part 3 cm in height, 2 cm broad with a small coronoid and a condyle

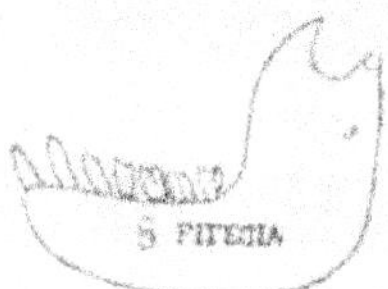

not quite so high as the latter Fig. 8. The angle is replaced by a curved border which runs into the posterior border above and into the lower border of the ramus below. Each ramus gets narrower as one traces it forwards, the lower border ascends. The two halves of the lower jaw are united by bone and the symphysis is 1.2 cm long. The upper jaw reaches back for a short distance underneath the jugal so as to form a portion of the arch, of which the jugal forms two thirds.

The outer surface of the ascending portion of the ramus is but slightly hollowed. The inner surface is hollowed, and the curved border is raised into a salient margin. The oblique ridge at the base of the last molar runs up towards the condyle and down obliquely to the symphysis. The articular surface of the condyle is elongated laterally and forms an elliptical surface of which the long axis runs inwards and backwards. The shovel-like appearance of the lower incisors will be remembered.

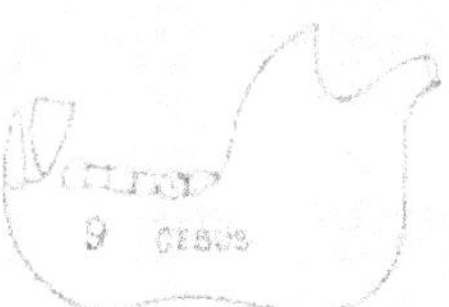

In Cebus (sp. Fig. 9) the jugal touches the parietal, so also does the sphenoid. The jugal reaches across the zygomatic arch

for half its length. The specimen which has got only five back
teeth (2 molars) has a moderately arched zygoma. The two halves
of the lower jaw are joined by a bony symphysis which is nearly
at right angles to the lower border of the jaw. The length of the
lower jaw is 4.8 cm, the depth near angle 1.7 cm, and in front
of ascending portion 1.2 cm, whilst of the coronoid process
is 2.5 cm above the lower border, the condyle is about 1 mm
less distant, and the angle which is not prominent is less than a
right angle. A well-marked impression is to be seen outside the
coronoid process, and a larger one reaching between the ridge
below and behind this and the angle. The impression on the
inner surface of the angle has a ridge and an elevated posterior
margin. The condyles have articular facets elongated outwards
and forwards. The notch which is wide and shallow in Marmo-
sets and small behind the hooked coronoid of Pithecia is shallow
and small in Cebus.

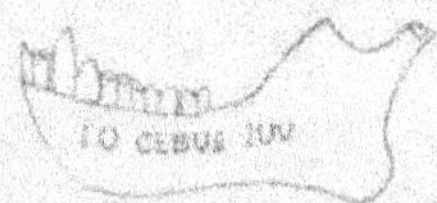

A Cebus (sp.) (Fig. 10) with a complete dentition and cranial
sutures partly obliterated has a jugal which forms more than half
of the arched zygoma and articulates with the parietal.

The lower jaw is very strong, the symphyses obliterated by
bone, and the ascending ramus very conspicuous with a large
round projecting angle which reaches downwards and backwards
from the ascending portion of the mandible.

The outer surface is hollowed behind the anterior border, but
is convex between this hollow and the angle, the bone here is
much hollowed and thinned internally, and ridged for muscle
attachment. The inner surface of the coronoid process, which is
of small elevation, is depressed, the notch between the coronoid
process and the still lower condyle is small and shallow. The
length of the ramus is 7 cm. The symphysis is 2.3 cm and oblique. The depth at the second premolar is 1.8 cm, and at second
molar about the same. The coronoid rises 4.4 cm above the
hollowed lower margin, and the breadth of the lower jaw from
anterior border to angle is 3.5 cm. The posterior border is straight
for 1 cm below the condyle, it then curves back and down and

forwards, and finally forwards and upwards making a curve 4 cm in length, which is followed by a hollow curve 2 cm in front of this.

In Mycetes the jugal does not articulate with the parietal. The jugal forms a third of zygomatic arch. There is a deep mandibular ramus, the depth is most marked in the ascending portion and angle. The coronoid process is prominent and strong. The angle is nearly equal to a right angle. Lagothrix has a larger lower jaw than Cebus, and is somewhat like that of Mycetes in the articulation of the vomer.

The bear of the Andes has a lower jaw like Mycetes. The large jaw besides protecting the soft parts (larynx, throat, vessels and air) will, in the pose assumed by these animals in a country of forests, be a shield against the crossing and springing branches.

The jaw ramus of Mycetes (sp.) has a large curved posterior border, raised up externally and internally. The length of the jaw is 9 cm, the length of symphysis is 3 cm, and receding. The depth at second premolar is 2 cm, and opposite second molar

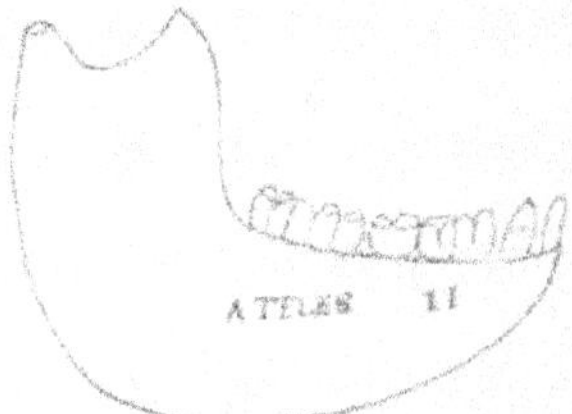

3 cm (Fig. 11). The depth of ramus is 8.5 cm, and its width 4 cm. There is a deep fossa below the small coronoid, and low condyle, a second fossa is still further down. The inner surface is deeply excavated and ridged.

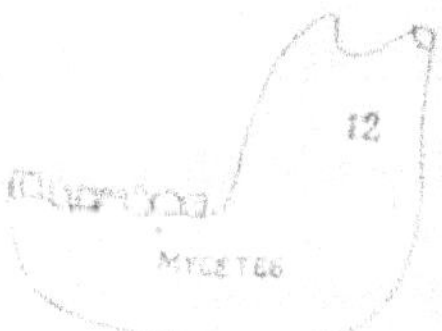

The coronoid in another and older skull is low. The outer surface of the ascending ramus has a marked impression above, but the lower part is bounded by a ridge posteriorly, the inner

surface (Fig. 12) is excavated and ridged below and behind, and is separated by an oblique ridge from the hollow on the inner surface of the coronoid. The symphysis bony and receding, and the jaw less deep in front than where it joins ascending part.

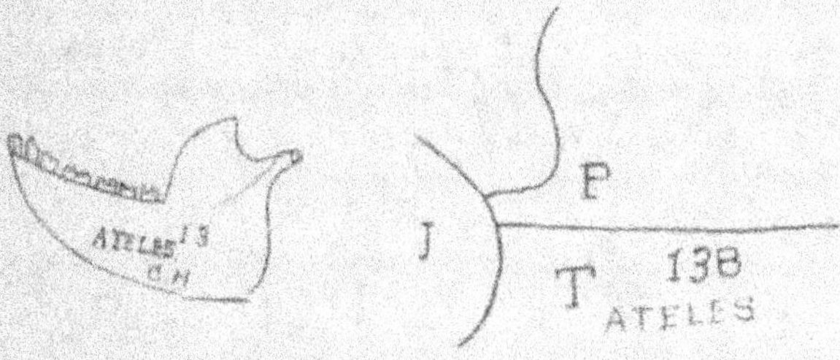

The Cercopithecidae (Fig 13) have in some groups, mandibles that are high, broad and flat, with a large facial angle. In others the dentary part of the lower jaw sometimes exceeds the ascending part.

Cynocephalus porcarius has a strong zygoma. The jugal does not reach the parietal which is cut off from the sphenoid by the temporal. This arrangement holds for Cynocephalus sphinx also, and for C. niger.

A Cynocephalus figured by Owen seems to have an ascending ramus about three times the height of the dentary part. The breadth of the ascending ramus is about two thirds of its height. The condyle is lower than the coronoid process.

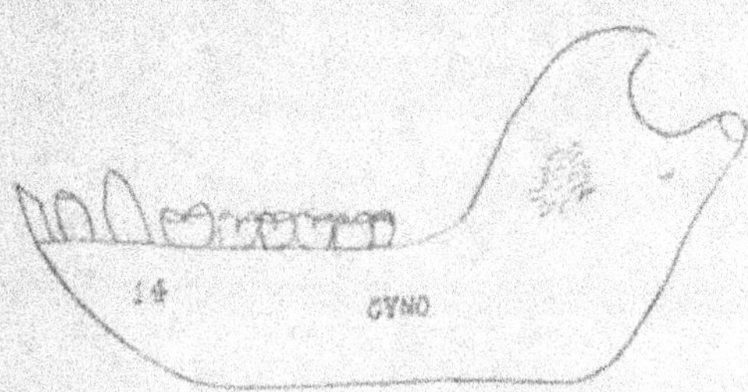

In Cynocephalus anubis (Fig. 14), the jugal is 2.5 cm from the parietal, which is separated from the sphenoid by the parietal. The jugal forms more than half the arch. The lower jaw is 12 cm long. The symphysis 4.5 cm and receding. The depth is 3 cm at second molar and less than 3 cm behind last molar. Depth at ascending ramus from coronoid to lower border 7 cm. There is a very large fossa below the coronoid process (which stands a centimeter higher than the condyle). The bone is excavated outside the angle and has three elevated rough impressions near the posterior border, and a depression on the inner side of the bone below the coronoid. The skull measures along the circumference from the parieto-temporal suture of one side to the corresponding suture of the opposite side 10.5 cm, and from the supraorbital eminence to the occipital protuberance in the middle line 9 cm (11.5 × 8.5 cm).

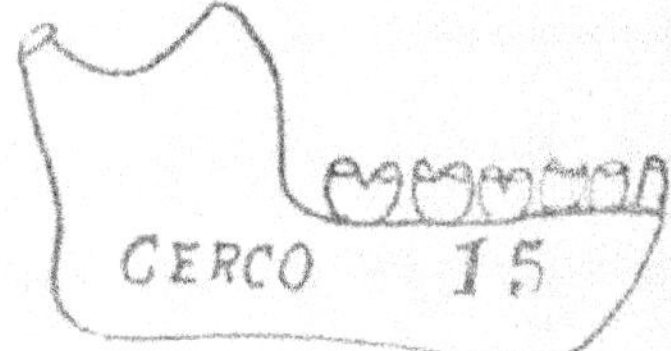

Cercopithecus (sp.) (Fig. 15) has a jugal that reaches quite half across the zygoma, but does not reach the parietal which is separated from it by the frontal.

The mandible is 9.3 cm long, the jaw is deeper opposite the first premolar (2.8 cm) than opposite the last molar tooth (2.4 cm). The ascending ramus rises 5 cm above the lower border of the jaw (from coronoid to lower border), the angle is obtuse. The coronoid process is not prominent. The incisor teeth stick out from the strong mandible. The outer surface is deeply sculptured below the coronoid process. The inner surface is hollowed and ridged near the angle. Cranial part (with callipers) $\frac{5}{4}$. Young

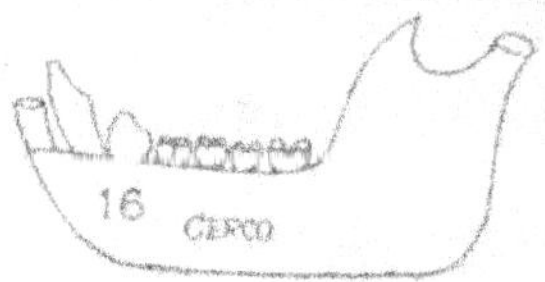

Cercopithecus (sp.) (Fig. 16), jaw 6 cm long, 1½ cm wide in front, same in front of ascending portion, and at coronoid 3.5 cm. Symphysis 2 cm. A skull of Cercopithecus sykesii, aet. 2 molars, has a parieto-sphenoid suture. The lower jaw has a receding symphysis. The external surface is grooved below the coronoid which is depressed inside, the posterior part of the angular surfaces internal to the angle is ridged. The condyles are elongated from side to side with a slight bend inwards and backwards, length 5 cm, breadth 1.2 cm.

Macacus innuus, has the dentary portion deeper in front than behind, and the ascending part of the ramus is broader than the dentary part. The height is double the breadth of the dentary portion.

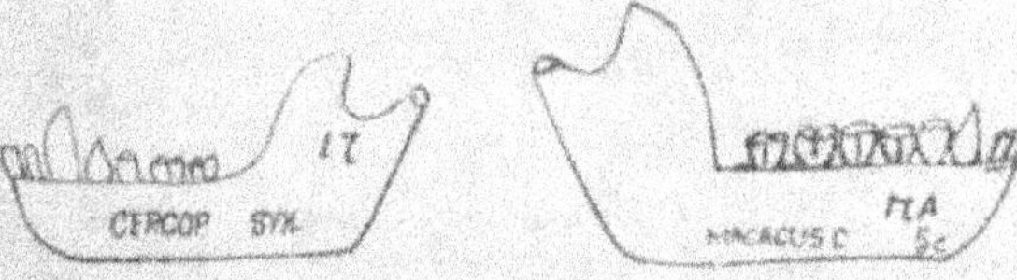

In Macacus cynomolgus (Fig. 17a) the jugal reaches beyond the middle third of the outer border of the orbit. The zygomatic process of the jugal reaches beyond the middle of the zygoma. The sphenoid intervenes between jugal and squamous.

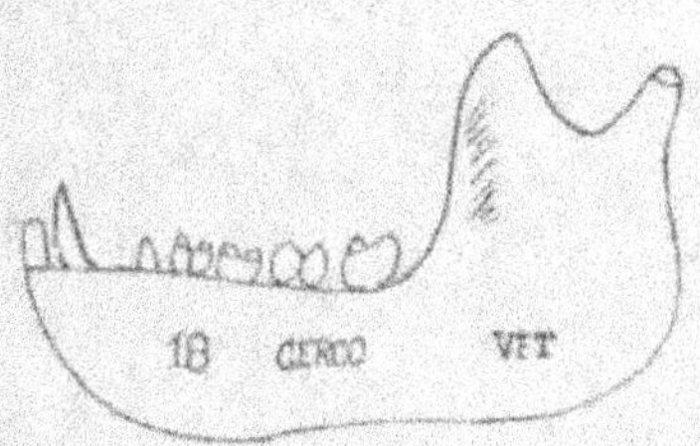

The mandible is broader in the anterior part than behind. The ascending ramus is much wider from before back than the breadth of the dentary portion of the jaw. The incisor teeth do not project much. A groove is found between the ascending ramus and the molar teeth.

A large space exists between the pterygoid process and the ascending part of the lower jaw.

The length of the mandible is 7 cm, symphysis 2.5, depth

at second premolar 1.8 cm and in front of ascending portion of mandible 1.4 cm. Depth from coronoid to lower border 4 cm and breadth 2 cm. The coronoid is a little higher than the condyle, the precondyloid notch is shallow. The coronoid process has a deep depression externally and a depression internally, the bone is very thin here. There is a hollow internal to the angle, and a raised irregular margin bounds this surface posteriorly. There is a finger-mark like impression outside the angle, which is obtuse, dentition complete.

Cercopithecus juv. (back teeth) (Fig. 18) has the mandible with a short ascending part 4.5 cm long, symphysis 1.5 cm, depth at first

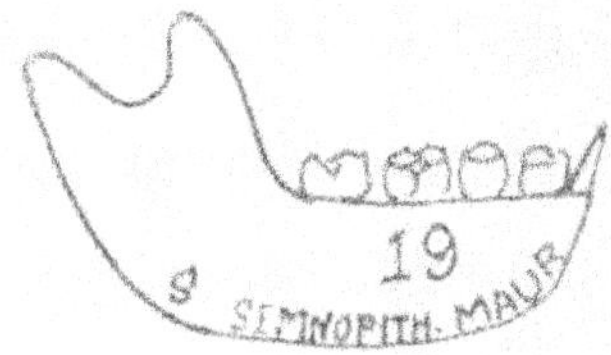

molar 1.3 cm, and in front of ascending part 1 cm, depth at coronoid 2 cm. The angle is obtuse, coronoid process hollowed external, angle surface hollow internally, convex from above down externally. Breadth of ramus 1.5 cm. Sphenoid reaches temporal.

Semnopithecus maurus (Juv) (Fig. 19) has a mandible with an obtuse angle, a receding symphysis, and a small coronoid, length 3 cm, depth at second p. m. 1 cm, and in front of ascending part 0.8 cm. Outer part of coronoid, and inner surface of angle hollowed. The inner part of coronoid is depressed. The jugal is separated from the squamous internally by a narrow sphenoid which touches the parietal, externally the jugal forms half the zygomatic arch.

The jugal of Hylobates reaches nearly half way across the slender zygoma.

The parietal was found in two or three specimens of Hylobates Mulleri to extend to the jugal. It will be noticed that this is mentioned as an unusual arrangement by Owen for the genus Hylobates.

Duckworth figures Hylobates Mulleri with the parietal removed from the jugal, as has been mentioned elsewhere for Hylobates Hainanus (Fig. 20). The ascending portion of the ramus is low. The height of the jaw in front of this is 1 cm, and the symphysis

is 1.7 cm. The length of the jaw is 6 cm, and the angle is nearly
a right angle (Fig. 21). The inner surface of the angle has the

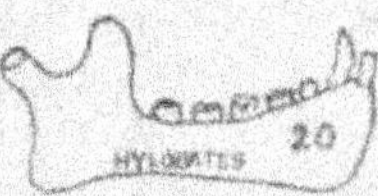

usual depression, and the impression on the coronoid is also
clearly seen. The symphysis in the Siamang (Hylobates syndacty-

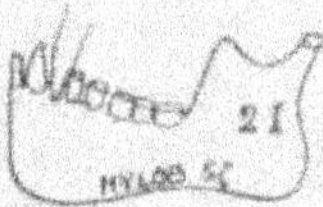

lus) is more vertical than in the Gibbons proper, hence the
«chin».

The depth of the ascending portion of the mandible opposite
the coronoid process is 2.5 cm, and the antero-posterior measurement is 2.2 cm. The depth at the coronoid is 2.4 cm, so that
the coronoid is not very prominent.

The ascending portion of the mandible in another Hylobates
(Sp. M.) is nearly square, the angle is inflected, or the surface is
so hollowed internally that the posterior inferior margin is rendered more conspicuous, or is added to by deposit. The incisors
and molar teeth are well worn down. The fossa on the inner part
of the coronoid process is conspicuous. The excavation on the
postero-inferior part of the outer surface does not reach the angle,
where the edge is somewhat raised.

The adult Gorilla has strong zygomas. The jugal and al-
sphenoids are separated from the parietal by the union of the
frontal with the squamosal. The mandible in the adult has no
true chin which is very long (Fig. 22). The dental part of the
mandible is 14 cm long, and 3 cm broad (deep). The angle between
the ascending and dentary parts of ramus is less than a right
angle. The ascending part of ramus is 9 cm $\times$ 6 cm, the former
is the height measurement and the latter the breadth.

The distance between the rami behind is less than the breadth of the skull.

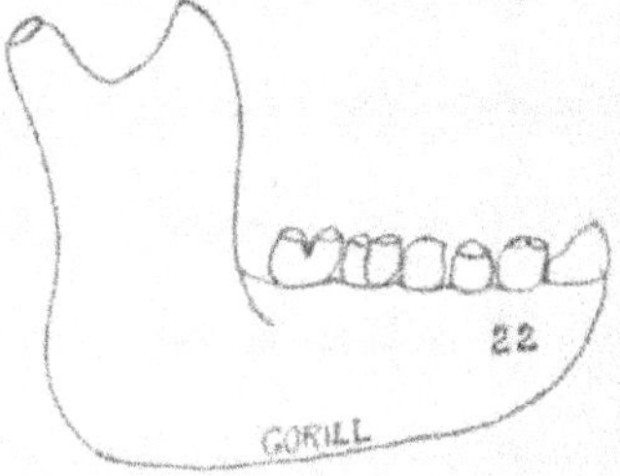

The coronoid depression is well-marked.

The young skull figured by Duckworth has apparently a much wider ramus proportionally than the older skull. Duckworth examined a great many skulls, but the one figured in the «Anthropology» seems to be a young adult. The fossa internal to the angle and the coronoid process are well-marked. The outer surface of the last-molar tooth is placed 1.5 cm internally distant from the outer surface of the ascending part of ramus. A deep and wide groove lies between the outer salient border of the bone and the tooth.

The *thickness* and *density* of the jaw is evidently due to the work that it performs. «Intermittent work produces hypertrophy». This is the cause, no doubt, of the stout condyles which have articular surfaces that are broadly elliptical with the inner ends but slightly back. The measurement from zygoma to zygoma, that is out to out is 14 cm. The skull increases enormously in weight

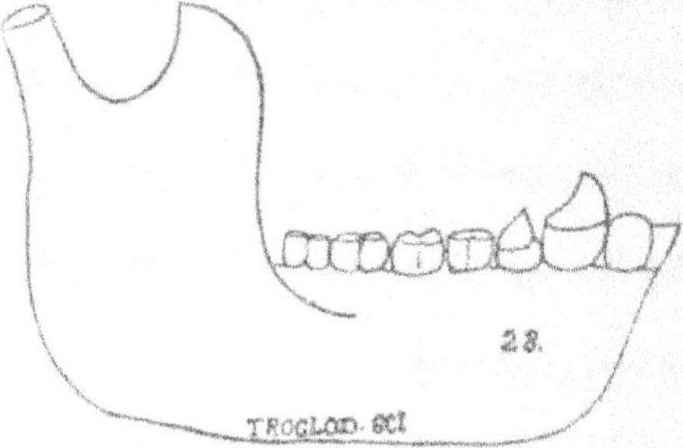

in relation to cranial capacity as age advances from birth to adult age.

In Troglodytes (sp.), Fig. 23, the angle of the lower jaw in three specimens, that have the milk dentition, is 125° in two, and 130° in one. The angle in an adult with a full mouth is 115°. The coronoid process is not high in any one of the four, but is broad in the adult skull. There is an almost vertical symphysis in the young skulls, a receding symphysis in the adult. The muscular impressions on the young jaws are not conspicuous, but the angle fossa is well marked inside and outside, and a depression on the interior of the coronoid process marks the adult skull. The distances between the rami (at the angle) on the one hand and the distances between the margins of the opposite auditory meati (lower borders), respectively, are for the former 9 cm. and for the latter 10.5 cm., the height of the ascending ramus is 6 cm, and that of the cranium 8.5 cm (this in the adult). The height of skull from lower border of maxilla is 11 cm, and the tip of the coronoid process is 4 cm above lower level of the jaw (young species).

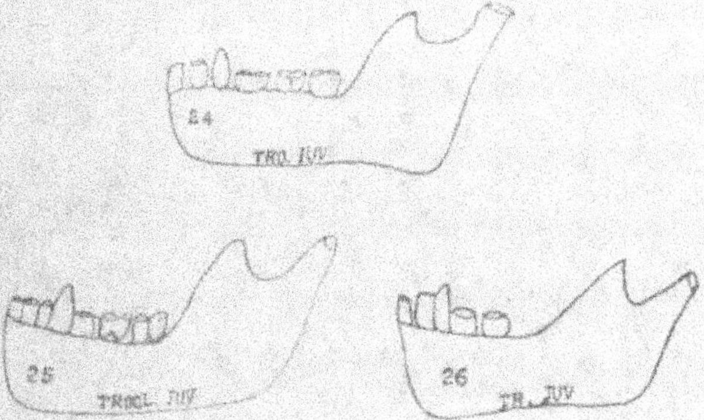

Fig 24. The length of the lower jaw from the posterior border of the ramus to the symphysis is 8 cm in the young. The symphysis is 2.5. The depth of jaw just in front of symphysis is 1.8 cm, and the antero-posterior diameter of the ascending portion is 3 cm. The lower jaw has a much less pronounced temporal ridge than the adult. The increase in the size of the coronoid process seems to show an extension of the ossific matter into the tendon, as the ridges that deepen the fossae show also.

In Young	Cranial length	taken from above and between supra-orbital prominences to	10 cm	= 1
	„ breadth	occipital protuberance	10 cm	
Adult	„ length	The skull recedes and the cranium is contracted behind orbits	11.5	= 0.86
	„ breadth		10.0	

The zygomata are much stronger and more prominent. In one young skull the calvarium has got very thick. The skull is nearly round on transverse section 10.2×9.2.

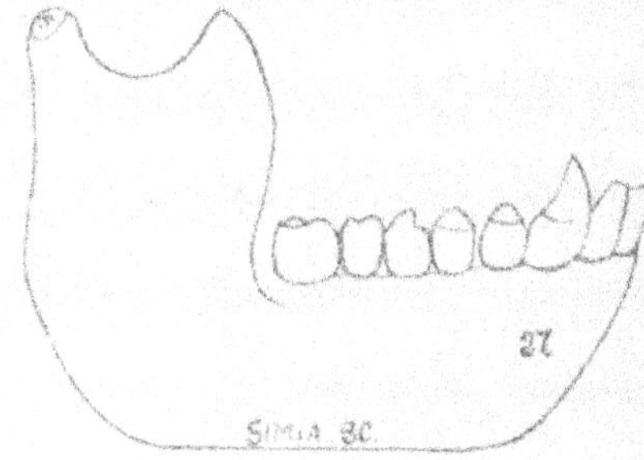

It seems from a consideration of these specimens that the main features, though influenced by the second dentition, are especially modified by the greater activity of the jaw, which has conspicuous ridges in the adult, although the ascending ramus is somewhat thinned in its central portion, as the temporal fossa also is near its upper part. The skull of one of the young specimens is thin above the supra-orbital ridges, this is not the case in the thick skulled specimen. The distance between the rami in a young specimen is 7.0 cm, which compared with a cranial breadth of 10 cm is interesting, the adult gives 9.5 cm from out to out behind the ramus a little below the condyle. The covering of the temporal fossa seems to remove the stimulus to bone formation which proximity to the surface (by blood supply) would secure for it.

The muscle ridges increase their bone, perhaps, at the expense of that absorbed from the fossa.

An adult Simia has a parietal-sphenoid articulation. The sphenoid is large. The jugal reaches one third across the zygoma. The upper jaw is very massive; moderately marked muscle impressions. Condyle a little higher than the coronoid, which is short and stout, the jaw is not much thinned where the muscles are. The temporal ridge is not well-marked. Zygomata arched.

    Length of cranium .... 11 cm
    Breadth .... 10 cm

The skull thins from behind the outer part of the orbital ridge to a point beyond middle of temporal fossa.

    Length of jaw .... 11.5 cm
          „ reaching symphysis .... 9 cm
    Depth of ascending part .... 7.3 cm
          „ dentary part .... 2.5 cm

There is a well marked depression inside coronoid process.

Fig. 27. The antero-posterior diameter of ascending portion is 4 cm. The distance from the summit of the skull to the lower border of the jaw is 15.5 cm. Compare with Troglodyte 15 high by 6.5 cm. for distance from coronoid to lower border.

The great length of the coronoid process in Cephalelaphus is

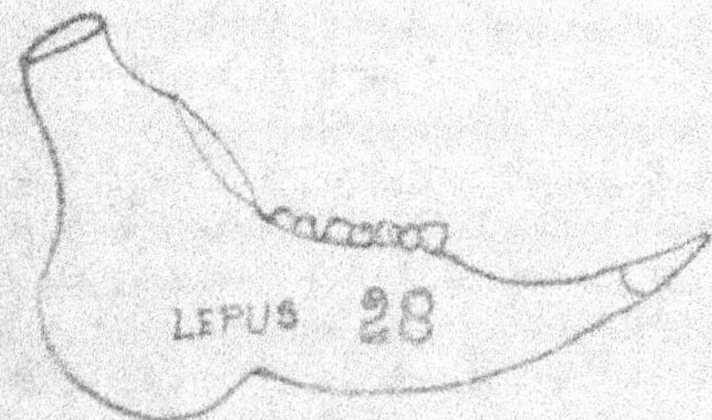

remarkable when compared to the same process in Primates; in no member of this latter group, except the Lemurs, is this process

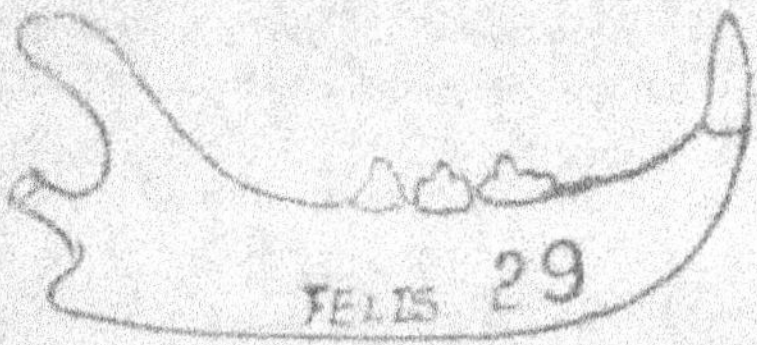

of considerable length. The process is of less importance in some rodents, inconspicuous in the rabbit, it is distinct, but not very pronounced in the Capabara, where it is external to the last molar tooth, and the jugal is shoved back also. The lower jaw angle is very strong in conformity with the rest of the skull.

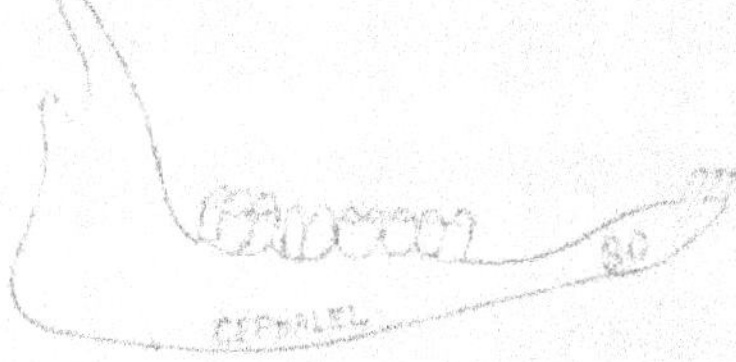

A deep groove runs forward outside the teeth. The angle resembles that of the lemurs, rather than that of the cat. The coronoid of the cat resembles that of the lemurs. The condyle is lower down and the outer surface of the condyle is much narrower, of course, the portion of the coronoid above the upper border of the dentary portion of the jaw really constitutes the ascending ramus in the cat. In the Simiadae, however, the coronoid is of small dimension and the size of the ascending ramus above the line of the dentary is partly due to the position of the condyle which is nearly as high as the coronoid process. The heavy bones have evidently to do with the support of the teeth. The ridges do not keep pace with the size of the bones, for the Orang has very heavy solid skull bones, with slight muscular impressions and a not very considerable zygoma. The skull is thin behind the orbits, and in parts of the temporal in Gorilla, and in a Troglodytes Niger thinning of the skull is also a feature. It is possible that the thickening of the bones of the jaw may be in response to the enlargement of the teeth; the skull is very weighty for the size, suggestive of a decadent type. The skull (without the lower jaw) of a Gorilla weighed more than the skull of a Veddah and less than the skull of European. Some other human skulls weighed a fourth more.

Racial types in Connaught with special reference to the Basque Type

Par M. Richard J. Anderson, Galway

There are so many detached facts and so many speculations built on historic records collected from time to time that it becomes difficult to decide upon the exact and early origin of many groups.

The historic record deals with times comparatively modern, and yet one sees how much greater difficulties would present themselves if we were deprived of the facts collected during the historic epoch. It has been suggested that the ancestors of our "Libyans, Egyptians, Pelasgians, Iberians" inhabited the North Africa, and Mediterranean regions (Keane and Laborowski). We can account for the migration by the elevation of the Mediterranean sea floor, as M. Zaborowski does, during quaternary times.

Specialization of the groups, at least the special groups, seems a necessary assumption. Virchow and others were of a different opinion and with Virchow the greater number of anthropologists agree in holding the migrations were largely, if not solely, in modern times from. The statements that a Negrito type established itself at one time in the South, if not Central and West Europe, have reference to an earlier period, and there seems satisfactory evidence that a pigmy race was among the first if not the very first (Kollmann). It seems too satisfactorily established that the various races are in a measure represented in various places by individuals, more or fewer, who may represent the last of their race, or may be examples of people who have sprung from a mixed ancestry, and who have developed ancestral characters which had lain latent during several generations. The difficulty is increased by the changes in the history and habits of families, tribes and groups. Changes in the mode of life, food and occupation seem to bring into existence, or into prominence, features that were never suspected to exist in the parent stem. This tendency was at one time thought to be of the nature of a reversion to a primitive type, but although the position of the Atavists is to some extent accepted yet it does not follow that in every case a greater tendency exists to develop ancient rather than more recently perceived peculiarities. The environment seems to be an important factor.

It is, however, probable that animals lose their most recently acquired features first. It will be admitted that in all such cases one should have a record of pedigree, and a clear and satisfactory description suitable for anthropological as well as ethnological purposes. It is scarcely possible to deal in a satisfactory way with records of young people in large towns, without ample evidence with reference to their environment, which should supplement the most accurate and detailed anthropological measurements and weights, and other statistical notes. Some observers believe that an investigation of the lung power and strength would be a useful adjunct to the work of the anthropologist.

Having regard to the fact that a group of people may either become located in a district, and may ultimately occupy the entire land, or may settle, assimilate, and mix with the pre-existing types, or may, by changing their habits, alter their own distinctive characters, it will be of no little importance to record the features which are considered most interesting. It is not always easy to mention all the chief facts with regard to the individual, but this is certain, the more complete one makes the records of the full grown the better, and the character of the muscular development and the build should be especially noted. The head of the greyhound is developed in response to a series of conditions which have been met by the lithe form of the animal.

The dachshund has, perhaps, responded to other conditions, but it seems probable that several special breeds of dogs have descended from different ancestors, yet one usually admits the specific characters; and the relations of breadth to length in a good number were published several years ago. Hence the local environment, which may produce a race of strong short men in one place, may produce, by the survival of the fittest, light active undersized men in another district, one group may climb trees well, and the other may climb mountains. There are other conceivable influences such as rapidity of movement, suitability for riding.

No doubt the bones respond to the musculature, but although the influences of heredity seem to play an important part, yet any peculiarities which men have, or animals, that are spoken of as acquired, have less chance of having been inherited if they are removed much from their proper type, that is, they are pathological (W. Krause). And when one comes to deal with man, remembering that from a very early age his muscles are really or potentially active, in his attempts to imitate those in his vicinity of his own species, or perhaps the movements of some other animal, we find that a complication of operations seems to work on the individual skeleton to bring it within the mould which the sight and touch, as well as the muscle force and sense, have all conjoined to make. The change of location and habit may lead to a more efficient way of lengthening and strengthening our posterity than we should conceive possible. The features of children are said by L. Robinson to be those of the nurse, or perhaps those of the person who impresses the child most. But objects of various kinds influence the imitating children. So a robust immigrant race might influence the local tribes or home communities.

I gave, on a former occasion, records extracted from various tables to show the relative numbers of the blonde and the brunette types in the Claddagh schools, Galway. The cranial measurements in the young are not an exact criterion of the relative percentages of the sections in which we place the relative types of skulls in adult life; it seems, however, that the growth of the brain is primarily responsible for the shape of the skull where the latter has freedom of growth. The separation of the condyles is evidently in response to the broadening of the head. It will, no doubt, be admitted that the bones of the head take their places in conformity with the type of individual, and that the short stout type will then be more likely to favour the growth of a broad skull and a broad brain. Perhaps the latter more than the former because the increase of skin surface and muscles is attended with a corresponding growth of brain in Elephants and Whales. There comes in another consideration which the investigations of Prof. Schiefferdecker have done much to establish, viz. that a symbiotic relationship exists between tissues where one may least expect it, so whilst abundant surface nerves and muscles ought to give larger brain, so the tendency would be to make broader, if the parietal centres (association and all) were to enlarge the skull might get broader. But without comparisons which are dangerous and marked with spitgalls and non sequiturs one may point to the breadth of the Amphibian heads and Chelonian bodies, and the corresponding broadening of the viscera in the latter when compared with the tendency to elongation in Lacertilia and Ophidia.

It has been said that the ancient type known as Basque is related to the Ligurians who lived in Italy at one time, as well as in Corsica and Sardinia, and were apparently derived from the same stock as the Picts and Iberians, if we separate the latter from the Basques.

The Basques are related to the Berbers and ancient Egyptians and spread at one time along the shores of France and reached Great Britain and Ireland. This was long before Brittany received accessions to its Keltic population from the English Kelts of the 5th century. There is in North Spain a tall fairhaired long-headed type, as well as a broad stout type. The latter predominates and blue eyes are common. Professor Reclus was inclined to think that the Basque type as described is less prominent than some have led us to believe. It is evident that the nature of the type may, by different observers, be studied in different localities, and the region in one case be more extensive.

The Berbers of Tunisia, Algeria and Tripoli are related to the Egyptian type, whilst the Berbers of the Atlantic Border are mixed with Southern types.

There is ample evidence from the skeletons that two races lived in Egypt in close relationship, and lie together in the pyramids. It seems probable that one race was the predominent group, and the other an inferior and subordinate race.

There are remains of Palæolithic man in Tunis. One type like the Neanderthal, the other like the Cro-Magnon, Dolmen building type. These Quatrefages identified with Mauritanians and those of the Canary Islands, they were fair, and tall, with blue eyes.

The Megalith builders of Mauritania were of the same type as those of Egypt.

Several examples are known in Iberia where the names of rivers, mountains and tribes have come from the Basque language, just as many such in other parts of Europe have been traced to the Keltic group. That the Basques contributed largely to the population of France and Iberia as well as Britain and Ireland no one doubts. It seems probable that the Central European Keltic tribes were closely related to the Basques, as were no doubt the ancient Albanians.

The Kelts were of varied types. One type, and to these one might limit the term dark type, viz. the black haired and black eyed type, and then the Red Kelt would apply to another conspicuous group found in Wales and Brittany. These people were no doubt associated with others, but were descendents chiefly, or largely, of dark and light haired races which went westward. These were respectively users of the smooth stone and bronze impliments.

If, as was supposed at one time, the flow of the human streams was eastward, then one may admit that the assertion (in the Four Masters) is probably correct, that the westward moving tribes were derived from those that previously had moved eastward.

The Firbolgs who are thought to have still held land in the western part of Ireland, early in the Christian era, were derived from the south group of which the ancient Albanians formed possibly a part. But all this is changed now, the Firbolgs were forerunners of the red and dark races, who were immediately preceded by the Dedanaans.

The still earlier tribes seem to have been palaeolithic so far as one can tell anything about them. It is as like as not that the British Isles were connected with Europe by land and it is within the reasonable speculations of the Antiquarian or poet that an Atlantis continent existed in these early times. The presence of isolated plant types and certain invertebrate animals contribute some positive evidence to this theory. It seems also from the great size of the caves in Ireland, that have been excavated by the waters, and the presence of animal remains in these, that the times at which these animals lived must have been long enough ago to give time for the changes that have since taken place.

The primitive types were somewhat different. The very first were small and apparently slight, and suitable for forest life. The investigations of Prof. Kohlmann are quite in favour of a primitive pigmy type. Such people could live in forests, build houses in trees, and take shelter there from their enemies. The Shetlanders thought the Picts were pigmies.

Between the times when these people lived and the time of the Dedanaan and Firbolg, other tribes, no doubt, found a home in West Europe and perhaps Atlantis, and amongst these the Partholon, a somewhat unfortunate group, and the Nemedians may be reckoned. It is probable that the giant race, that legends speak of, were either mythological, suggested by rocks in impassible gorges, and those outstanding rocks near the coast enswathed by fogs, or by the appearance of some scouts of a migrant group who harbingered the approach of others dangerous and deadly. Fairies evidently were suggested by people at a distance; distance is not understood by children or primitive peoples.

The Cornish, Welsh and Breton traditions speak of pigmy men, but the Irish mention fairies, no doubt referring to the disappearance of the Partholon which in some districts was so sudden and so complete, owing to disease, that the supernatural agency of fairies was suggested as at once the cause of the disappearance of these and then it was said that they became fairies.

Some Keltic names still record the places where the plague was said to have filled pits and trenches with these very ancient men of Europe.

The following figures from Topinard will give the relations of Irish and Berber and other types.

```
Height of Irish     =  1.697 metre
   "     "  Berbers =  1.655   "
   "     "  Germans =  1.667   "
   "     "  Chinese =  1.630   "

Cephalic Index

(Inland) Bretons  =  81.9
Coast Bretons     =  83
Berbers           =  76.7
English           =  78.1

Relation of length of line from )  Irish   = 101.6
  tip to tip of middle finger to )  Berbers = 101.2
  stature taken as 100)          )  Arabs   = 101.3

If height = 1, Gorilla is     =  1.651
               Chimpanzee     =  1.428
```

Grey, greenish, and tinted eyes are found in Irish.

Hair:

	Sandy & Fair	Intermediate & Chestnut	Brown
Irish	46.3	21.2	31.9
Bretons	20.0	22.7	57.3
Ligurian	17.0	16.0	67.0

		Chestnut	Eyes Blue	Eyes Brown
Cymric	55.0	44.9	56	41.8
Celtic	21.8	78.0	50	50

Yet black hair is common in Basques and Iberians. The Berbers were always remarkable for their adaptability to place and mode of life. They have been described as having a brown ground work, which became modified by fusion with Negroes, Arabs, and light Northern types.

The Berber type gives a large cranial capacity which is developed still further in the European extensions, 1523 cc records a good cranial capacity.

```
The European types are   blonde in the North,
                         brunette in the South,
     and central German States have intermediate types.
The first are dolichocephalic and blue eyed.
The last are brachycephalic with dark eyes.
```

(W. Krause)

It will remembered that residence in large towns in England seems to make the blondes brunettes, and tends to develop nerve

affections, whilst heart affections are less common in the darker
types. The increased warmth is probably the cause (Report of Anthropological committee).

One record from a special district in Navarre gives:

The majority examined had black hair, some were light, and
some red or chestnut.

One third of the number had blue eyes, one sixth had grey
(?) and half dark.

Half the Irish in Dublin were found by Sir Wm. Wilde to
be light-haired. The percentage of red, yellow and chestnut vary
in different parts of the British Islands as has been proved.

Eyes gave   24 p. c. blue
             9 p. c. brown
            65 p. c. black

The stature of the Berber derivatives is above the average,
and the proportions good.

The skin is fairer in children than in the adult.

The skull is Dolichocephalic, Leptorhinal and Orthognathous.

The nose is somewhat elongated, but not quite aqueline,
and the face is oval, the ear of the Berber wants, often, the
lobule and is in many prominent and stands out from the
head.

The Ibero-Keltic substratum was, in the British Isles, nowhere completely effaced. The Kymry migrated, Keane thinks, to
Brittany and the Gaels to Ireland. It seems that there is some reason for holding the doctrine that the Gaels preceded the Kymry.
The central bog of Ireland must have presented great difficulty
for migrants. Thus it has happened that the older inhabitants of
Connaught were represented for a long time after people of a
similar race seem to have disappeared in the Eastern parts of
the Island (Keane chiefly).

There have been difficulties, which are now disappearing, in
obtaining evidence of the presence of Palæolithic man in Ireland,
although there are few who doubt the statement that early man
found his way to or through Connaught when Atlantis formed a
continent, of which Galway was a portion.

Neolithic stone hammers have been found in Connemara,
(by Beager) and smooth stone implements near Menlough Castle,
within three kilometres of Galway city.

Even in Palæolithic times the task would have been easy, if the soft stone of the district was used for the manufacture of celts on the rough stone type. It seems clear that the population was not large, and the simplest and most ready tools would be used.

Hence it is not safe to assume that the absence of quartzite celts is proof of the absence of early man.

The time of the smooth stone period is believed to have been very long in the West of Ireland. The smooth stone weapons may have overlapped the Palæolithic period as far as the earlier times. The Dolmen builders arrived in Ireland during Neolithic times; whether Neolithic implements were used in the East, as well as in the West in these times, it is difficult to say; but there is no reason for doubting that the smooth stone period overlapped the Palæolithic, and that the Bronze age overlapped the smooth stone age is proved by the barrows.

There is some historical evidence of the migration of the Basque to Ireland, amongst which the following is quoted «Hibernia Basclensibus s. Iberis incolenda datur» (Geoffrey of Monmouth, quoted by Keane) and again «de Gargunio Brytonum rege qui Basclenses in Hiberniam transmisit et eandem ipsis habitandam concessit».

Keane after Webster quotes from Geraldus Cambensis. One cannot lose sight of the fact that featural peculiarities are modifiable by the objects around, as I have endeavoured to show elsewhere, and this susceptibility is essentially human. Just as the mimicking musculature destinguishes the Mammalian group, as Wiedersheim long ago suggested, so Primates are exceptionally gifted in this respect, and man possesses the power of using his face muscles in the highest degree. The features of many men can be pulled about like Indian rubber, so that it is not surprising that a response may arise in the skeleton to impressions of the kind, if it be within the history of the race that such features were ever possible. It is highly probable that some, if not many, of the apparently racial characters are modified by imitation of pose, form and feature by young children of those around them.

If a glance at the features enables one to gain an accurate idea of the emotions of the man, so one may readily admit that, if the emotions be induced in the children by the aid of mimicry, the pose, form, and feature, can be established or modified. It is not necessary to assume that acquired features are hereditary. It is denied that satisfactory proof has ever been given of this. The imitation, however, always remains. What comes out in breeding animals, has been latent on the ancestor. The weight of gorilla skull.

There is much research required in order to decide upon the origin of each particular type found in isolated districts. There are examples of very many types in Galway, Mayo and other western counties. The origin is not so easily arrived at. Tradition points to an early emigration from Ireland. The inhabitants had already come from the great plain. One portion of these had moved eastward and southward and were perhaps to be identified with the «long-haired Achæans», indeed prior to the times concerning which Homer writes a race lived in Ireland, which seems to have had some customs in common with the earliest Greeks, and generally speaking a history of the performances, weapons, armour, etc. of the one nation would do at a particular period for the other; due allowance being made for the embellishments which the bard historian introduced into his story. The first Irish group probably conquered the then dwellers in Greece, whilst those who found their way later may have become associated or perhaps enslaved to their predecessors. This latter race seems to have returned to Ireland, accompanied, perhaps, by the former. It is questionable, however, whether the Greek type can be properly located by feature, seeing that the featural peculiarities of man enable him to mould himself on the rigid and strict nature type of the Greek, or its complementary architectural type, the square temple form. The imitative blended with the emotional is a common peculiarity of the Grecian pose, which seems to be therefore a type easily induced.

The Egyptians were, of course, much influenced by the Greeks, and one cannot have any doubt but that the later immigrants gained in a most round about way their customs from the early Hibernians.

There is no doubt that the impressions gained from early associations have been modified by the subsequent immigrants, and some cases of the Iberian type may be referable to the earlier intercourse with Greece. The black-haired dark-eyed type seems to be derived chiefly from the Iberians inhabiting the Basque countries. Some time ago I took a group, forming a class in the Queen's College, and found that half the number had brachycephalic or subbrachycephalic heads, these were not all dark haired and dark eyed; some were dark with blue eyes. One can indeed in West Ireland have no difficulty in selecting a dark-haired, blue-eyed man or woman with a light coloured complexion which becomes absolutely brown without freckling on exposure to the first week or two of summer sun.

There are those whose skin is naturally of a darker tint, but whose eyes are also dark, brown or hazel, and who do not get much darker by exposure; these seem to approach more closely to the Celtic type pure and simple. I have noticed the absence of the ear lobule in several. It is absent or modified very frequently in the Berber type.

Light sandy-haired types with blue or grey eyes are known in Ireland. In some of these freckling is common, and they are found tall with high cheek bones, and small, undersized, and strong. I have examined some with ears without lobules, an with brachycephalic heads, these approach the Xanthochroic, and are, as near as one can put the statement, of the Lapp or Eastern type.

Some time ago on noting the cerebral features of a native of the West of Ireland, I was surprised to find certain peculiarities of face, colour and feature with a dolichocephalic head. The man in question told me his mother came from the south of France. A student with a subbrachycephalic head said he was of French ancestry. Another native was of German extraction, and had a brachycephalic head and was decidedly South German.

One cannot say absolutely that build has everything to do with the shape of the head. Two of the most decidedly brachycephali were 175 cm in height, whilst four subbrachycephali were 165 cm in height. The latter were muscular and broad. The former were strong and decidedly Basque in feature and build.

Of the latter one had reddish brown hair.

There are many Connaught people with elongated features that suggest to one long heads, but this combination is not always met with. The tendency to form these features is due perhaps largely to the «Gothic» influence in architecture, and the tendency that obtains to tone down the rigidity of the Greek, or to further modify the Roman type. The divergence seems to arise chiefly from these influences.

The Greek build of the schoolroom, which is well seen in many educational institutes, is corrected by the Gothic form of the churches. The simple everyday house is compromised by the

Roman window, whilst the more gorgeous Greek mansion is relieved by the Gothic church or monument.

It seems, however, that the racial peculiarity is damned, if not obliterated, by the immense influence of such animals as the horse; the military pose and bearing are really impressed by the features and pose of the equine model. One often sees in those who spend much of their time with horses (in riding and training) that a feature decidedly artificial is acquired, there is the peculiarity of the mouth referred to by Robinson, but the entire pose is altered. This must concern the Anthropologist, for race features are easily disguised in that way. It will be only necessary, therefore, to give some lists that are instructive.

The colour of the hair and eyes are given in detail. The dolichocephali exceeded the number of brachycephali in the first set. The hair was 10 per cent black or brown black. There were 90 per cent ligth, 13 per cent eyes were brown, 45 per cent dark blue, the remainder were light (grey, grey blue or yellow). There are more than 20 per cent that show complexions that darken in the first weeks of sunshine. Twelve out of twenty nine had broad features.

Industrial Schools Galway.

	Name	Age	Place of Birth and Occupation	Colour Hair	Colour Eyes
1	Haverty Patrick	12	—	light	light blue
2	Holloran James	10	—	light	— —
3	Hogan James	11	—	light br.	grey
4	Darcy Hugh	13½	—	brown	hazel
5	McDermott Patrick	14	—	light	yellow grey
6	McDonnell Wm	15	—	brown	blue
7	Boucher Edward	15½	—	brown	blue
8	Kennedy M	14	—	brown	blue
9	McCormac Jno	14	—	brown	blue
10	Gardner Michael	13	Galway	red	yellow
11	Clarke Paul	15	Midlands	light	blue
12	Connolly Patrick	14	—	brown	blue
13	McDonagh Thos	15	—	light	blue
14	Golding Wm	14	Galway	sandy	blue
15	Joyce Patrick	15½	Galway	black	grey
16	McDonnell Patrick	15½	Galway	black	dark blue
17	Conolly Path	15½	Galway	brown	brown
18	Byrne Thos	15	Castlerea	brown	blue
19	Connolla George	15½	—	red	dark blue *
20	Conachan Patrick	14	Clare	light	blue
21	Frayne Patrick	16	Mayo	brown	green grey
22	Naughton Stephen	14	Clifden	light brown	blue
23	McDonnell Antony	11	Galway	light brown	blue
24	Delnor John	12	Galway	brown	dark blue
25	Naughton John	15	Galway	dark brown	light green
26	Lenahan Fr	13	Gort	[illegible]	dark green
27	Faby Patrick	15	Galway	brown	blue
28	Boylan John	11	Mayo	brown	blue
29	Ryan Harry	15	Dublin	brown	brown
30	Golding Thos	12	—	light red	blue
31	Keats Patrick	14	Dublin	brown	blue
32	Crane James	15	Mayo	brown	light blue
33					
34	Regan Antony	14	Mayo	light	blue
35	McCaffrey Thos	13	Mayo	brown	dark blue
36	Teed R	7	England	brown	blue
37	Shiel Francis	8	Loughrea	light	light brown
38	Carrol Path	9	Tipperary	black	brown
39	Gapp Thos	6	W. Meath	sandy	blue
40	McCann Michael	11	Ballinasloe	light	light blue
41	Connuchan Michael	11	Clare	light	blue
42	Stephens Path	9	Athlone	light	brown
43	Madden John	14	Dublin	dark	light brown
44	Carroll Michael	9	Tipperary	light	blue

	Names	Age	Place of Birth and Occupation	Colour Hair	Colour Eyes
45	Brosnahan Martin	9	Clare	light	blue
46	Garry Lawrence	7	W. Meath	light	blue
47	Bignan Patrick	7½	Galway	light	brown
48	Ryan Martin	7	Loughrea	brown	blue
49	Gore John	13½	Galway	brown	blue
50	Corley Martin	9	Ballina	light	brown
51	Rafferty Thos	10	Roscommon	light	blue
52	Cavan James	11	Mullingar	brown	light blue
53	King John	11	Moate	light	brown
54	Garry Christopher	9	Mullingar	light	blue
55	Boyle Patrick	8	Kellseller	light	grey
56	Lyons Thos	8	Roscommon	light	dark blue
57	Cavan George	9	Mullingar	sandy	grey blue
58	O'Hara Martin	7	Swinford	brown	grey
59	Murray Thos	8	Ballina	light	grey
60	Marshall Robt	8	Ballina	brown	dark grey
61	Ryan John	7	Loughrea	black	dark brown
62	Reilly Martin	7	Galway	brown	light blue
63	Noone James	7	Athenry	brown	light grey
64	Malony John	10	Ennis	red	
65	Quinn James	11	Castlerea	light brown	blue
66	Clute Albert	14	Dublin	brown	dark blue
67	M'Donagh John	15	—	black	grey
68	Grealy Thos	14½	Oranmore	dark	grey blue
69	O'Donnell Jos	14½	Gort	dark	blue
70	M'Garry John	15	Mayo	sandy	blue
71	Mannion Fr	14	Mayo	dark	light blue
72	Dyer John	15	Tobermurry	dark	blue
73	Skinners Dan'	14	Dublin	brown	blue
74	Brosnan Patk	11	Clare	light	dark blue
75	Donnellan John	9	Athlone	light	blue
76	Griffin Patk	10	Ballina	brown	brown
77	Lensky Patk	14	Boyle	light	blue
78	Parsons Thos	12	Mayo	brown	blue
79	Ryan Thos	13½	Dublin	brown	brown
80	Noonan Michael	13	Portumna	light	grey
81	Redmond John	11	Wexford	brown	dark blue
82	Brehen Geo	12	Athlone	brown	blue
83	Robinson John	15	Glasgow	light	dark blue
84	Burke Francis	12	Roscommon	light brown	blue
85	Farrell Michael	10	Roscommon	light brown	blue
86	O'Neill Chas	15	Ballinaslee	brown	blue
87	Conelly Patk	13	Galway	.	dark blue
88	Kelly Patk	9½	Galway	red	brown
89	O'Hare James	10	Mayo	light	blue

	Name	Age	Place of Birth and Occupation	Colour Hair	Colour Eyes
90	Keveny John	13½	Galway	brown	grey
91	Keveny Thos	10	Galway	brown	blue
92	Geoghan Terence	14	Galway	brown	blue
93	Behoon John	11	Athlone	light	blue
94	Tiffany John	13	Loughrea	brown	grey
95	Murray Michael	11½	Ballina	light	brown
96	Chapman Archibald	10	Oughterard	brown	blue
97	McDonnell James	13	Galway	brown	blue
98	Browne Wm	14	Dublin	light	brown
99	Mulligan Francis	12	Ballyhaderreen	light	blue
100	Welly John	11	Tipperary	brown	blue
101	Burke Francis	14	Ballyhaderreen	light	blue
102	White James	11	Athlone	brown	dark blue
103	Doran Michael	14	Athlone	brown	brown
104	Burke Bernard	13	Roscommon	brown	blue
105	Mannion John	12	Galway	black	dark blue
106	Mulligan John	14	Ballyhaderreen	sandy	grey
107	Geraghty Nicholas	13	Galway	brown	dark blue
108	Kilaller James	15	Roscommon	brown	brown
109	Byrne Wm	11	Dublin	black	dark blue
110	Brady John	12	Portsmouth	light	light blue
111	Lacy Lawrence	11	Arklow	dark brown	blue
112	Walsh Patrick	13	Limerick	brown	blue
113	Mulvay Wm	12	Galway	red	blue
114	Doherty Patrick	13	Tuam	brown	grey
115	Roache Edward	13	Galway	black	brown
116	Keogh Alfred	15	Athlone	black	grey
117	Leonard Thos	13	Kinvara	light brown	blue
118	Fuery Charles	16	Loughrea	brown	blue
119	Byrne Patk	16	Galway	brown	brown
120	Donahue Peter	15	Roscommon	-	.
121	Hehir Michael	15	Athlone	black	grey
122	Flaherty Thos	14	Galway	brown	blue
123	Fox Edward	15	Mullingar	sandy	grey
124	Neville Martin	16	Clare	brown	grey
125	Hogan Joseph	15	Portumna	brown black	brown
126	Cosgrove Thos	14	Eyrecourt	light	blue
127	Wolfe Michael	14	Tipperary	light	blue
128	Fuery Walter	15	Loughrea	light	blue
129	O'Connel Thos	15	Sligo	brown	blue
130	Brown Michael	14	Kerry	brown	blue
131	Burke Wm	15	Gort	black	brown
132	Flynn Michael	15	Roscommon	brown	grey
133	McCormack Edward	13½	Roscommon	brown	light blue
134	Peyton Jos	14	Mayo	brown	dark blue

	Name	Age	Place of Birth and Occupation	Colour Hair	Colour Eyes
135	Hickey Patrick	15	Galway	light	blue
136	Reilly Wm	15	Galway	red brown	blueish
137	Doherty John	13	Tuam	brown	dark blue
138	McCormick James	14	Roscommon	dark	brown
139	Davis Francis	13½	Ennis	brown	brown
140	Kelly Hubert	15	Castlebar	brown	blue
141	Kilkelly M	9	Galway	light	grey
142	Lacy Patrick	11	Arklow	brown	blue
143	Lloyd Martin	12	Portumna	reddish brown	blue
144	Collins Peter	12	Ennis	brown	blue
145	Gore Thos	11	Galway	dark	blue
146	Harwood Robt	13	Athlone	brown	blue
147	Leary Thos	13	Castlerea	dark	brown
148	Fallon Sylvester	12	Roscommon	brown	"
149	Reilly John	13	Galway	red	grey
150	Flaherty Martin	11	Galway	brown	blue
151	Meehan Thos	15	Ballymoe	brown	tbrnish brown
152	Cosgrove Martin	14	Eyrecourt	brown	dark grey
153	Twoomy D	14	Dublin	brown	blue
154	Francis James	13	—	brown	blue
155	Fleming Michael	13	Ballyhaunreen	brown	grey
156	Samuel Henry	12	Galway	brown	brown
157	Finneran Thos	14	Galway	brown	grey
158	Horan Patrick	14	Galway	brown black	blue
159	Sweeny John	15	Castlebar	black	grey
160	Devany Wm	15	Loughrea	light	grey
161	Durane John	13	Costemara	light	grey
162	Savage James	16	Dublin	light sandy	"
163	Lynsky Thos	14	Boyle	brown	blue
164	Carroll Martin	15	Loughrea	brown black	brown
165	Kelly John	11	Roscommon	brown	"
166	Emmeran Michael	10	Galway	brown	grey
167	Campbell John	9	Galway	brown	grey
168	Duane Patk	10½	Portumna	brown	brown
169	Whelan J	12	Galway	light	blue
170	Moore P	12½	—	light	light blue
171	Heffernan Patk	8½	Mullingar	light	grey
172	Kelly Martin	8	Galway	brown	light blue
173	Stanton Thomas	11	Mayo	brown	blue
174	Murray Thos	12	Ballina	black	dark grey
175	Thompson Michael	13	Clare	brown	blue
176	Whelan M	15	Galway	red	brown
177	Brsen M	12	Strokestown	brown	brown
178	Pigott Michael	15	Athlone	brown	brown
179	White D	10	Athenry	light	grey

No.	Name	Age	Place of birth and Occupation	Colour Hair	Colour Eyes
180	Carroll Thos	15	Tipperary	light	grey
181	O'Donnell Jos	11	Gort	brown	brown
182	Trod Jos	11	Eyrecourt	light	blue
183	Connor Patk	12½	Boyle	light brown	light blue
184	Walsh Martin	13	Ballinasloe	black	brown
185	Davis Thos	10	Ennis	brown	brown
186	Hogan John	12	Gort	light	blue
187	Halpin Wm	10	Galway	brown	grey blue
188	Flannery Michael	12	Galway	brown	blue
189	Geraghty Martin	13½	Galway	black	brown
190	Rafferty John	11½	Roscommon	sandy	blue
191	Trod Henry	7½	Eyrecourt	brown	blue
192	Kenny Michael	11½	Portumna	light	blue
193	Kelly John	12	Galway	yellow	grey brown
194	Ganning Edward	12½	Roscommon	light	blue
195	Kearns Thos	11	Galway	sandy	blue
196	Golding Francis	11	Galway	light brown	grey
197	Marr James	11	Athlone	brown	grey
198	Robinson John	11	Roscommon	light brown	blue
199	Mulvany Martin	11	Galway	red	grey
200	Chute Michael	14	Dublin	black brown	brown

A detailed analysis of the list gives light hair and eyes (light blue) as 54 percent. Red or sandy hair occur in 10 per cent in all with grey or blue eyes, remembering that black hair is in many cases simply very dark red; one can see how a relationship may have existed between the black haired and even the yellow-haired types. A small percentage of black haired individuals appears in this list. 12 p. c. one half of these had brown eyes, the other half dark grey or dark blue. It will be noticed that some of the students and a few industrial boys come from other parts of Ireland.

The explanations given by Mendel and Cossar Ewart are of great value in studying race types. An attempt is made to divest the possible causes of nigrescence of the accidents that are associated with a town life, and overstrain. There are few if any cases of progressive paralysis in Galway and the neurotic affections are easily explained. There are no large towns in the West of Ireland as has already been mentioned. So causes that in large cities give rise to changes in the hair, eyes, and skin, lungs etc., may be exclude. The present railway from Galway to the Western shore of Ireland is open less than 12 years and the railway to Dublin is open a little more than sixty (60) years. Very few of the greatly populous districts of the County of Galway in West of Galway have ever been in Galway city which is 132 kilometres distant, it rarely ever happens that one goes to Dublin which is 139 kilometres from the West Coast. Very few people who are scattered over the hundreds of square kilometres West of Galway have ever seen the Eastern Coast. Sailing vessels before the time of steam came Westward to the meridian of Galway before proceeding Southward to the Iberian coast, and mariners seemed anxious to avoid the dangerous if not inhospitable coast that lay between West Ireland and Gibraltar. It was easy to go to backwards to Ireland or Southwards by simply keeping the Polestar ahead or by letting it shine on the stern.

It may not be unexceptable to mention that reference may be made to the works of Virchow, Topinard, W. Krause, Kohlmann, Keane, the valuable manual of Duckworth, the works of Quatrefages and the papers of C. Browne, who has taken the records of several important groups in the West of Ireland. The references to Broca, Quatrefages and Reclus are in many works. I would only add that the influence of Architecture is more potent than that of Painting and Sculpture, for the greater number. The latter strike deeper if not so wide. The consideration of the influences of the steam carriage and the steam boat on the children of sixty years ago is not taken into account, it is too soon to estimate the value of these in neutralizing old or developing new characters. A short account of a discussion on muscular anomalies will be found in the *International Monatsschrift* for 1901.

RICHARD ANDERSON

	Age	Place of Birth	Father's Place of Birth	Mother's state of Birth	Colour Skin
1	21	Glasgow	Glasgow		L
2	19	India	Cork		L
3	18	Roscommon Connaught	Roscommon		L
4	18	Tyrone	Antrim		L
5	17	Waterford	Kings County		L
6	18	Derry	Derry		L P
7	19	Mayo	Mayo		Br
8	18	W. Clare	W. Clare		L S
9	21	Tyrone	Tyrone		L P
10	21	Galway	Galway		L P
11	18	Galway	Mayo		L S
12	19	Galway	Galway		R Br
13	21	Ballymena	Ballymena		L F
14	21	Armagh	England		L
15	18	Galway	Galway		Br Yellow
16	20	Derry	Derry		L
17	50	Monaghan	Monaghan		L P
18	30	Armagh	Armagh		L
19	20	Limerick	Limerick		L
20	20	Sligo	Sligo	Marseilles	Ruddy
21	24	Tyrone	Tyrone		L Pale
22	22	Cork	Cork		L F
23	20	Dublin	Tyrone		R brown
24	13	Tipperary	Tipperary		Dk.

L P = pale
L S = sand
L F = sun

ry classes

	Head measurements			Ear		Height	Weight (kilos)
	Length	Breadth	Height	Length	Breadth		
	7.3	5.7	—	5.5	4.5	173	78
	7.7	6.0	—	6.5	3.0	175	75
	7.7	6.0	—	7	3.5	175	83
	7.7	6.0	—	6.8	2.5	177	78
	7.5	5.6	—	6.5	4	173	70.5
	7.70	6.0	—	6.3	4	172	78
	7.5	6.5	—	6.5	4.5	175	84
	7.7	6	—	6.	4.5	160	75
	7.8	6.5	—	7	5.4	180	88
	8.0	6.5	—	6.5	4	172.5	83
	7.75	6.25	—	6.5	4.5	172	71
	7.0	6	—	6.0	4.5	175	71
	7.5	5	—	6.5	4	177	82
	7.6	5.6	—	6.5	4	166	73
	7.6	6.0	—	6.5	3	164	63
	7.7	6.0	—	7	4	170	71
	8.0	5.9	—	6.5	3.0	187	100
	7.7	6.0	—	6.5	3	166	72
	8.0	6.2	—	6.5	3.5	180	85
	8.	6.2	—	7	3	175	77.5
	mm	mm					
	190	150		6.5	3.2	165	63.4
	198	152		6.5	3.5	170	68
	196	154		6.3	4.0	170	73
	190	154		6.0	3.5	162	66

= brown
= black
= blue
= yellow

À propos de l'involution accidentelle du thymus

Par MM. R. Collin et M. Lucien, Nancy

On sait depuis longtemps que des facteurs d'ordre divers tels que le surmenage, les maladies infectieuses, les intoxications, les troubles de la nutrition générale, etc., sont susceptibles de faire varier le poids du thymus. C'est cependant en grande partie à l'influence méconnue ou mal interprétée de ces facteurs que paraissent dus les résultats contradictoires obtenus par les auteurs en ce qui concerne l'évolution pondérale du thymus.

Dans deux mémoires remarquables parus en 1905 (¹) J. Aug. Hammar a de nouveau appelé l'attention sur les causes susceptibles d'abaisser le poids de la glande en dehors de l'involution normale due à l'âge. Il a donné le nom d'involution accidentelle aux modifications de structure du thymus déterminées par l'influence des facteurs dont nous faisions précédemment mention; l'involution accidentelle se traduisant macroscopiquement par une réduction parfois très notable du volume et du poids de l'organe. Pour Hammar, volume et poids du thymus sont fonction du nombre de lymphocytes qu'il renferme. Le nombre de ces leucocytes vient-il à augmenter sous l'influence de certaines circonstances, il se produit un de ces états connus sous le nom d'hypertrophie ou d'hyperplasie du thymus. Le nombre des lymphocytes vient-il au contraire à diminuer par suite du ralentissement ou de la suppression de la multiplication cellulaire, l'involution accidentelle s'installe. — On ne peut donc considérer comme normaux les thymus d'individus morts de maladie, et si l'on veut obtenir des renseignements exacts sur l'évolution de cette glande, il faut se borner à faire cette recherche sur des sujets morts accidentellement et rapidement. Hammar, qui s'est mis, semble-t-il, à l'abri des causes d'erreur habituelles, est arrivé aux conclusions suivantes: Le thymus s'accroît jusqu'à la période de la puberté qui a été souvent considérée comme celle de la régression et de la dégénérescence de l'organe, puis il diminue lentement de poids,

---

(¹) J. Aug. Hammar, Zur Histogenese und Involution der Thymusdrüse, mit 20 Abbildungen. Anat. Anzeiger, XXVII B., N° 1, 2, 3 Juin 1905.
Ueber Thymusgewicht und Thymuspersistenz beim Menschen. Verhandlungen der anatomischen Gesellschaft. Premier congrès fédératif international d'anatomie. Genève, 6-10 Août 1905.

mais fonctionne jusqu'à quarante ans. Vers 50 ou 60 ans, il perd toute activité en même temps que se produit la disparition du parenchyme glandulaire. Les thymus que nous avons eus à notre disposition provenaient, pour la plupart, d'enfants ayant succombé à l'hôpital au cours d'affections diverses, de durée variable. La plus grande partie d'entre eux pouvaient être considérés comme ayant subi l'involution accidentelle. Nous avons cependant utilisé ce matériel de la manière suivante, qui, si elle ne donne pas des résultats absolument rigoureux, permet cependant de tirer des conclusions très voisines à coup sûr de la réalité.

Avec la moyenne des poids absolus établie pour les différents âges et pour tous les thymus sans distinction d'origine, nous avons établi une première courbe générale. Pour nous rapprocher autant que possible des vues de Hammar, nous avons ensuite construit une seconde courbe en éliminant les facteurs d'involution accidentelle. Pour atteindre ce résultat sans laisser place à une opinion personnelle plus ou moins arbitraire, nous avons décidé de mettre de coté les thymus de tous les enfants n'atteignant pas au moins les quatre cinquièmes du poids moyen du corps à l'âge considéré [1].

Si l'on compare les deux courbes ainsi obtenues, on est frappé de leur grande ressemblance, et leur parallélisme apparaît tout à fait évident au moins pendant la première année de la vie.

La courbe établie avec la totalité des cas montre que le thymus s'accroît régulièrement pendant la vie intra-utérine pour passer par un maximum au moment de la naissance.

Le poids moyen à cette époque, évalué sur six cas, est de 12 gr. 88. Il représente la $\frac{1}{611}$ partie du poids total du corps.

Pendant les dix premiers jours de l'existence, le poids moyen de l'organe diminue dans des proportions considérables. Cette chute se continue jusque vers le deuxième mois sans toutefois être aussi accentuée que pendant les premiers jours après la naissance.

Jusqu'à deux ans, le poids moyen du thymus oscille entre 3 et 5 grammes. Au delà de cette période il se relève un peu jusqu'à atteindre 7 grammes.

La courbe construite avec les seuls thymus ne paraissant pas

---

[1] P. Courts et M. Lucien. Sur l'évolution pondérale du thymus chez le foetus et chez l'enfant. *Bibliographie anatomique*, 1906, T. xv, fasc. 1, avec un graphique.

avoir subi l'involution accidentelle montre, comme la précédente, une chute brusque du poids de l'organe après la naissance. Dès le premier mois, le poids moyen est d'environ 5 grammes et conserve une valeur sensiblement égale jusqu'à un an.

Comme on le voit, la différence entre ces deux courbes réside essentiellement dans la valeur moyenne du poids du thymus pendant les premiers mois de l'existence. Toutes deux montrent que cette glande passe par un maximum pondéral à la naissance, cette haute valeur étant du reste assez éphémère. L'involution accidentelle est exprimée par la différence des poids moyens dans l'une et l'autre courbe.

Cette différence n'est guère sensible du reste que pendant les huit premiers mois de la vie. Elle s'explique par le fait que cette période est celle où les affections cachectisantes de la première enfance sont le plus fréquentes. On sait de plus que quelques auteurs ont vu dans l'atrophie du thymus, non pas un effet des troubles de nutrition générale, mais au contraire la cause de ces troubles.

Quoiqu'il en soit, l'involution accidentelle qui, à la vérité, abaisse le poids moyen du thymus, ne semble pas être un facteur suffisant pour troubler l'évolution générale de la glande. De toute façon, le thymus passe par un maximum pondéral au moment de la naissance et son involution normale, autant du reste que les résultats fournis par les pesées peuvent le faire préjuger, commence également à cette époque.

L'involution accidentelle modifie surtout la valeur absolue du poids moyen du thymus à une époque déterminée et à ce point de vue on doit en tenir le plus grand compte.

Les données que nous avons tirées de l'examen comparatif de l'ensemble de nos cas et de ceux où l'involution accidentelle peut être mise hors de cause sont corroborées par l'examen d'une troisième courbe qui représente le poids relatif moyen du thymus (rapport entre le poids de l'organe et le poids total du corps).

Cette dernière courbe, comme les précédentes, montre en effet d'une façon manifeste que le thymus possède une très grande importance pendant la vie intra-utérine et au moment de la naissance et que cette importance va en diminuant régulièrement à partir de cette époque.

DÉMONSTRATION

Mlle. Marie Lavez démontre une série d'excellentes préparations d'ovaires de reptiles, où l'on voit d'une façon très nette la part que prennent les cellules folliculaires à la formation du vitellus, en envoyant à l'intérieur de l'œuf des produits de sécrétion; ceux-ci forment au début de petits noyaux dans la zone périphérique de l'œuf et deviennent ensuite des globules vitellins. Le corps vitellin contribue aussi à la formation du vitellus.

Les préparations que Mlle. Lavez a présentées se rapportent à son travail «Sur le développement du corps vitellin des œufs méroblastiques à gros vitellus», publié dans les *Archives d'Anatomie microscopique*, vol. VIII, 1905-06.

SÉANCE DU 24 AVRIL

(10 h. du matin)

Présidence: MM. K. Benda et W. Waldeyer

Sont présents: MM. Celestino da Costa, Mlle. Bunn, MM. Feyo e Castro, Kamon, Mlle. Lavez, MM. Mann, Athias, Paes Leme, Parra, Pinto de Magalhães, Silva Tavares, etc.

Ueber die anatomischen Ursachen der Hernien

Par M. Wilhelm Waldeyer, Berlin.

In der für den verstorbenen Generalstabsarzt der Königlich Preussischen Armee, R. v. Leuthold bestimmten Festschrift (Berlin, 1906, Verlag von A. Hirschwald) habe ich eine Reihe von Erfahrungen mitgetheilt, welche dafür sprechen, dass für die Unterleibsbrüche bestimmte anatomische Zustände vorhanden sind, die zu ihrer Entwicklung disponiren. Es ist dies, wie wir alle wissen, keine neue Erkenntniss: in jedem Lehrbuche der Chirurgie und in jeder Spezialabhandlung über Unterleibsbrüche im Allgemeinen und über die einzelnen Abarten derselben im Besonderen, sind diese praedisponirenden Momente erwähnt und mehr oder weniger eingehend besprochen. Ich würde diesen Gegenstand auch nicht weiter verfolgt und abgehandelt haben, wenn mich meine Erfahrungen nicht dahin geführt hätten zu behaupten, dass es gar keine Hernien am Abdomen — un wahrscheinlich auch an allen übrigen

Körpergegenden, wo Hernien überhaupt vorkommen — gibt, bei
denen nicht eine *anatomische Praedisposition* vorhanden gewesen
wäre. In dieser Ausschliesslichkeit ist bisher die betreffende Frage
nur von wenigen — ich verweise bezüglich der Literatur auf die
eingangs erwähnte Festschrift — beantwortet worden; in den meis-
ten Lehrbüchern und Sonderabhandlungen wird eine solche anatomische Praedisposition nur als ein mehr oder weniger häufiges
Vorkommniss angesehen. So glaubte ich, da es sich um eine
äusserst wichtige Sache handelt, mich mit dem, was ich beobachtet
hatte, zu der Frage äussern zu sollen.

Ich bringe die Angelegenheit hier abermals vor, weil erfahrungs-
gemäss die in Gelegenheits- und Festschriften niedergelegten
Arbeiten häufig nicht bekannt zu werden pflegen, und weil ich sie
auch vor ein anatomisches Forum bringen möchte, einmal weil es
sich um eine anatomische Praedisposition handelt und dann, weil
mir daran liegt, das von mir Behauptete weiter erhärtet zu sehen.
Gerade die Anatomen haben so häufig Gelegenheit Hernien genauer
zu beobachten und sorgfältig praepariren zu lassen, dass ich ihre
Aufmerksamkeit auf den beregten Gegenstand durch diesen mei-
nen Vortrag an dieser Stelle lenken möchte.

Die Beobachtungen, auf welche ich mich bei meiner Behaup-
tung stütze, sind folgende:

1. Die grosse Häufigkeit leerer peritonealer Bruchsäcke an
den bekannten Bruchpforten. Hiermit ist die anatomische Disposition gegeben; nun kann eine Gelegenheitsursache oft ganz leicht,
ohne dass die Entwicklung einer Hernie von dem Betreffenden
nur empfunden wird, einen Bruch zu Stande bringen.

2. Das so sehr häufige Vorkommen mehrfacher Brüche bei
einer und derselben Person und das Vorkommen von ein oder
zwei, selbst von mehr leeren Bruchsäcken neben einer ausgebil-
deten Hernie.

3. Das häufige Vorkommen *weiter* Bruchpforten auch ohne
leere Bruchsäcke, entweder für sich oder mit einer bereits beste-
henden Hernie vergesellschaftet.

4. Das Vorkommen aller dieser Dinge auch bei Feten und
Neugeborenen in bemerkenswerter Häufigkeit; auch intraabdomi-
nale Hernien Brösike hahe ich schon zu wiederholten Malen bei
ganz jugendlichen Individuen beobachtet; hier ist übrigens die
anatomische Praedisposition eine *conditio qua non!*

Diese Thatsachen zwingen, so meine ich, zu dem Schlusse,
dass eine anatomische Praedisposition das Erste und Wesen-

tlichste für das Zuiztandekommen einer Unterleibshernie ist. Gern möchte ich mit dieser kurzen Mittheilung die Aufmerksamkeit der anatomischen Fachgenossen auf diesen Gegenstand hingelenkt und zu weiteren Beobachtungen angeregt haben.

DISCUSSION

M. BENDA: Mes expériences confirment parfaitement l'opinion de l'orateur. Moi aussi j'ai vu souvent la combinaison de plusieurs hernies ou de plusieurs conditions de hernie dans un même individu. Je me souviens principalement d'un cas, qui est conservé dans ma collection, où il y avait d'un côté une hernie du basseau obturateur, qui était complète et gangréneuse, pendant que l'autre côté montrait seulement une excavation circonscrite de la même région, sans doute la condition de la même hernie. Surtout la multiplicité des hernies est la preuve la plus importante qu'en général les conditions génétiques des hernies préexistent, comme M. Waldeyer l'a indiqué.

Pourtant, quant à la signification pratique de cette constatation il faut délimiter que l'acquisition des hernies est prouvée pour les hernies cicatricielles. Pour cela nous sommes forcés d'admettre, à propos du jugement de questions d'assurance, la possibilité d'une acquisition des hernies, car l'anamnestique du cas ne résiste pas à cette opinion.

Distribution of the afferent Nerve Supply to the Leg of Rana virescens brachycephala, Cope

Par Mlle. ELIZABETH HOPKINS DUNN, Chicago.

The purpose of the experiment reported at this time was to produce degeneration of all the efferent nerve fibers innervating one leg of a frog, leaving the supply for the opposite side intact, and then to study, by enumeration, the fibers present at various levels on the two sides. The frog used was a female, lenght 229 mm, corrected weight about 61 grams.

The material was stained with 1% osmic acid solution, embedded in paraffin and cut 4 micro in thickness.

The conclusions presented at this time are as follows.

1. The distribution of the afferent fibers to the thigh and shank has been determined. 774 afferent fibers pass to the muscles, 1527 fibers to the skin of the thigh. The muscular afferent supply is then about one-third that to the entire thigh, and one-half the supply to the skin. The numbers found for the shank are 303 for the muscles, 1078 for the skin. For the shank the number of muscular afferent fibers is about one-fourth the number to the entire shank, one-third that for the skin covering the shank,

2. The afferent supply for the muscles was found to be about one-half the total nerve supply to the muscles. Seven muscular nerve branches for the thigh gave for the operated side 484 fibers, for the intact side 982 fibers. For the shank, eight branches gave on the operated side 303 fibers, on the intact side 601 fibers.

3. The efferent and the muscular afferent nerve supply to the segments of the leg are distributed according to the weights of muscle in the segments. From a study of the weight values for the muscles of the thigh, shank and foot respectively, made by Donaldson and Schoemaker in 1900, we find that the percentage values of the muscles for the three segments are, for the thigh 63,9% of the entire weight of muscle in the leg, for the shank 24,4% and for the foot 11,7%. The number of efferent or of afferent fibers to the muscles of the leg is 1915. If we distribute these according to the weights of muscle and compose with the numbers found by count in the various branches, we find the percentage relation between the estimated and the counted to be practically the same for both the thigh and the shank. The distribution to the foot is in excess of the weight of muscle and indicates a richer afferent and efferent supply to the muscles of this segment.

4. The distribution of the afferent fibers to the skin was found to be proportional to the area of the skin covering the segment.

The percentage values of the cutaneous covering of the various segments of the leg of the frog were determined in connection with an investigation published by Donaldson in 1903. The percentage values were found to be, for the thigh 35,9% of the total area of the skin of the leg, for the shank 25,7%, and for the foot 38,1%.

The number of fibers entering the leg which pass to innervate the skin is 2682. If this number is distributed to the segments according to their cutaneous areas, we find that these estimated numbers bear the same percentage relations to the counted fibers in both the thigh and the shank. This relation holds true also in the foot.

DISCUSSION

M. GUSTAV MANN suggests that a recount of the muscle fibers of the different muscles in the thigh, leg and foot in relation to the number of nerves might yield interesting results.

Sur la conservation des sujets pour les études anatomiques.
L'embaumement par le Formol

Par M. BRANT PASS LEME, Rio de Janeiro.

Le Formol semble être, au moment actuel, l'agent le plus avantageux pour la conservation des sujets destinés aux études anatomiques. Il est bon marché, d'une technique très simple pour l'usage, conserve merveilleusement les sujets, plus même qu'il ne serait peut-être nécessaire, parce que, si l'on n'est pas sobre dans la proportion des solutions, il les momifie facilement, et surtout il a le grand mérite de rendre stérile le milieu en faisant disparaître les dangers des salles d'anatomie; il rend inoffensives les piqûres anatomiques. Nul doute que la priorité du procès des grandes injections formalinées pour la conservation des sujets appartienne à Gerota (de Berlin) qui a fait sur la question, il y a déjà quelque temps, au moins que je sache, des publications détaillées.

L'auteur de la présente communication veut faire connaître, ce qui peut avoir intérêt en Europe, les résultats magnifiques qu'il obtient aussi au delà de l'Atlantique, à Rio de Janeiro, avec cet agent dans la proportion maxima de 10 %, et surtout les résultats en vue de l'impunité des piqûres anatomiques, ce qu'il n'a pas vu suffisamment signalé, jusqu'à présent, dans les publications ou communications faites.

Dans ses premières expériences, l'auteur a voulu constituer une formule complexe, capable non seulement de conserver les sujets, mais aussi de retenir la coloration naturelle aux organes, particulièrement aux muscles. Ainsi il a adopté la classique et ancienne formule Le Prieur, en la complétant par l'adjonction du *formol*. Les résultats furent bons; la couleur des muscles restait admirable; mais ensuite, en jugeant que le petit bénéfice de la conservation de cette couleur, simple affaire pour ainsi dire esthétique, ne valait pas le surcroît de prix de l'injection, vu en outre l'inconvénient de la cristallisation des sels qui s'opérait au niveau des coupes, etc., etc., l'auteur, en simplifiant petit à petit sa technique, s'est tenu aux simples formules d'eau avec le *formol* dans la proportion de 10 %, absolument comme Gerota.

La question, à Rio de Janeiro, avait une bien plus grande importance qu'en Europe, à cause des conditions de la température du pays, en moyenne 20° à 25°, mais pouvant aller à 34°, 35°, 36° à l'époque des cours. Tous les procédés connus, toutes les formules avaient déjà échoué là-bas où l'on était contraint, avec les plus grandes difficultés et dépenses, à la conservation par la glace, si problématique quand il faut aller et venir avec les cadavres des glacières aux salles des travaux, les exposant aux conditions de température les plus rudes et les plus opposées.

Ainsi, à Rio de Janeiro, le *formol* a marqué un vrai progrès dans les études d'anatomie descriptive et anatomie médico-chirurgicale, cette dernière sous la direction particulière de l'auteur de la présente communication.

Chaque sujet exige d'habitude 3 à 5 litres d'injection selon sa corpulence, injection qu'il faut faire passer convenablement par la carotide, de préférence. Pour le tronc et la tête, aucun doute que la conservation est toujours très bien obtenue. Nous avons même fréquemment des sujets en commencement de décomposition, qu'il est possible de faire arrêter. Pour les membres, principalement les inférieurs, on a quelquefois des injections supplémentaires à faire, à la fin de 24, 48 heures, si par hasard on voit par là quelque plaque de putréfaction; et tout est fait, c'est-à-dire, la conservation pour les études et la besogne, si on le voulait, de l'embaumement, au coût minime de 2 fr. au plus; rien n'est meilleur marché!

L'habitude de travailler avec le formol fait rapidement disparaître le petit inconvénient qu'on ressent les premiers temps du côté des organes visuels et olfactifs. Les salles d'anatomie perdent absolument l'odeur cadavérique, ordinairement si insupportable même quand on emploie l'acide phénique et d'autres agents conservateurs.

Ce qu'il faut tâcher pourtant d'éviter, c'est la *dureté* des sujets, qui quelquefois peut nuire aux travaux. De fait ils ont une manifeste tendance à *sécher*, c'est-à-dire, à se momifier. C'est la vertu et le mal du *formol*. Pour cela il faut ne pas employer les fortes solutions; au *maximum* elles ne doivent être supérieures à 10 %, et il faut aussi *manier* les sujets, faire mouvoir les articulations, rendre la mobilité à tout le corps.

Comme Gerota, l'auteur a expérimenté la glycérine dans sa formule à cet effet, mais il croit suffisantes la malaxation et la mobilisation dont il vient d'être question; cela évite d'augmenter le prix de la conservation.

Comme dernier mot, l'auteur tient à faire connaître que, de-

puis qu'on emploie à Rio le formol, on n'a jamais plus observé
le moindre accident dans les cas fréquents de piqûres parmi les
élèves et le personnel du laboratoire. D'ailleurs cela est d'accord
absolument et avec les résultats de la conservation qu'il obtient,
et avec les expériences de laboratoire, cultures et inoculations
multiples qu'il a faites maintes fois avec les produits cadavériques,
moelle des os, liquide péritonéal, etc., etc., toujours sans aucune
conséquence.

Une nouvelle classification des articulations

Par M. Porfirio Parra, Mexico

SOMMAIRE

Quelques considérations préliminaires — Exposition de la nouvelle classification.
— Les groupes fondamentaux — Les groupes secondaires. — Parallèle entre
l'ancienne et la nouvelle classification. — Tableau de la classification.

Décrire pour faire connaître les choses, classifier pour faire
connaître les groupes ou classes qui, au moyen des choses, peuvent être formés; voilà les deux étapes que fait l'esprit de l'homme en parcourant le chemin des sciences concrètes et descripti-
ves parmi lesquelles l'Anatomie joue un rôle important.

Dès les lointains temps que Galien et les anatomistes de
l'école d'Alexandrie ont illustrés, on peut remarquer déjà de bien
visibles traces de descriptions et classifications qui avaient été
accomplies par ceux qui désiraient connaître la machine humaine. Au fur et à mesure que les organes étaient décrits, ils étaient
en même temps classifiés; le développement de la science anatomique enseigne que les deux opérations s'entre-aident, influant
l'une sur l'autre.

Dans la complexité du corps humain les articulations forment un vaste système, dont la connaissance exacte a beaucoup
d'intérêt au point de vue multiple de l'Anatomie, Physiologie, Thé-
rapeutique et Médecine opératoire. Elles sont le moyen d'union
qui, en unissant les pièces osseuses, constituent le squelette et
donnent à ses parties, soit une grande mobilité, soit une grande
solidité, selon leur fonction, afin que la charpente osseuse rem-
plisse la fonction d'organe locomoteur passif.

Les articulations sont très nombreuses et sont en plus très
variées. Nous y trouvons les très simples qui s'appellent sutures,
qui lient très solidement les os du crâne; nous y trouvons aussi
celles très compliquées, au moyen desquelles le fémur ou l'hu-

mérus s'unissent respectivement à l'omoplate ou à l'os iliaque en leur donnant tous les degrés de mobilité sans nuire à leur solidité. C'est ainsi que le squelette poussé par la contraction musculaire, laquelle à son tour est provoquée par l'action du nerf, peut exécuter les très divers mouvements propres à la dynamique humaine.

Pour le progrès des sciences il est donc nécessaire de classer les articulations, et ce besoin on l'a éprouvé de plus en plus au fur et à mesure que la connaissance du corps humain a progressé à travers les siècles. Nous trouvons dans les livres didactiques, et avec les caractères du classique, une classification très ancienne sans doute, puisqu'on en aperçoit des traces dans Galien; mais cette classification, si vénérable qu'elle soit, est tout à fait insuffisante et défectueuse, les groupes ne sont pas bien définis, les noms qui dénotent ces groupes ont quelque chose d'arbitraire, et sont dépourvus de ce cachet du langage scientifique qu'on remarque si bien dans la terminologie botanique ou dans la nomenclature chimique.

Nous avons estimé qu'une dénomination significative et convenable et une classification bien faite des articulations étaient une tentative utile à la science, et nous avons publié quelques mémoires sur ce sujet, si important à notre avis, et que nous ne croyons pas avoir épuisé. Voilà pourquoi nous appelons l'attention du XV Congrès International de Médecine sur la nouvelle manière de grouper les articulations que nous avons trouvée.

Pour former les groupes fondamentaux nous prenons pour base la mobilité ou l'immobilité. Nous avons d'une part des articulations tout à fait immobiles, et en face d'elles nous en avons d'autres de mouvements plus ou moins amples. Les os du crâne appartiennent au premier groupe, et les articulations du tronc et des membres au deuxième. Nous avons nommé statiques les articulations immobiles parce qu'elles remplissent les conditions d'équilibre et résistance, tandis que nous appelons dynamiques les articulations mobiles parce que, dans le fait, elles réalisent les conditions des divers mouvements de la dynamique animée.

Si nous comparons, quant aux groupes fondamentaux, notre classification et celle classique, nous trouvons cette différence remarquable: Dans le vieux classement ces groupes sont trois: Les articulations immobiles appelées synarthroses, les articulations demi-mobiles qui s'appellent symphyses ou amphiarthroses, et les articulations mobiles qui portent le nom diarthroses.

Le groupe d'articulations semi-mobiles est très vague, tellement que pour distinguer ce groupe de celui des diarthroses la seule mobilité ne suffit pas, et il faut considérer l'anatomie de l'articulation et donner pour caractère aux diarthroses l'existence d'une membrane synoviale.

Dans notre mode de grouper les articulations nous avons fait, pour éviter ces imperfections, une seule classe avec les articulations mobiles, si petit qu'en soit le mouvement, et en faisant ainsi, le groupe est très bien constitué puisqu'il n'y a pas de contraste plus grand que celui que l'esprit aperçoit entre la présence et l'absence, l'existence ou la non existence d'une certaine qualité.

Mais le groupe des articulations mobiles ainsi formé devient immense, puisqu'il résulte de la réunion des deux vieux groupes des amphiarthroses et des diarthroses, lesquels, quoiqu'ils se ressemblent, restent toujours distincts, et on doit les séparer pour former les groupes secondaires qui subdivisent la classe principale.

Mais comment faire pour marquer la différence qui sépare ces groupes secondaires? Prendrons-nous la donnée anatomique d'une synoviale? Avouerons-nous que pour faire cette distinction la donnée physiologique de la mobilité est tout à fait épuisée? Non. D'abord la cavité synoviale n'apparaît pas tout à coup et formée de toutes pièces dans les diarthroses, elle se montre peu à peu, lentement, pour ainsi dire, à travers les amphiarthroses; la partie centrale des disques intervertébraux est molle, et ce ramollissement du fibrocartilage à son centre est regardé avec justesse par les anatomistes comme une tendance à la formation d'une cavité; la symphyse pubienne nous montre déjà une véritable cavité dans l'épaisseur du disque interpubienne; à l'articulation sacro-iliaque, non seulement il y a une cavité, mais encore la dite cavité est doublée d'une synoviale; voilà pourquoi les anatomistes ont hésité pour classer cette articulation; les uns, Boyer entre autres, la rangeaient parmi les synarthroses; tandis que Blandin voyait en elle une arthrodie serrée, c'est-à-dire, il en faisait une diarthrose; la plupart des auteurs l'ont placée parmi les amphiarthroses, et Sappey déclare que cette articulation ne rentre, en réalité, dans aucune des classes, mais qu'elle est intermédiaire entre les articulations mobiles et semi-mobiles, et placée justement sur la ligne divisoire qui sépare les deux groupes.

D'autre part, le principe de la mobilité ne s'épuise pas, et il est capable de faire distinguer les sous-groupes contigus des articulations mobiles; il va nous servir pour en marquer la différence; s'il s'agit des anciennes amphiarthroses les mouvements sont indéfinis, c'est-à-dire, il n'est pas possible de les réduire à des lignes, des plans ou des surfaces courbes douées d'un axe, tandis que les mouvements des amphiarthroses sont définis.

Donc, nous divisons ainsi la grande classe des articulations mobiles: celles de mouvements indéfinis et celles de mouvements définis; les premières comprennent non seulement les amphiarthroses de la vieille classification, mais aussi d'autres qui ont formé jusqu'ici un groupe flottant et mal défini, que quelques auteurs désignent sous le nom d'articulations à distance; dans ce groupe les os qui s'unissent restent à une certaine distance les uns des autres en se liant au moyen de ligaments en forme de cordes ou de membranes, comme on voit aux articulations des lames des vertèbres, de leurs apophyses épineuses, de l'occipital avec l'apophyse odontoïde de l'axis, de l'apophyse transverse de la cinquième vertèbre lombaire et la crête iliaque.

Le groupe des articulations à distance nous force à subdiviser en deux la sous-classe des articulations de mouvements indéfinis: les synostéoses et les dialostéoses. Les os des premières ont des surfaces articulaires très solidement unies par un fibrocartilage interosseux; les os des dialostéoses, n'arrivant pas au contact, n'ont plus de telles surfaces articulaires, et un ligament ou une membrane lie tout simplement les os.

Si nous comparons les articulations de mouvements définis, nous remarquerons entre elles de grandes différences, dont la principale est celle-ci: dans quelques-unes les mouvements ont lieu autour d'un ou plusieurs axes de rotation fixes; aux mouvements des autres il n'est pas possible d'attribuer d'axes, ou ils ne sont pas fixes. Nous appelons axiles les articulations qui se trouvent dans le premier cas, et abaxiles celles du second; ces dernières correspondent aux arthrodies de la classification usuelle.

Le nombre d'axes fixes qu'on peut attribuer aux mouvements d'une articulation, lequel peut varier depuis un jusqu'à trois, nous donne le moyen de diviser, selon le nombre des dits axes, la classe des articulations axiles en uniaxiles, biaxiles et triaxiles.

Les uniaxiles, leur nom l'indique bien, sont celles dont les mouvements ont toujours lieu autour d'un seul axe, et constituent le ginglyme ou charnière des auteurs, genre mentionné déjà dès le temps de Galien, et qui a été subdivisé en deux par Winslow au commencement du XVIIIe siècle: le ginglyme angulaire, dont le type est l'articulation du coude, et le ginglyme latéral ou articulation en pivot, comme l'articulation radio-cubitale supérieure; Fallope l'appela trochoïde ou ginglyme latéral.

La direction de l'axe de rotation nous donne le moyen de distinguer les ginglymes entre eux; si l'axe de mouvement est à peu près perpendiculaire à l'axe de figure des os mobiles, nous aurons un ginglyme angulaire qui, dans notre plan de classification, porte le nom d'articulations uniaxiles transversales. Si l'axe de mouvement est parallèle, ou à peu près, à l'axe de figure des os articulés, ou si tous les deux ne font qu'un, nous aurons les articulations uniaxiles longitudinales, qui correspondent au ginglyme latéral de Winslow et à la trochoïde de Fallope.

Ce dernier groupe offre encore deux sous-types importants; il est toujours constitué anatomiquement par une tige osseuse reçue en un anneau ostéo-fibreux; mais parfois, comme à l'articulation radio-cubitale supérieure, l'anneau est immobile et la tige osseuse tourne; en d'autres cas, comme à l'articulation alloïdo-odontoïdienne, le pivot ou tige osseuse est fixe, et c'est l'anneau ostéo-fibreux qui tourne autour du pivot, comme une bague qu'on fait tourner sur le doigt qui la porte. Dans notre classification nous appelons uniaxiles longitudinales d'axe mobile les premières, et uniaxiles longitudinales d'axe fixe les secondes.

Les articulations, dont les mouvements ont lieu autour de deux axes perpendiculaires entre eux, forment notre groupe d'articulations biaxiles; les métacarpo-phalangiennes des quatre derniers doigts se rangent dans ce groupe. Si nous ne regardons qu'à la mobilité, tel groupe reste indivisible; mais si nous faisons attention à la configuration des surfaces articulaires, la classe sera divisible en deux autres, dont chacune correspond à un groupe de l'ancienne classification.

Dans une d'elles les surfaces ont une forme cylindrique à génératrice courbe, laquelle est engendrée à l'un des os par la convexité, et à l'autre par la concavité de la génératrice. Ce groupe est celui qui dans l'ancienne classification s'appelle par emboîtement réciproque; nous les appelons bi-cylindriques pour constater que les surfaces articulaires se rangent parmi les cylindriques; ou bi-concavo-convexes pour rappeler que chacune des surfaces articulaires est concave suivant une direction et convexe à l'opposée. L'articulation trapézo-métacarpienne du pouce en est le type.

Le second groupe qu'on peut former dans les articulations biaxiles en regardant la forme des surfaces articulaires, est formé par les articulations de la classification ordinaire qui s'appellent condyliennes. Ces surfaces ne peuvent être définies géométriquement puis qu'elles ne réalisent pas toujours un seul et même type; le plus qu'on en peut dire c'est que leurs diamètres sont inégaux, et que l'une d'elles est concave et l'autre convexe; pour consigner ce dernier fait, proposons de les appeler concavoconvexes. Ainsi constitué le groupe, on le subdivise en regardant chacune de ces circonstances: au mode de formation de la surface articulaire, sa nature, ses rapports fonctionnels de l'articulation d'un côté et de la symétrique du côté opposé.

Pour ce qu'on rapporte à la composition des surfaces qui forment l'articulation, chacune d'elles peut être constitué par une seule ou par plusieurs pièces osseuses; les articulations métacarpo-phalangiennes des quatre derniers doigts sont des exemples du premier cas, l'articulation radio-carpienne en fournit un du second; nous appelons concavo-convexes simples ces articulations dans lesquelles chaque surface articulaire n'est formée que d'un seul os, et composées ces autres dont l'une ou les deux surfaces sont taillées sur plus d'une pièce osseuse.

En général, les surfaces articulaires concavo-convexes sont osseuses et revêtues du très connu cartilage d'encroûtement; mais il arrive parfois qu'une seule des surfaces est osseuse, tandis que l'opposée est fibro-cartilagineuse; cela arrive aux articulations appelées de ménisque. Nous les appelons ostéo-fibro-cartilagineuses; l'articulation temporo-maxillaire en est l'exemple et le type.

De très respectables auteurs forment avec les articulations de ménisques un groupe qu'ils nomment: *articulations à surfaces discordantes*. C'est ainsi qu'on voit à l'articulation temporo-maxillaire la surface convexe du condyle s'opposer à une autre surface convexe, celle de la racine transverse de l'apophyse zygomatique, et en conséquence les deux surfaces ne peuvent s'emboîter; mais cette interprétation ne s'accommode pas bien à la réalité, puisque le ménisque inter-articulaire, interposé entre les surfaces osseuses, en rétablit l'accord et dédouble l'articulation, qui réellement est formée de deux articulations superposées, celle de la racine transverse et le ménisque, et celle du ménisque et le condyle.

En général l'articulation d'un côté du corps est indépendante de celle du côté opposé, l'articulation du côté droit peut fonctionner, tandis que la symétrique du côté gauche reste en repos; à l'articulation temporo-maxillaire arrive le contraire, puisque la relation fonctionnelle la plus étroite lie les articulations des deux côtés. Pour exprimer cette intime dépendance nous appelons conjuguées les articulations respectives.

Si les axes de mouvement sont trois et perpendiculaires entre eux, nous aurons le groupe d'articulations triaxiles, lequel est indivisible et correspond aux énarthroses de la classification vulgaire. L'articulation scapulo-humérale et la coxo-fémorale sont les seuls exemples bien caractérisés de ce groupe.

Pour finir nous copions ici les lignes suivantes d'un mémoire que nous avons publié sur ce sujet y a quelques années:

En résumé, la mobilité des articulations pouvant être étudiée avec plus de précision, le concept d'axes de rotation y aidant nous permet d'en former le tableau suivant. On y peut remarquer que le principe de la mobilité sert à former les groupes primaires, la plus grande partie des secondaires et même des tertiaires, et quelquefois le seul principe de la mobilité nous sert à arriver jusqu'aux groupes les plus bas. Quand ce principe est épuisé, nous faisons ce qu'on fait dans toute classification, nous prenons une autre base, par exemple, la forme de la surface articulaire. Nous tenons pour impossible, et même pour contraire à la méthode scientifique, de faire une classification, tant soit peu compliquée, sur une seule base. Ce serait comme si l'on demandait à un chimiste de faire toutes les opérations, pour reconnaître la nature d'un corps, au moyen d'un seul réactif. Quand le chimiste reconnaît l'impuissance d'un réactif, il en prend un autre; de même le classificateur, après avoir épuisé un principe en emploie un autre.

Voici le tableau dont il s'agit:

I. Articulations statiques.

II. Articulations dynamiques.

Ce deuxième groupe se subdivise en deux autres:

1. Articulations de mouvements indéfinis, subdivisé encore en synostéoses et dialostéoses.

2. Articulations de mouvements définis.

Ces dernières se décomposent en deux groupes:

A. Articulations axiles, caractérisées par un ou plusieurs axes de rotation.

B. Articulations abaxiles, auxquelles on ne saurait assigner d'axe de rotation.

Le groupe des articulations axiles se divise en trois sections d'après le nombre des axes qui peuvent être assignés aux articulations y comprises, à savoir:

a. Uniaxiles, qui ont un seul axe.

b. Biaxiles, qui en ont deux perpendiculaires l'un à l'autre.

c. Triaxiles, qui en ont une infinité; mais tous ces axes peuvent être réduits à trois dont chacun est perpendiculaire aux deux autres.

Les articulations uniaxiles se divisent en deux groupes:

a. Uniaxiles transversales dont l'axe est perpendiculaire à l'axe longitudinal des os articulés. Ce groupe comprend le ginglyme angulaire ou trochlée des auteurs; les articulations phalangiennes en sont le type.

b. Uniaxiles longitudinales, dont l'axe de rotation est parallèle à l'axe de figure des os articulés ou au moins de l'un d'eux équivalent au ginglyme latéral ou trochoïde des auteurs. L'articulation atloïdo-odontoïdienne en est le type.

Ce groupe admet deux variantes:

a. Uniaxiles longitudinales à axe fixe: articulations atloïdo-odontoïdienne et radio-cubitale inférieure.

b. Uniaxiles longitudinales à axe mobile, telles que l'articulation radio-cubitale supérieure.

Les articulations biaxiles, d'après la forme de la surface se divisent en deux groupes:

a. Bicylindriques ou bi-concavo-convexes, formées par deux surfaces cylindriques à génératrice courbe, engendrées l'une par la concavité, et l'autre par la convexité de la génératrice. Chaque surface est concave en un sens et convexe dans le sens perpendiculaire, et la concavité ou convexité de l'une s'adapte à la convexité ou concavité de l'autre. Ces articulations équivalent à celles qui sont appelées par emboîtement réciproque, dont le type est la trapézo-métacarpienne du pouce. Ce groupe ne se divise pas.

b. Les concavo-convexes: surfaces à diamètres inégaux, l'une concave, l'autre convexe, qui ne peuvent être définies géométriquement; elles correspondent aux condyliennes et peuvent être divisées ainsi:

a. Concavo-convexes simples. Chaque surface articulaire est taillée dans un seul os, exemple: les métacarpo-phalangiennes des quatre derniers doigts.

b. Concavo-convexes composées. La surface articulaire est formée par plus d'un os: articulation radio-carpienne.

Les articulations concavo-convexes, si l'on considère la nature des surfaces articulaires, seront encore divisées en deux groupes :

a. Concavo-convexes bi-osseuses : chaque surface est taillée sur un os.

b. Concavo-convexes ostéo-fibro-cartilagineuses : l'une des surfaces est taillée sur un fibro-cartilage. Ce dernier groupe correspond aux articulations à ménisque des auteurs. La temporo-maxillaire et la sterno-claviculaire en sont le type.

Les articulations concavo-convexes donnent lieu encore à cette division :

a. Indépendantes. L'articulation d'un côté fonctionne indépendamment de celle du côté opposé.

b. Dépendantes, ou conjuguées. L'articulation d'un côté est sous la dépendance fonctionnelle la plus étroite de celle de l'autre côté.

La temporo-maxillaire et l'occipito-atloïdienne sont des exemples d'articulations conjuguées, et elles sont même les seules qu'on puisse observer dans le groupe entier des articulations axiles ; mais si l'on y comprend aussi les articulations abaxiles et celles de mouvements indéfinis, on pourra trouver plusieurs exemples d'articulations conjuguées : telles sont celles des côtes, des apophyses des vertèbres, et celles des lames vertébrales.

Enfin, les articulations triaxiles forment un groupe indivisible, lequel embrasse les énarthroses des auteurs. Il n'y en a que deux exemples bien caractérisés : la scapulo-humérale, et la coxo-fémorale.

Sur l'anthropométrie médicale

Par M. João Carlos Mascarenhas de Mello, Lisbonne.

L'étude de la croissance qui fait partie de l'anatomie du développement a assez d'intérêt non seulement pour le médecin et l'hygiéniste, mais aussi pour l'éducation physique et intellectuelle des adolescents.

Ce qui pourra accorder quelque valeur à ce travail, c'est la manière dont il a été organisé, car il est fait sur l'examen d'un grand nombre d'enfants appartenant à la classe moyenne de la société portugaise.

Ceux-ci en effet, se trouvant dans le même collège, ont pu

être suivis depuis 10 à 18 ou 19 ans, et cette circonstance, qui a permis d'étudier la marche de la croissance individuelle, est importante.

Matériel existant au Collège militaire et règles adoptées pour mesurer les écoliers.

Au commencement et à la fin de chaque année scolaire on prend les mesures anthropométriques de chaque élève. Cette opération est faite à l'aide des instruments ci-dessous:

ruban métrique,

dynamomètre de pression et de traction,

étalon et anthropomètre de Collin,

balance,

pneumomètre de Mathieu.

Cette opération ou examen anthropométrique a pour but la détermination des indications suivantes: stature, poids, rapport entre le poids et la stature, périmètres thoraciques (supérieur, moyen et inférieur) autant pour l'inspiration que pour l'expiration, forme géométrique des thorax, capacité pulmonaire, force de pression des deux mains, force de traction, et quelques autres renseignements qui puissent ajouter quelque chose à la perfection de l'examen.

Le résultat de cet examen est écrit dans une table, d'où découle l'évolution physique de chaque élève.

Pour évaluer la hauteur, les élèves sont mesurés les pieds nus.

Pour évaluer le poids, les élèves portent seulement la chemise, le caleçon et les bas.

Pour les périmètres thoraciques: le supérieur est mesuré au bord inférieur des muscles de l'aisselle; le moyen aux mamelles; l'inférieur, à la taille, tout près de l'épigastre. Autant les inspirations que les expirations ne doivent pas être exagérées. Les élèves, pendant qu'on les mesure, ont les bras levés et les mains appuyées sur la tête.

Outre les mesurages ci-dessus indiqués, réglementaires au collège et dont je me suis servi dans cette communication, je cherche à augmenter le nombre des mesures à prendre et le matériel à employer, afin de mieux compléter mes études, dans quelques années.

Conditions des élèves.

Le nombre d'élèves existant au collège était de 222 en 1900, mais à présent il atteint 268. Ils sont divisés, selon leur provenance, comme suit : 179 fils d'officiers de l'armée de terre, 23 fils d'officiers de la marine, et 20 de la classe civile.

Dans mes rapports annuels j'écris en détail pour chaque élève les mesures anthropométriques, tempérament, constitution et les maladies qu'il a eues au collège pendant l'année.

Les élèves, dont les mesurages ont servi pour les conclusions que je vous ai présentées, sont : 40 de 10 ans, 177 de 11 ans, 238 de 12, 223 de 13, 204 de 14, 172 de 15, 153 de 16, 115 de 17, 51 de 18, 12 de 19 ans. Total 1385.

Les tempéraments sont, pour la plupart, mixtes et lymphatiques; la constitution est, selon les cas, considérée bonne, régulière, passable et mauvaise.

Dans le registre clinique de chaque élève on mentionne les antécédents morbides et héréditaires, etc.

Je dois remarquer que, dans l'examen médical auquel les élèves sont soumis, lorsqu'ils se présentent candidats à l'entrée au collège, je reconnais tout de suite les fils des veuves, parce qu'ils sont généralement chétifs et maigres, ce que je crois pouvoir attribuer aux circonstances précaires dans lesquelles vivent les veuves d'officiers.

Les maladies qui dominent au collège depuis 1898 jusqu'à 1904 sont indiquées dans la table ci-dessous, résumé des tableaux nosographiques publiés annuellement :

Abrégé des tableaux nosographiques des élèves

Maladies	[illegible]	[illegible]	[illegible]	[illegible]	[illegible]	[illegible]	[illegible]	Totaux
Maladies infectieuses — fièvres éruptives — Érysipèle		2	1		2	1	1	7
Roséole	19	1		2	1	5	8	36
Rubéole					7	1		8
Rougeole			1	8		8		17
Scarlatine					1			1
Varicelle	3	4		3	1			11
Variole	1							1
» » — non éruptives — Diphtérie		4			5		1	10
Fièvres intermittentes	1	1	2					4
Fièvre typhoïde — Coli bacillose						5		5
Grippe ou influenza	9	6	21	7	1	9	7	72
Oreillons				29		12		41
Rhumatisme		3		2	1	1	1	8
Maladies du tube digestif — Stomatites				2	2			4
Angines aiguës	16	9	31	19	30	3	6	120
Autres maladies de l'amygdale ou du pharynx	3	2	2	1	5	2	3	18
Troubles gastriques	15	13	5	13	7		7	60
Entérites	4	4	2		3		4	17
Vers intestinaux					1			1
Constipation		2	2					4
Autres maladies du tube gastro-intestinal	5	3	1	1		2	1	13

The column group "Années scolaires" spans the seven dated year columns (headings illegible) that precede the "Totaux" column.

							Totaux
Laryngites striduleuses	2		3			1		6
Bronchites	8	2	7	3	6	3	3	32
Pneumonies	2	1			3			6
Pleurésies				1				1
Tuberculose pulmonaire		1					1	2
Autre maladies de l'appareil respiratoire	5	4	1	1		1		12
Maladies du système nerveux — Neurasthénie	3	3	1	1				8
Névroses (chorée, hystérie, etc.)		1	1		1	2	2	7
Méningites					1		1	2
Dermatoses	4	2	2	6	2			16
Maladies vénériennes			2		1		4	7
Manifestations syphilitiques	1	5						6
Maladies des organes des sens — Blépharites	1			1		1		3
Conjonctivites	5	1		2	5			13
Kératites, etc.		1		1				2
Otites et otalgies		1	1	3	3			8
Maladies chirurgicales — Abcès	1	1		1	1	1	1	6
Plaies contuses et contusions	1		1	1	3		1	7
Luxations	1	1	2	3	3	2		12
Fractures	1	1	2			1	1	6
Ulcères		1	1					2
Furoncles	1	1						2
Observés	20	6	5	2				33
Convalescents	9	15	8	6	137	182	144	501
Totaux	143	106	105	122	254	246	205	1481

Régime du collège (suivant l'horaire de l'année scolaire de 1898 à 1899)

Diane — 6 heures du matin
Retraite, pour les 3 premières classes 8h.30
         pour les autres classes 9h.15

La distribution du temps se fait selon le tableau ci-dessous

Distribution du temps		Pour les 3 premières classes	Pour les autres classes
Travail intellectuel	Temps de classes......	3h.45	3h.45
	Temps d'études......	2h	3.30
	Total............	5h.45	7.15
	Maximum admis......	6h	8
	Exercices physiques	0.45	1
Repos complet	Selon l'horaire......	9	8
	Maximum admis......	9	8

Nota. — Quelques exercices physiques sont exécutés pendant le temps consacré aux classes qui ne sont pas destinées aux leçons.

La nourriture jusqu'à 1901 se composait de quatre repas: déjeuner à 8h.15 du matin (un plat, du café au lait et du pain beurré); lunch à 12h.25 (repas léger); dîner à 4 heures (du potage, un ou deux plats de viande ou de poisson, du vin et dessert; souper à 8 heures, pour les 3 premières classes, et à 8h.45 pour les autres classes (du thé et du pain beurré).

Pour la composition de ces repas on a organisé des cadres qui ont été publiés et qui, comme condition physiologique, se basaient sur ce que la ration des élèves ne devrait jamais être inférieure pour les principes alimentaires aux proportions suivantes:

Albuminoïdes . . . . 120 grammes
Graisses 80   —
Hydrates de carbone 470   —

L'année passée, après de nouvelles études et après une augmentation du budget, l'alimentation fut modifiée de façon que le dîner n'eût jamais moins de deux plats. Par la suite on a supprimé le lunch, en donnant le matin un petit déjeuner composé de café, café au lait, ou du cacao et des biscuits, et alors plus tard le déjeuner. Vers la fin de l'année scolaire on a remplacé le repas du soir qui se composait de thé et de pain beurré, par du thé et du lait et du pain beurré aussi.

Conditions hygiéniques

L'édifice où est installé le Collège Militaire Royal est situé à Luz, paroisse de Carnide, à six kilomètres NW de Lisbonne; c'est un lieu qui a toujours joui de la meilleure réputation de salubrité. À son origine, cet édifice était destiné à servir d'hôpital pour les moines pauvres; il fut fondé par l'infante D. Marie, fille du roi D. Emmanuel, et terminé en 1618; il était administré par l'ordre du Christ, qui possédait tout près un couvent et une église somptueuse. Tout cela fut fortement endommagé à l'occasion du tremblement de terre de 1755.

En 1814, après quelques réparations, l'édifice de l'hôpital fut destiné à l'installation du Collège Militaire Royal. De l'église, seulement une partie de la nef et le maître-autel échappèrent, et ils méritent d'être visités pour leur somptuosité.

Ce qui existe du couvent est connu aujourd'hui sous la désignation de «quarteis velhos» (vieux quartiers) et sert de dépendances du collège.

Les conditions spéciales où se trouve ce collège et les vastes terrains annexes, sa situation en plein air, tout cela contribue à sa salubrité.

Mensuration des élèves

Pour bien faire comprendre les résultats que j'ai obtenus sur la mensuration des élèves, je les ai représentés par des graphiques, et ci-dessous je transcris les conclusions auxquelles je suis arrivé:

10 ans

1898 1899	1899 1900	1900 1901	1901 1902	1903 1904	Moyenne générale
27	2	5	5	1	40
27	2	5	5	1	40
27	2	5	5	1	40
27	2	5	5	1	40

11 ans

							Moyennes générales
Taille							
N. d'élèves mesurés	37	31	33	40	21	15	177
Poids							
N. d'élèves mesurés	37	31	33	40	21	15	177
Périmètre thoracique moyen							
N. d'élèves mesurés	37	31	33	40	21	15	177
Spiromètre							
N. d'élèves mesurés	37	31	33	40	21	15	177

12 ans.

	1898 1899	1899 1900	1900 1901	1901 1902	1902 1903	1903 1904	Moyenne générale
Stature							
N. d'élèves mesurés	31	43	39	37	25	63	238
Poids							
N. d'élèves mesurés	31	43	39	37	25	43	238
Périmètre thoracique moyen							
N. d'élèves mesurés	31	43	39	37	25	43	238
Spiromètrie							
N. d'élèves mesurés	31	43	39	37	43	43	238

13 ans

	1898 1899	1899 1900	1900 1901	1901 1902	1902 1903	1903 1904	Moyenne générale
Stature							
N. d'élèves mesurés	26	37	41	37	38	40	223
Poids							
N. d'élèves mesurés	26	37	41	37	38	40	223
Périmètre thoracique (au repos)							
N. d'élèves mesurés	26	37	41	37	38	40	223
Segment...							
N. d'élèves mesurés	26	37	41	37	38	40	223

14 ans

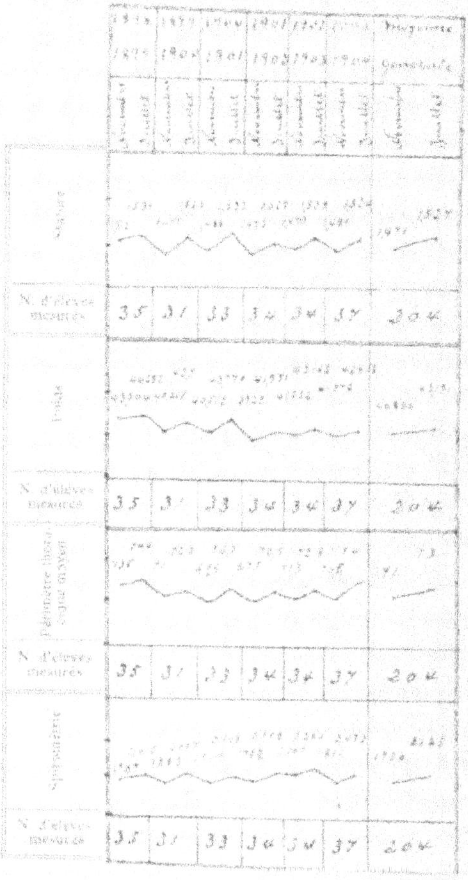

1895 1898	1899 1900	1900 1901	1901 1902	1902 1903	1903 1904	Progressive Cumulative
Taille						
N. d'élèves mesurés	35	31	33	34	34	37	204
Poids						
N. d'élèves mesurés	35	31	33	34	34	37	204
Périmètre thoracique moyen						
N. d'élèves mesurés	35	31	33	34	34	37	204
Spirométrie						
N. d'élèves mesurés	35	31	33	34	34	37	204

16 ans

	1873 1899	1874 1900	1900 1901	1901 1902	1901 1903	1902 1904	moyenne générale
Taille							1573 1590
N. d'élèves mesurés	25	21	27	31	35	33	178
Poids							
N. d'élèves mesurés	25	21	27	31	35	33	178
Périmètre thoracique au repos							
N. d'élèves mesurés	25	21	27	31	35	33	172
Spiromètrie							
N. d'élèves mesurés	25	21	27	31	35	33	172

16 ans

	1898 1899	1899 1900	1900 1901	1901 1902	1902 1903	1903 1904	Moyennes Générale
Stature							
N. d'élèves mesurés	21	28	19	22	29	34	153
Poids							
N. d'élèves mesurés	21	28	19	22	29	34	153
Périmètre thoracique moyen							
N. d'élèves mesurés	21	28	19	22	29	34	153
Spirométrie							
N. d'élèves mesurés	21	28	19	22	29	34	

17 ans

	1878 1879	1899 1900	1900 1901	1901 1902	1902 1903	1903 1904	Moyenne générale
Stature							1635 1641
N. d'élèves mesurés	11	20	17	16	22	29	115
Poids							53257 53091
N. d'élèves mesurés	11	20	17	16	22	29	115
Pression thoracique inspiration							479 80
N. d'élèves mesurés	11	20	17	16	22	29	115
Spiromètrie							2341 2502
N. d'élèves mesurés	11	20	17	16	22	29	115

18 ans

	1898 1899	1899 1900	1901 1902	1902 1903	1903 1904	Moyenne générale
Taille						
N. d'élèves mesurés	7	5	16	13	10	51
Poids						
N. d'élèves mesurés	7	5	16	13	10	51
Capacité thoracique moyen						
N. d'élèves mesurés	7	5	16	13	10	51
Périmètre						
N. d'élèves mesurés	7	5	16	13	10	51

19 ans

1902 1903	1903 1904	Moyenne générale
Taille		1695
N. d'élèves mesurés 4	8	12
Poids		
N. d'élèves mesurés 4	8	12
Périmètre thoracique moyen		88.4
N. d'élèves mesurés 4	8	12
Spiromètre		2775
N. d'élèves mesurés 4	8	12

Moyennes générales

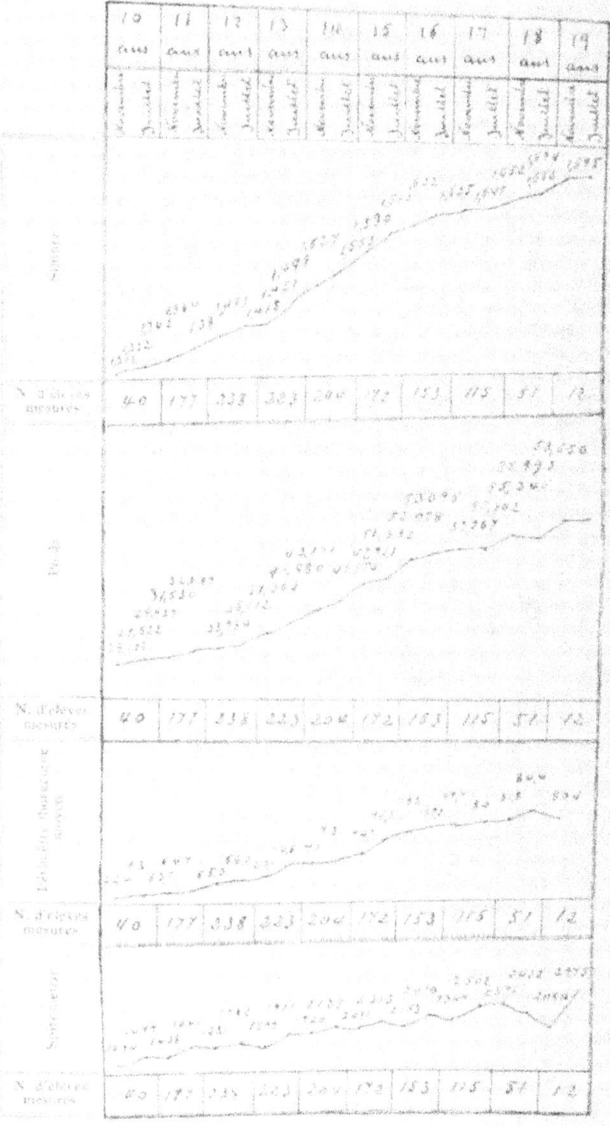

Les conclusions de mon mémoire sont analogues à celles des observateurs étrangers, et je trouve ce fait d'autant plus remarquable que les conditions ethniques portugaises sont différentes de celles des populations où ces études anthropométriques ont été faites.

Les tableaux ci-dessous, où mes observations sont résumées, me permettent d'établir les conclusions suivantes:

1. Le *poids*, la *stature*, et le *périmètre thoracique moyen* augmentent dans la même progression de 10 à 18 ans.

2. Cette augmentation est graduelle et progressive de 10 à 14 ans, diminue de 14 à 16 ans, et grandit une autre fois de 16 à 18 et 19 ans.

3. C'est de 14 à 16 ans que la crise de la croissance physique se manifeste, c'est-à-dire que la puberté arrive généralement.

4. Les moyennes de la *capacité pulmonaire* indiquées par la spirométrie croissent de 10 à 18 ans, sans une progression régulière comme il arrive pour les trois phases des autres mesures physiques, dont je me suis occupé dans la deuxième de mes conclusions.

	Moyennes du poids		Moyennes ne tenant pas compte des fractions	Moyennes de croissance	Phases de croissance
à 10 ans	en novembre (commencement de l'année scolaire)	28k,200	29		
	en juillet (fin de l'année scolaire)	29k,822		1,5	
» 11 »	en novembre	29k,959	30,500		
	en juillet	31k,820		2,5	
» 12 »	en novembre	32k,689	33		a
	en juillet	33k,984		3,5	
» 13 »	en novembre	35k,612	36,300		
	en juillet	37k,362		5,5	
» 14 »	en novembre	40k,880	42		
	en juillet	43k,191		5	
» 15 »	en novembre	46k,154	47		
	en juillet	47k,921		4,5	
» 16 »	en novembre	51k,092	51,500		b
	en juillet	52k,078		1,5	
» 17 »	en novembre	53k,095	53		
	en juillet	53k,267		2,5	
» 18 »	en novembre	56k,102	55,500		
	en juillet	55k,316		3	
» 19 »	en novembre	58k,098	58,500		c
	en juillet	58k,864			

Moyennes de stature

Âge		Moyenne en tenant compte des fractions	Moyennes de croissance	Phases de croissance
à 10 ans	en novembre 1m,312	1,320		
	en juillet 1m,332		0,020	
» 11 »	en novembre 1m,342	1,350		
	en juillet 1m,360		0,040	a
» 12 »	en novembre 1m,380	1,400		
	en juillet 1m,417		0,040	
» 13 »	en novembre 1m,418	1,430		
	en juillet 1m,451		0,070	
» 14 »	en novembre 1m,491	1,500		b
	en juillet 1m,527		0,070	
» 15 »	en novembre 1m,553	1,570		
	en juillet 1m,590		0,050	
» 16 »	en novembre 1m,610	1,620		
	en juillet 1m,632		0,010	
» 17 »	en novembre 1m,635	1,630		
	en juillet 1m,644		0,020	
» 18 »	en novembre 1m,652	1,650		c
	en juillet 1m,682		0,040	
» 19 »	en novembre 1m,691	1,690		
	en juillet 1m,695			

3 — Moyennes du périmètre thoracique moyen

Âge		Moyenne en tenant compte des fractions	Moyennes de croissance	Phases de croissance
à 10 ans	en novembre 62,4	62,5		
	en juillet 63		1,5	
» 11 »	en novembre 63,7	64		
	en juillet 64,7		2	
» 12 »	en novembre 65,3	66		a
	en juillet 66,3		3	
» 13 »	en novembre 67,1	69		
	en juillet 70,8		3	
» 14 »	en novembre 71	72		
	en juillet 73		3,5	
» 15 »	en novembre 74,7	75,6		
	en juillet 76,5		3	
» 16 »	en novembre 78,2	78,5		b
	en juillet 79,2		1,5	
» 17 »	en novembre 79,9	80		
	en juillet 80		1,5	
» 18 »	en novembre 81,8	81,5		
	en juillet 81,6		1	
» 19 »	en novembre 81,4	82,5		
	en juillet 80,4			

Moyennes de la quinconce		Moyennes relatives par rapport des tranches	Moyennes de croissance
à 10 ans	en novembre	1294	1386	
	en juillet	1427		155
» 11 »	en novembre	1498	1540	
	en juillet	1641		160
» 12 »	en novembre	1631	1709	
	en juillet	1788		100
» 13 »	en novembre	1809	1860	
	en juillet	1911		250
» 14 »	en novembre	1926	2020	
	en juillet	2125		173
» 15 »	en novembre	2075	2196	
	en juillet	2313		85
» 16 »	en novembre	2353	2380	
	en juillet	2410		180
» 17 »	en novembre	2349	2460	
	en juillet	2562		10
» 18 »	en novembre	2576	2500	
	en juillet	3432		20
» 19 »	en novembre	2684	2520	
	en juillet	2975		

N. B. Les élèves sont reçus au Collège militaire à l'âge de 10 ans et en sortent à 18 ans; ce n'est qu'exceptionnellement qu'ils y sont reçus à l'âge de 11 ans, et en sortent à 19 ans.

Anatomie du membre anormal d'un pygomélien étudiée par la radiographie

Par MM. Feyo e Castro et Augusto de Vasconcellos (Lisbonne)

J'ai l'honneur de vous présenter, au nom de M. le prof. Augusto de Vasconcellos et au mien, le rapport d'un cas de polymélie pelvique.

Il s'agit d'un enfant du sexe masculin, âgé de 19 mois, bien développé, présentant vers la partie inférieure de l'abdomen, au-dessus du pubis et un peu à gauche de la ligne médiane, un appendice simulant un troisième membre inférieur.

Les photographies, bien mieux que la description, font voir la conformation de ce membre tératologique, dont le prof. Vasconcellos a fait l'amputation; l'enfant, on le voit sur une des photographies, est resté parfaitement normal.

Des radiographies faites avant l'opération démontrèrent que

les organes abdominaux n'avaient aucun rapport avec ce membre
et qu'il n'existait pas d'altération au squelette du pelvis; son insertion se faisait au-dessus de la branche gauche du pubis.

On remarque aussi, sur ces mêmes radiographies, qu'il existait à l'extrémité supérieure du membre quelques pièces osseuses
qui paraissaient appartenir à un segment pelvien; au-dessous, à
la cuisse, on voyait un os rappelant un fémur, bifurqué à son
extrémité inférieure; à la gauche, deux tibias; au pied, deux
métatarsien et aux doigts trois phalanges sur l'un, deux sur
l'autre.

Après l'amputation, le membre a été envoyé au Laboratoire
d'analyses cliniques de l'Hôpital de S. José où il a été observé
avec plus de soin.

Dans la coupe du pédicule, qui était circulaire et mesurait 3
cm de diamètre, apparaissait l'extrémité d'une pièce cartilagineuse et, tout autour, au milieu d'un tissu fibro-graisseux, on remar-
quait des petits vaisseaux dont le calibre n'était pas supérieur à
2 mm.

L'articulation du genou avait très peu de mobilité et la jambe, abandonnée à elle-même, formait avec la cuisse un angle de
120°.

La mobilité de l'articulation tibio-tarsienne était aussi très
bornée; l'angle des deux axes de la jambe et du pied était à peu
près de 60°.

Le poids du membre était de 530 gr; sa longueur, selon une
droite allant de la partie supérieure à la pointe du pied, dans la
position naturelle, atteignait $0^m,23$; depuis l'extrémité supérieure
jusqu'au genou il mesurait $0^m,16$, du genou à l'articulation tibio-
tarsienne $0^m,09$; le pied mesurait $0^m,06$.

Deux radiographies, prises en deux plans perpendiculaires —
frontal et sagittal — nous renseignent sur la disposition du squelette;
on voit à l'extrémité supérieure trois pièces osseuses, qui paraissent
correspondre à un segment pelvien, d'après leur forme et leur
situation. A la cuisse, un os bifurqué en haut et en bas, formé
par la soudure de deux os parfaitement symétriques; à la jambe
deux os ressemblant à deux tibias, celui de droite plus court; le
pied portait deux métatarsiens, en rapport avec deux doigts, pos-
sédant l'un d'eux trois phalanges, l'autre seulement deux.

Des trois pièces qui composaient le segment pelvien, une,
celle d'en haut, était allongée, à peu près cylindrique, mesurant
$0^m,015$ de longueur et $0^m,003$ d'épaisseur et se terminait par

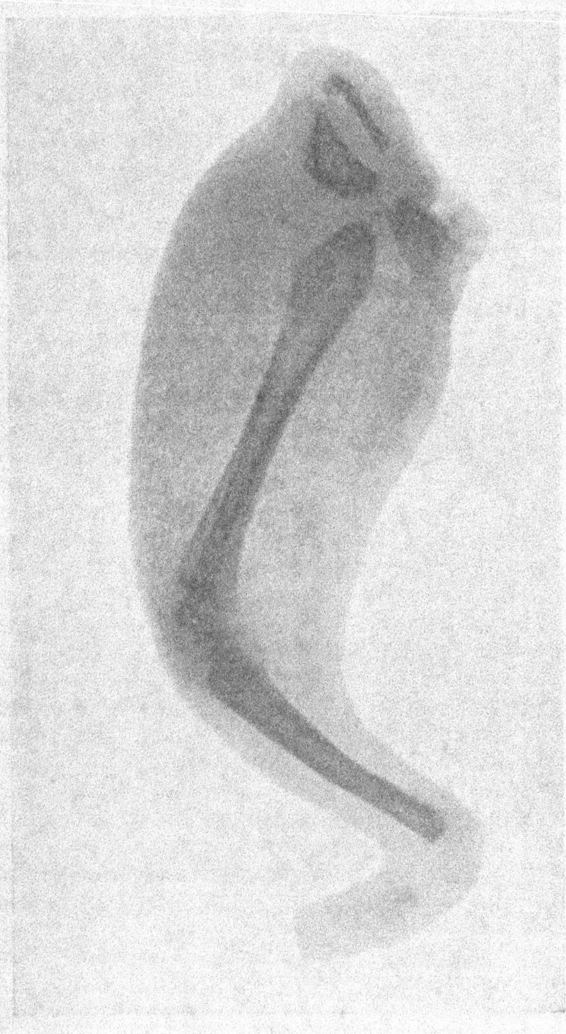

Fig. 1.

deux petites portions d'os sphériques, comme deux épiphyses; elle se dirigeait obliquement de haut en bas, de droite à gauche et d'avant en arrière.

Immédiatement au-dessous de cette pièce se trouvait une autre qui, en projection transversale, ainsi que sur la radiographie au plan frontal, se présentait sous la forme d'un croissant, presque en demi-cercle, à diamètre parallèle à l'axe de la pièce précédente.

La radiographie, en plan sagittal, montre que cette pièce avait environ $0^m,02$ de largeur, se terminant en bas par une crête antéro-postérieure, située entre deux dépressions latérales symétriques.

La troisième pièce, située au-dessous et en arrière de celle-ci, se montre sur la radiographie au plan sagittal sous l'aspect d'un cœur d'une carte à jouer, elle porte en haut une dépression médiane en correspondance avec la crête de la pièce antérieure; en bas elle se termine par une pointe qui accompagne la partie postérieure de l'os de la cuisse dans une extension d'un centimètre et demi.

La radiographie, dans le plan frontal, montre dans le sens antéro-postérieur une section qui rappelle un triangle à angles arrondis, dont l'un est antéro-supérieur, l'autre postérieur et le troisième inférieur.

L'angle antéro-supérieur s'adaptait à la pièce précédente; le postérieur correspondait au pédicule d'insertion du membre; à l'angle inférieur aboutissant un bord antéro-inférieur, situé dans le plan de la crête de la pièce antérieure et, limitant les deux, une échancrure, servant d'articulation à l'extrémité de l'os de la cuisse portant, lui aussi, une échancrure dans un plan perpendiculaire.

L'os de la cuisse, vu dans un plan sagittal sur la radiographie, rappelle un Y renversé. Son extrémité supérieure échancrée dans le plan transversal, *s'amincit* dans le sens antéro-postérieur; au plan transversal l'épaisseur de l'os va en diminuant graduellement de haut en bas, jusqu'au tiers médian; au plan antéro-postérieur l'épaisseur augmente rapidement, atteignant un maximum de $0^m,015$ au-dessous de l'extrémité supérieure, et diminuant ensuite d'une façon régulière jusqu'à proximité du tiers inférieur.

La tendance à se diviser se montre sur cet os déjà à partir de son extrémité supérieure. De l'échancrure supérieure part une ligne qui se dirige longitudinalement dans le tiers supérieur de la diaphyse, s'efface à proximité du tiers moyen et apparaît de

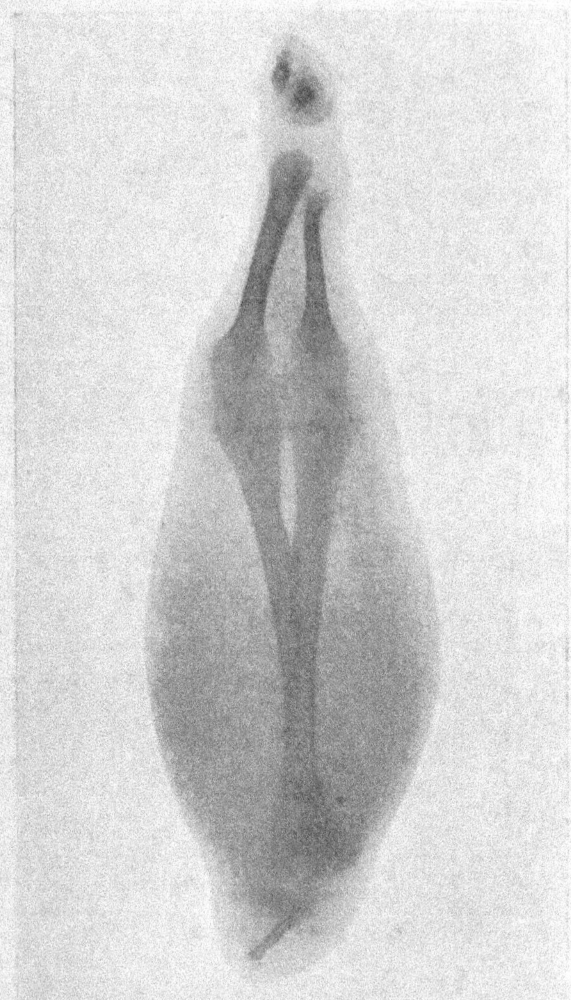

Fig. 2

nouveau à partir de celui-ci; au tiers inférieur les deux parties de l'os deviennent indépendantes, divergent en formant un angle très aigu; leur écartement va jusqu'à 0^m,004, mais ils se réunissent au moyen d'un petit pont osseux, par lequel les deux diaphyses se rallient à leur partie inféro-postérieure.

À son extrémité inférieure on voit deux épiphyses indépendantes, semblables à celle du fémur normal.

Les os de la jambe rappellent, comme nous l'avons dit, deux tibias; leur articulation avec l'os de la cuisse ne porte pas de rotule; on note deux épiphyses supérieures bien développées; des deux diaphyses, celle de droite est la plus courte et s'incurve en dehors à sa partie inférieure. L'os de droite ne montre pas d'épiphyse inférieure; à celui de gauche on note un point microscopique d'ossification qui lui correspond.

On ne voit guère de traces de squelette ossifié au tarse.

Au métatarse on voit deux os longs qui ressemblent à deux métatarsiens; celui de droite est plus épais.

Aux doigts on note deux phalanges chez celui de droite qui est le plus gros et ressemble à un gros orteil, trois phalanges chez celui de gauche, la première déjà ossifiée et les deux dernières représentées par deux points d'ossification très petits.

J'ai essayé de faire l'étude du système artériel par l'injection d'une substance opaque aux rayons X et en faisant la radiographie du membre en différentes positions.

Je préfère le mercure, par son homogénéité, fluidité et par la simplicité de technique, à tous les autres liquides employés, composés, pour la plupart, d'une poudre métallique en suspension dans un véhicule liquide ou pouvant se liquéfier par échauffement.

J'ai suivi un procédé pareil à celui de l'injection des lymphatiques — un entonnoir avec du mercure rallié à une canule par un tube en caoutchouc. — Après pénétration de la canule dans un vaisseau artériel, j'ai porté l'entonnoir à une hauteur d'environ 0^m,30 au-dessus de la canule et je l'ai laissé dans cette position pendant 24 h. Aussitôt que j'eus soulevé l'entonnoir, le mercure se montra dans les vaisseaux très minces ouverts dans la coupe du pédicule, et j'ai été forcé de faire 15 ligatures afin d'empêcher le reflux. J'ai fait ensuite des radiographies dans les plans frontal et sagital, permettant de se rendre compte de la disposition générale des vaisseaux. L'ampoule a été placée à une grande distance — un mètre — de façon à obtenir une image nette et à éviter les déformations dans la projection.

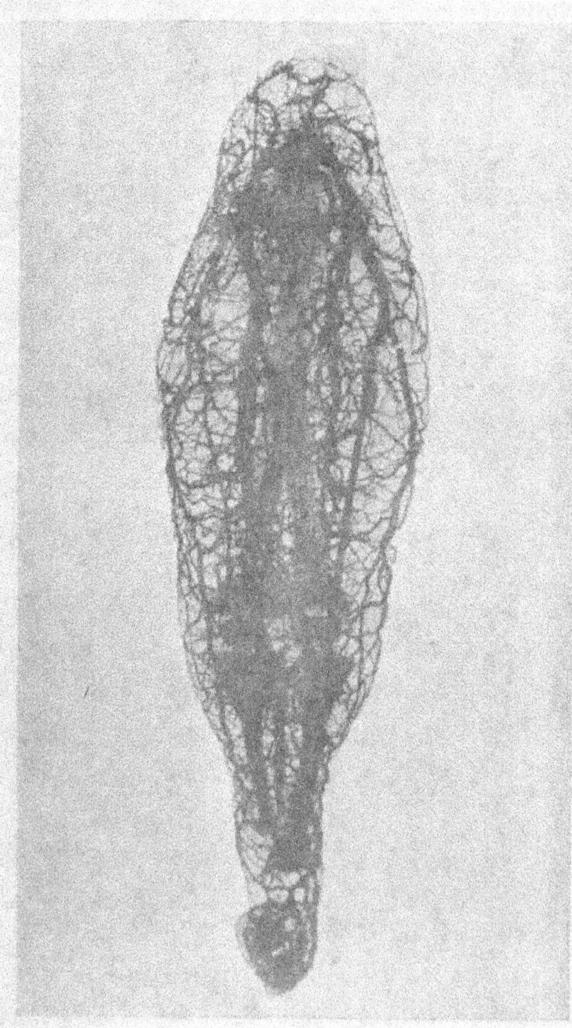

Fig. 3

On voit, d'après ces radiographies, que la vascularisation est extrêmement développée, et que la distribution des vaisseaux se fait d'une façon symétrique à l'axe du membre, ce qui vient confirmer ce fait, déjà indiqué par la disposition du squelette, qu'il s'agit, en effet, non d'un membre simple, mais de deux membres, qui se sont fondus en un seul.

On voit, à partir du niveau du pédicule, et de chaque côté, un gros vaisseau qui se dirige en haut et en dedans et va s'anastomoser par inosculation avec son homologue du côté opposé; ils donnent origine à une arcade, d'où partent quelques branches se dirigeant vers l'extrémité supérieure. Un de ces vaisseaux, celui de droite, a servi à l'injection du mercure, ainsi que l'indique, sur les radiographies, l'ombre de la canule.

Au-dessous du pédicule, les deux vaisseaux se continuent dans une extension de $0^m,01$ — un de chaque côté, sensiblement dans le même plan de l'os — ; après un court trajet ils se bifurquent, donnant origine à deux autres branches de chaque côté. Les deux branches secondaires se dirigent verticalement, se bifurquent $0^m,025$ plus bas et donnent origine à quatre branches de chaque côté de l'os.

De ces quatre vaisseaux, le plus externe se distribue à la surface; on peut suivre ses ramifications jusqu'à la jambe et au pied.

Celui immédiatement en dedans a un trajet plus profond; il va en ligne droite jusqu'à la partie inférieure du genou où il semble souffrir une inflexion en arrière vers la partie postérieure de chaque os de la jambe, et se continue jusqu'au pied.

Des deux branches latérales restantes, la plus interne semble se distribuer à l'os, la plus externe suit presque en ligne droite jusqu'au genou, passe en arrière de l'articulation et s'anastomose, à la partie supérieure de la jambe, avec la branche du côté opposé.

A partir de l'anastomose, jusqu'au pied, fait suite un seul vaisseau médian.

Au pied, ses deux bords sont longés par deux branches qui s'anastomosent à la partie antérieure du métatarse et forment une arcade d'où partent d'autres branches se dirigeant vers la région antérieure du pied.

Aux doigts, deux collatérales paraissent exister tout comme aux doigts normaux.

L'examen des coupes en série (perpendiculaires à l'axe du membre dans la région correspondante) montre dans cette pièce,

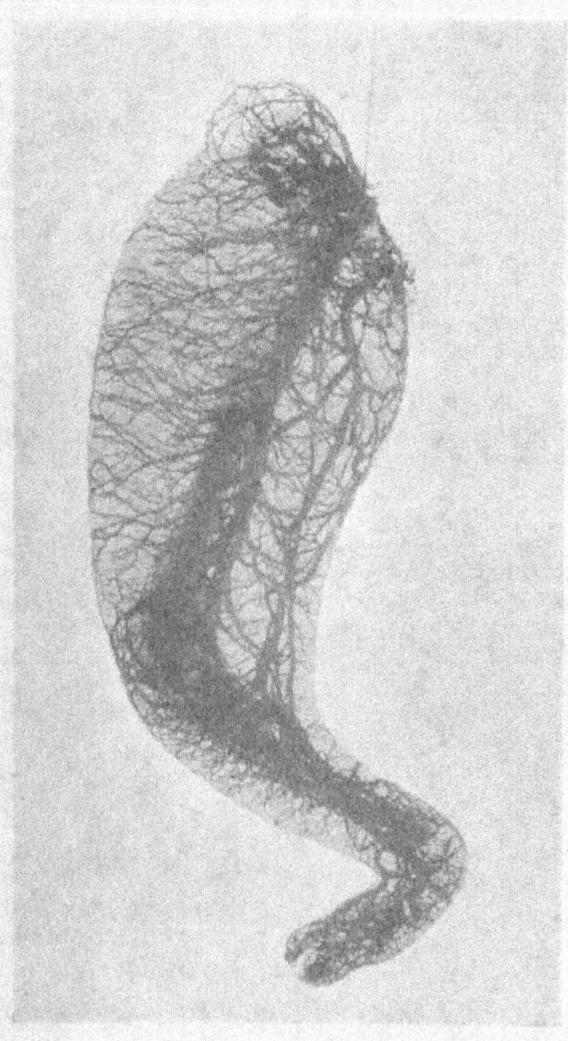

Fig. 4

RADIOGRAPHIE DANS UN CAS DE PYGOMÉLIE 373

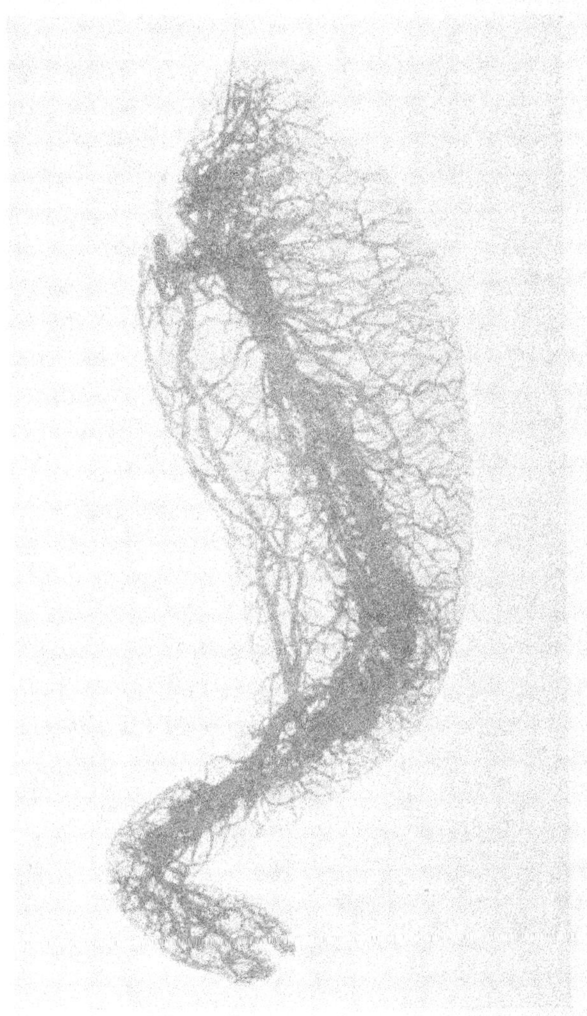

relativement au squelette, la même disposition que nous indiquent les radiographies. On voit dans la partie correspondant au tarse, deux pièces cartilagineuses, en situation astragalo-calcanéenne.

Tout autour des sections des os, quelques groupes musculaires.

Au pelvis, sur la quatrième coupe, 3 groupes distincts se montrent, bridés par une aponévrose et séparés par l'os; un antérieur et deux postéro-latéraux, fondus dans les coupes suivantes en un seul antéro-latéral.

À la cuisse, quatre groupes commencent à se distinguer; deux antérieurs et deux postérieurs, symétriquement placés en rapport au plan sagital; les antérieurs, plus développés, se terminent à la partie inférieure de l'os de la cuisse.

Tout près de la jambe, à la partie inférieure de la cuisse, un groupe antérieur commence à se montrer; il se continue dans la jambe, séparé par un ligament interosseux d'avec un autre groupe qui apparaît entre les os et devient un peu antérieur.

Voilà tout ce que j'ai à dire au sujet de ce curieux exemplaire.

SÉANCE DU 26 AVRIL.

(à 10 heures du matin)

Présidence: M. RAMON

Sont présents, MM. Benda, Cajal, Cacrarido, Celestino da Costa, Ramon, Mik, Loyez, Marck Athias, Mattoso Santos, Paes Leme, Pinto de Magalhães, Silva Tavares, Waldeyer, etc.

Station biologique maritime

Avant l'ordre du jour, M. K. BENDA propose que la section émette le vœu qu'il soit créé en Portugal une station biologique maritime, où des savants portugais et étrangers puissent trouver les matériaux et la place nécessaires à la poursuite de recherches scientifiques sur les animaux et végétaux marins.

M. MATTOSO SANTOS remercie M. Benda de sa proposition, qu'il accepte avec plaisir.

M. WALDEYER s'y associe également et propose que l'on demande que ce vœu soit émis par le Congrès et non pas uniquement par la section d'Anatomie.

M. CAJAL fait ressortir l'importance que la création de cette station peut avoir et pour le Portugal et pour l'Espagne.

Après une courte discussion à laquelle prennent part aussi MM. SILVA TAVARES et CARRACIDO, la proposition est approuvée par toute l'assemblée; le vœu est signé par tous les Congressistes présents des sections I et II.

Classification, origine et rôle probable des leucocytes

Par M. GUGLIELMO ROMITI, Pise (v. page 13), et M. LOWELL GILLAND, Édimbourg (v. page 178)

Phénomènes histologiques de la sécrétion, particulièrement dans les glandes à sécrétion interne

Par M. SWALE VINCENT, Winnipeg (v. page 1)

Origine, nature et classification des pigments

Par M. MARCK ATHIAS, Lisbonne (v. page 132)

Sur les phénomènes de sécrétion des cellules des corps jaunes vrais

Par M. MARCK ATHIAS, Lisbonne.

Presque tous les histologistes inclinent actuellement à admettre que le corps jaune possède une fonction sécrétoire; cette idée, émise il y a quelques années par Podvissotzky, Beard, Prenant, etc., a trouvé un appui considérable dans les recherches cytologiques de Regaud et Policard (1) et de Cohn (2). Ces auteurs ont en effet pu mettre en évidence dans les cellules des corps jaunes de quelques Mammifères des formations particulières, qui doivent être indubitablement en rapport avec des fonctions sécrétoires. Regaud et Policard ont vu chez une femelle de Hérisson des gouttelettes de sécrétion colorables par la méthode de Weigert pour la myéline et des filaments ergastoplasmiques dans les cellules du corps jaune; ils signalent aussi l'existence de gouttelettes de sécrétion semblables chez le Lapin, le Cobaye et le Rat, sans toutefois donner assez de détails sur leurs caractères morphologiques et leur distribution.

(1) Cl. Regaud et J. Policard—Notes histologiques sur l'ovaire des Mammifères.—Comptes rendus de l'Association des anatomistes, 5e session, Lyon, 1901.

(2) F. Cohn—Zur Histologie und Histogenese des Corpus luteum und des interstitiellen Ovarialgewebes.—Arch. f. mikr. Anat.—62. Bd. 1903.

Cohn a rencontré dans les cellules du corps jaune du Lapin des inclusions cellulaires colorables par la méthode de Plossen-Rabinowicz, ayant une forme sphérique et constituées par une couche corticale qui se montre bien colorée et une portion centrale qui se teint faiblement. Des formations semblables à celles décrites par Cohn ont été plus récemment observées par Celestino da Costa (1) chez le même animal, à l'aide de l'hématoxyline ferrique.

Au cours des recherches que je poursuis actuellement sur quelques points de la structure de l'ovaire des Mammifères, j'ai eu l'occasion de retrouver des formations qui correspondent à celles qui ont été vues par les auteurs précédents, dans des préparations provenant d'ovaires de Lapin et de Cobaye fixées par le liquide de Zenker et colorées par l'hématoxyline ferrique de Heidenhain. Dans cette note préliminaire je désire surtout ajouter quelques détails d'ordre morphologique à la description que les auteurs cités plus haut donnent de ces inclusions des cellules qui constituent les corps jaunes et en même temps signaler quelques autres particularités de structure que j'ai pu observer dans ces éléments.

Aussi bien chez le Lapin que chez le Cobaye, les cellules des corps jaunes vrais ayant atteint leur développement complet sont des éléments volumineux, de forme irrégulièrement polyédrique; elles sont pourvues d'un gros noyau vésiculeux, ordinairement excentrique, limité par une membrane très nette, et contenant un ou deux corpuscules nucléaires.

Dans le cytoplasme de la plupart de ces cellules, l'hématoxyline ferrique met en évidence de petits corpuscules de forme sphérique, plus ou moins irrégulière, qui, examinés à un fort grossissement, offrent presque toujours une zone corticale fortement colorée et une partie centrale claire; les dimensions de ces corpuscules sont très variables. Les plus petits ne présentent pas de centre clair et prennent une teinte bleu noirâtre plus foncée. Les plus volumineux sont bien plus pâles, et parfois la couche corticale plus colorée ne forme pas un anneau complet. A côté de ces corpuscules arrondis il y en a souvent qui ont des formes très différentes et se montrent comme de petits bâtonnets irréguliers, plus ou moins incurvés, sinueux ou verruqueux, etc. Ces

---

(1) A. Celestino da Costa — Sobre alguns pormenores de estructura da cápsula supra-renal dos Mammiferos — Medicina Contemporanea, Lisboa, 1905; Glandulas supra-renaes e seus homologos — Lisboa, 1906.

formations sont souvent situées à la périphérie du cytoplasme (fig. 1 à 4). Quand le noyau est placé au centre de la cellule, elles existent sur toute la périphérie du cytoplasme, disposées sur une ou plusieurs rangées; dans les cellules de forme allongée, ces inclusions se montrent souvent accumulées aux extrémités du corps cellulaire. Dans quelques cas, elles remplissent plus ou moins complètement la cellule, deviennent confluentes et donnent à la portion qu'elles occupent l'aspect d'une masse spongieuse, à travées fortement colorées et à mailles claires. Cette disposition est surtout accentuée dans les cellules du corps jaune de la femelle du Cobaye. Dans ces cellules, il y a souvent des vacuoles circulaires entourées d'une couche colorée d'une façon assez intense par l'hématoxyline ferrique; ces vacuoles contiennent probablement une substance qui a été dissoute par les réactifs par lesquels ont passé les pièces; on dirait que les travées du cytoplasma qui séparent les globules de cette substance, probablement la lutéine, sont imprégnées d'une matière qui prend une couleur bleue plus ou moins foncée par la méthode de Heidenhain (fig. 2, 4). De même que Regaud et Policard, je n'ai jamais rencontré, dans le cytoplasme des cellules du corps jaune du Cobaye et du Lapin, des filaments ergastoplasmiques semblables à ceux que ces savants ont vus chez la femelle du Hérisson.

Les inclusions cellulaires que l'hématoxyline ferrique colore dans les corps jaunes en pleine activité offrent une analogie morphologique frappante avec les *corps sidérophiles* décrits par Guieysse et retrouvés par de nombreux auteurs dans les cellules de la portion corticale des glandes surrénales du Cobaye. Du reste, on avait déjà signalé la ressemblance qu'il y a entre la disposition et la forme des cellules de ces deux organes, qui probablement jouent tous les deux un rôle important dans les processus qui se passent dans l'organisme pendant la gestation.

Dans quelques cellules du corps jaune de la Lapine, j'ai rencontré une autre sorte d'inclusions cytoplasmiques. Ce sont des masses sphériques, la plupart très régulières, ayant un aspect tantôt parfaitement homogène, tantôt, mais moins souvent, finement alvéolaire, qui sont toujours logées dans des vacuoles creusées dans le corps cellulaire. Ces sphérules se colorent en rouge par l'éosine, en gris par l'hématoxyline ferrique. Il y en a une ou plusieurs dans chaque cellule, situées d'ordinaire au voisinage du noyau; les vacuoles dans lesquelles elles se trouvent sont également circulaires, à bords nets et presque toujours réguliers. Les

dimensions de ces masses homogènes sont très variables; les
unes sont plus petites que les globules rouges du sang; d'autres,
bien plus volumineuses, sont parfois plus grandes que le noyau
de la cellule. Entre ces tailles extrêmes il y a tous les intermédiaires (fig. 2 et 3). Au premier abord, à un faible grossissement,
on les prendrait pour des hématies, à cause de la coloration rouge
que leur donnent l'éosine et l'érythrosine, de leur forme circulaire
et de leur aspect homogène; mais les différences dans la grosseur
et leur situation intra-cytoplasmique, facilement reconnaissable à
l'aide d'objectifs plus puissants, font écarter immédiatement cette
hypothèse.

Partout, où il n'y a pas d'inclusions colorables, on constate
que le cytoplasme des cellules des corps jaunes présente une disposition nettement alvéolaire qui ressemble beaucoup à celle des
cellules de la couche corticale de la glande surrénale, mais qui est
cependant moins marquée. Dans ces portions du cytoplasme il y
a parfois de petites cavités vides dans les préparations qui n'ont
pas été fixées par des réactifs contenant de l'acide osmique; elles
renfermaient sans doute de petites gouttelettes de cette substance grasse bien connue sous le nom de lutéine. Mais, ainsi que le
font remarquer Regaud et Policard, les gouttelettes de graisse
sont très peu abondantes dans les corps jaunes, dont les cellules
sont riches en formations colorables par les méthodes de Weigert
et de Heidenhain.

Les formations cytoplasmiques que nous avons plus haut décrites n'existent pas dans les cellules des corps jaunes pendant
toute la durée de leur évolution. Dans un ovaire de Lapine dont
l'utérus renfermait des embryons macérés, les cellules des corps
jaunes ne présentaient aucune formation colorée par l'hématoxyline ferrique. Par contre, il y a dans ces préparations un plus grand
nombre de cellules creusées de cavités vides et celles-ci sont le
plus souvent plus volumineuses que celles qui existent alors que
les cellules renferment des inclusions sidérophiles. De même chez
une Chatte qui portait quelques fœtus mesurant 0^m,048 à 0^m,051
de longueur, le corps des cellules des corps jaunes, criblé de vacuoles vides, plus ou moins grandes, ne montrait pas la moindre
particule colorable par l'hématoxyline ferrique.

Il y a donc absence de formations colorables dans les cellules des corps jaunes vrais d'un certain âge, alors qu'elles se montrent chargées d'une plus grande quantité de substance grasse;
il semble que dans l'évolution de ces cellules il y a deux phases

successives d'élaboration, premièrement d'un produit de nature inconnue se présentant sous forme de particules décelables par l'hématoxyline après mordançage par un sel de chrome (méthode de Weigert) ou par un sel de fer (méthode de Heidenhain), secondairement d'une substance de nature grasse, sous forme de gouttelettes. Les observations faites jusqu'à présent ne sont guère suffisantes pour pouvoir affirmer s'il y a un rapport entre ces deux substances ; néanmoins, on serait tenté de le croire à cause de l'existence de ces anneaux colorés limitant des espaces qui étaient vraisemblablement remplis de lutéine et qui se montrent vides dans les coupes de pièces qui n'ont pas subi l'action de l'acide osmique.

Quoiqu'il en soit, ce qui résulte nettement des recherches de Regaud et Policard, de Cohn, de Celestino da Costa et des miennes, c'est que les cellules des corps jaunes vrais présentent à un certain moment de leur évolution des formations semblables à celles que les mêmes méthodes de coloration mettent en évidence dans des éléments dont la nature glandulaire est incontestable et que l'on considère comme étant en rapport avec leur fonction sécrétoire. Elles viennent donc appuyer l'opinion de Podvissotzky, Beard, Prenant, et bien d'autres pour lesquels le corps jaune représente une glande à sécrétion interne. En face de ces faits, la théorie défendue par quelques auteurs et notamment par Paladino [1], d'après laquelle cet organe fournirait "un classique processus de cicatrisation et de réparation de l'ovisac après sa rupture", n'est plus soutenable ; le corps jaune doit avoir une signification bien autrement importante que celle qu'il aurait d'après ces derniers savants.

[1] Voir le dernier travail de Paladino — La lutéine dans le corps jaune, et les récentes controverses sur la signification de cette formation — Archives italiennes de Biologie, T. XLIII, fasc. II, 19...

Travail du Laboratoire d'histologie de l'École de Médecine
de Lisbonne

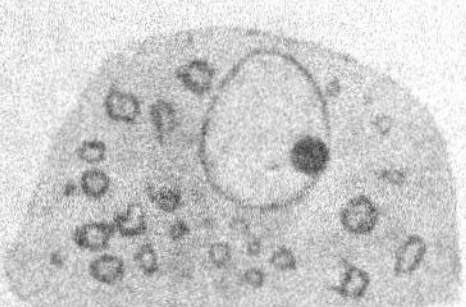

Fig. 1 — Cellule du corps jaune de
la Lapine.

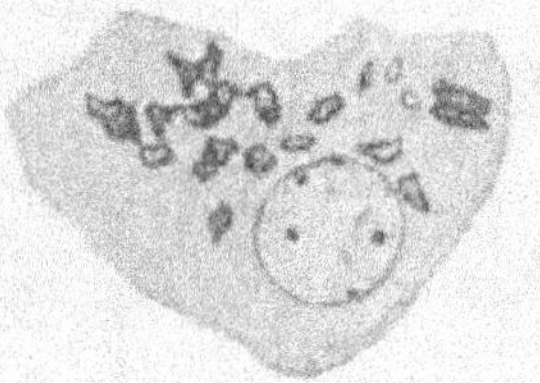

Fig. 4 — Cellule du corps jaune du Cobaye.

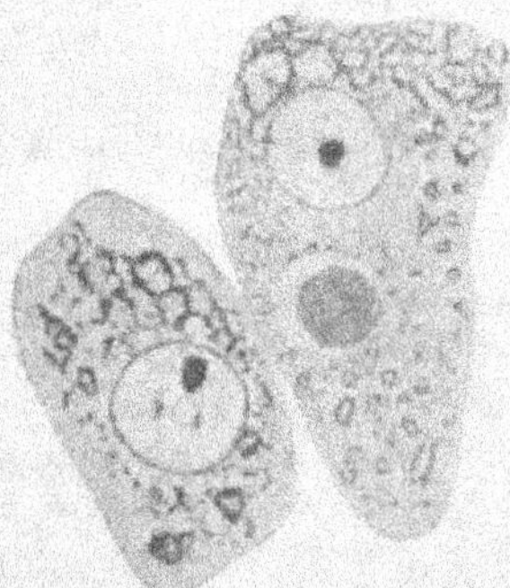

Fig. 2 — Deux cellules du corps jaune de la
Lapine.

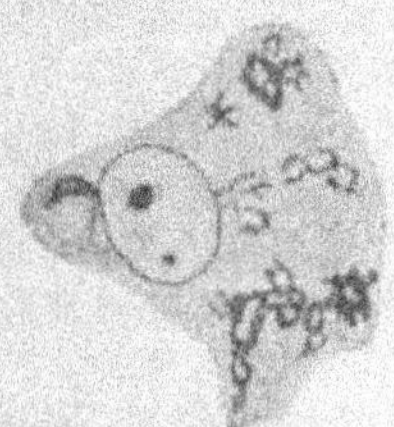

Fig. 3 — Cellule du corps
jaune du Cobaye.

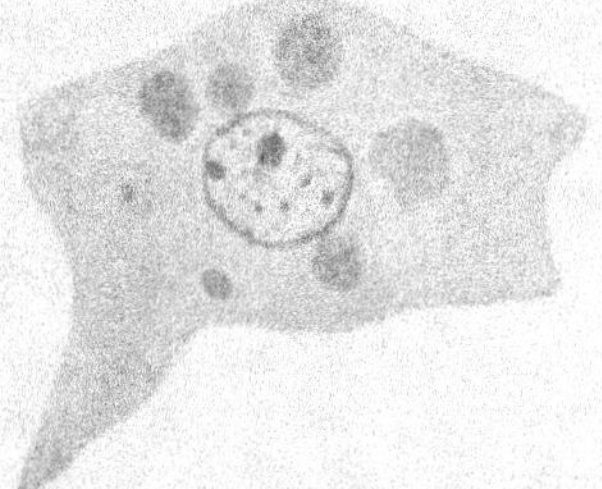

Fig. 5 — Cellule du corps jaune de la Lapine.

Notes cytologiques sur les cellules corticales des glandes surrénales

Par M. A. CELESTINO DA COSTA, Lisbonne.

Depuis quelques années, je m'occupe de l'étude des glandes surrénales et en particulier de la cytologie des cellules du cortex de ces organes.

Quelques-uns des résultats de ces études ont été déjà publiés dans deux mémoires parus en 1904 et 1905. Je crois utile de les rappeler brièvement et d'y ajouter les faits nouveaux que j'ai obtenus depuis lors.

Je m'occuperai des sujets suivants: structure des cellules corticales; corps *sidérophiles* et autres inclusions cellulaires; phénomènes de division nucléaire.

I.—Le corps cellulaire des cellules cortico-surrénales a une *architecture* alvéolaire spongieuse. Il ne s'agit pas d'une structure vraie, mais d'une pseudo-structure due à la dissolution des enclaves graisseuses contenues dans ces cellules. Ce fait, déjà remarqué par Koelliker en 1856, admis par Hultgren et Andersson, a été récemment démontré par Mulon pour les cellules dites *spongieuses* du cobaye (partie externe de la couche fasciculée) et de la glomérulaire du chien.

Ayant étudié le cobaye, le chien, le chat, le hérisson et le lapin, j'ai soutenu que cette texture n'était pas spéciale à des zones limitées du cortex, mais était *caractéristique* de la *cellule corticale* dont je fis un type spécial. Je suis allé ainsi à l'encontre de l'opinion de Guieysse qui a décrit quatre types cellulaires dans le cortex.

La graisse de nature toute particulière que les glandes surrénales contiennent existe chez tous les animaux étudiés, au niveau de toutes les zones corticales. Ce sont les cellules de la couche moyenne ou fasciculée, celles qui en contiennent en plus grande abondance; mais on la rencontre aussi dans les couches externe et interne.

Les cellules de la zone interne ou glomérulaire sont complètement remplies de graisse, tout comme les cellules de la fasciculée des autres animaux (chez le cobaye, zone *spongieuse*, d'après Guieysse). Chez les autres animaux les cellules de la glomérulaire contiennent aussi de la graisse, bien qu'en moins grande quantité et en gouttelettes de petites dimensions. Leur dissolution fait aussi apparaître l'aspect spongieux, plus difficile à déce-

ler ici cependant, à cause de la grande minceur des travées du
cytoplasme.

Dans la zone interne il y a quelques rares cellules qui n'ont
que dix ou douze gouttelettes graisseuses; d'autres en sont remplies, comme dans la zone moyenne; la plupart ont des gouttelettes graisseuses, mais seulement dans une partie de la cellule,
ce qui donne aux éléments cellulaires, lorsque les réactifs ont
dissout la graisse, l'aspect particulier que j'ai décrit sous le nom
d'*état spongieux partiel*.

Donc, nous rencontrons dans toutes les zones du cortex la
même structure fondamentale; la graisse est bien la seule caractéristique constante de toutes les cellules corticales, et semble
en constituer le produit principal d'élaboration chez tous les animaux. C'est pourquoi j'ai déjà émis l'opinion que nous sommes
en présence d'une seule espèce de cellules, dont l'activité et l'importance ont des degrés différents suivant la couche où elles se
trouvent, et je l'ai définie comme cellule épithéliale, spécialement
consacrée à l'élaboration ou à l'emmagazinement d'une substance
adipeuse.

Bonnamour admet cette opinion et la défend dans son travail d'ensemble. Mulon soutient aussi qu'il y a un type unique:
la cellule corticale, à évolution centripète, au moins chez le
cobaye:

1) cellule de la couche glomérulaire (stratum germinatif)
2) cellule de la couche graisseuse (zone fasciculée)
3) cellule de la couche pigmentée (zone réticulée).

Je soutiens encore l'unité du type cellulaire. On ne rencontre
pas de différences tranchées entre les cellules des diverses couches et on passe de l'une à l'autre par des transitions presque
insensibles. Cela se voit même chez le cobaye où la présence des
corps sidérophiles dans les cellules de la zone interne leur donne
un cachet spécial; il y a toujours des formes de passage.

Donc, je ne peux pas accepter les opinions de Guieysse qui
décrit quatre types cellulaires chez le cobaye, de Marrassini qui,
tout récemment, en décrit trois, de Ciaccio qui en décrit plusieurs; de même que dans les vertébrés inférieurs il y a un seul
type de cellule corticale, chez les mammifères la différenciation
porte sur des caractères secondaires, sans détruire l'unité du
type.

II — Guieysse a décrit en 1901, dans les cellules de la couche
fasciculée de la surrénale du cobaye, des corps différenciés colo-

rés en noir par la méthode à l'hématoxyline ferrique de Heidenhain. «Ces corps se présentent sous la forme de lignes hérissées
de ramifications, de masses disposées près du noyau, de disques
plus clairs au centre». Il les nomma corps sidérophiles, en décrit l'augmentation dans les surrénales des cobayes gravides et
les interpréta comme des formations *ergastoplasmiques* au sens
donné à ce mot par Ch. Garnier.

Ce fait et cette interprétation ont eu des défenseurs parmi
lesquels Bernard et Bigart, etc. Ciaccio a aussi décrit dans la zone
interne du cortex des *masses sidérophiles polaires* qu'il considère
aussi comme une substance prégranulaire ou prézymogène.

D'un autre côté, Bardier et Bonne, Delamare, Diamare considèrent ces formations des produits artificiels. Pour les premiers
elles sont dues à une précipitation de l'hématoxyline ferrique en
des points mal fixés de protoplasma rétracté.

Bonnamour est aussi d'avis que les corps sidérophiles sont
des produits artificiels; il croit que la structure alvéolaire polaire
de Ciaccio est due à la coloration du contour des vésicules graisseuses.

Mulon, qui a tout récemment étudié ces formations, les considère tout simplement comme des artéfacts; cependant ces artéfacts «traduisent en effet une réalité», car la substance qui est
cause de ce que les fixateurs divers produisent sur le protoplasma
de ces cellules ces figures, est une substance de nature graisseuse
existant à l'état d'imprégnation dans le cytoplasma des cellules de
la zone interne (pigmentée de Mulon).

La sidérophilie de ces corps gras, il l'explique par une combinaison avec l'adrénaline dont Abelous, Soulié et Toujan ont récemment affirmé l'existence dans le cortex. L'adrénaline est, on le sait,
capable de réduire l'alun de fer et les autres sels ferriques, et de rendre ainsi colorable par l'hématoxyline la cellule où elle se trouve.

Depuis mon premier mémoire de 1904, j'ai confirmé la découverte de Guieysse. J'ai rencontré ces corps sidérophiles chez
tous les cobayes examinés, j'en ai décrit la situation presque toujours polaire et la répartition topographique dans toute la zone
interne (fasciculée et réticulée de Guieysse). Les résultats alors
obtenus je les ai confirmés l'année suivante et aujourd'hui encore
je suis convaincu de leur exactitude.

Les corps sidérophiles se présentent en général comme des
masses alvéolaires, des réticules à la coupe optique, dont les parois sont énergiquement teintées par l'hématoxyline ferrique.

On les rencontre, en plus que dans les pôles cellulaires, autour du noyau lui formant une espèce de couronne, ou à la périphérie cellulaire constituant une bordure.

La forme la plus commune est celle d'une masse alvéolaire, spongieuse, constituée par une certain notabres d'alvéoles, formant quelquefois, disposées en ligne, une bordure, d'autres fois des masses globuleuses. Il y a des cellules où il n'y a que des lignes hérissées de prolongements situés sur l'un des bords de la cellule; sur le contour cellulaire prennent insertion les travées cytoplasmiques qui séparent les alvéoles de la partie marginale de la cellule.

D'autres fois, ce sont des disques, des anneaux à contours sombres, en nombre variable, 4 ou 5 au plus, situés dans l'intérieur de la cellule, d'autres fois encore ce sont des masses noires, compactes, ayant les formes les plus extraordinaires.

Un examen soigneux nous montre que les corps sidérophiles sont toujours dus à l'existence dans le cytoplasme d'une substance *sidérophile*. La forme dépend des endroits où elle existe et de cette façon on peut voir tout ce polymorphisme qui dépend, d'une part, de la quantité de cette substance; de l'autre, de l'architecture du corps cellulaire. Il y a des cellules qui en sont remplies; chez d'autres la substance sidérophile n'imprègne que quelques travées cytoplasmiques et le reste de la cellule conserve son aspect alvéolaire, caractéristique de toute cellule corticale.

On observe ces cellules dans les pièces fixées au Zenker; le formol et aussi les liqueurs de Flemming et Holtgren et Anderson le montrent aussi. Je ne les ai rencontrées que chez le cobaye.

A ces faits déjà publiés dans mes précédents mémoires, je vais en ajouter d'autres d'observation plus récente. J'ai continué à rencontrer des corps sidérophiles chez tous les cobayes examinés, sauf un; ce dernier est une femelle enceinte dont les capsules ont été fixées au Zenker. La coloration par l'hématoxyline ferrique ne m'a révélé nulle part des corps sidérophiles. Tout à l'heure j'indiquerai comment je crois pouvoir interpréter ce fait.

La surrénale d'un autre cobaye femelle m'a permis d'obtenir des résultats qui, selon moi, jettent une vive lumière sur la signification des corps sidérophiles. Les coupes de cette capsule fixées aussi au Zenker et colorées par la méthode de Heidenhain m'ont montré toute la couche corticale, y compris la glomérulaire, remplie de corps sidérophiles; c'est-à-dire, presque toutes les cellules corticales ont leur cytoplasme intensément coloré par l'hématoxyline ferrique qui dessine aussi admirablement les contours de leurs alvéoles et vacuoles. L'architecture alvéolaire du corps des cellules est on ne peut mieux mise en évidence et ces préparations sont à cet égard aussi démonstratives que celles des fixations au Flemming. L'aspect de ces cellules rappelle absolument celui des cellules qui ont été fixées au Flemming et dont la graisse osmiée a été dissoute par l'emploi de réactifs dissolvants, xylol, etc. On est ici en présence d'un cytoplasme *sidérophile*; le phénomène a deux maxima, l'un à la zone interne où l'on a les corps sidérophiles vulgaires, l'autre à la couche fasciculée ou spongieuse de Guieysse. L'hématoxyline cuprique donne des images identiques. Ce qu'on peut observer aussi, c'est que nulle part le contenu des alvéoles n'a été coloré.

Ce fait m'a confirmé dans mon opinion de l'existence dans le cortex du cobaye d'une substance sidérophile, c'est-à-dire susceptible d'être mise en relief par l'hématoxyline au fer.

En rapprochant ces faits de ceux de Mulon et Bonnamour, je suis amené à conclure en faveur des relations intimes existant entre cette substance et la graisse. Il s'agit probablement d'un stade préliminaire de formation de la graisse, mais non du produit définitif qui ne semble pas colorable par la laque ferrique et se présente sous la forme granulo-globuleuse.

Chez les mammifères autres que le cobaye (chat, chien, lapin, hérisson) je n'ai jamais décelé la substance sidérophile, à en excepter peut-être le lapin où j'ai pu voir, avec des fixations au Tellyesniczky, des traces de corps sidérophiles dans quelques cellules de la zone interne.

Il faudrait donc conclure que chez ces animaux le protoplasme en voie de formation de la graisse surrénale n'est pas sidérophile, qu'il ne l'est que chez le cobaye et dans la zone interne, à moins qu'il ne s'agisse de certaines conditions d'ordre inconnu qui permettent quelquefois de déceler le processus dans toute la portion corticale.

Chez les autres mammifères, le protoplasme de la zone interne est toujours plus fortement colorable que celui des zones externe et moyenne; il faut voir dans ce fait, je le crois du moins, l'équivalent de la sidérophilie des cellules du cobaye. Du reste, une seule fois j'ai constaté l'absence de sidérophilie. J'attribue ce fait, pour une grande part, à des causes d'ordre technique (lavage à l'eau trop prolongé [48 h.] et imprégnation insuffisante par l'hématoxyline [2 h. à peine]. D'ailleurs, le cytoplasme des cellu-

les de la zone interne était aussi coloré d'une façon bien plus intense et diffuse par le mélange hématoxyline-ferrique-érythrosine,
comme s'il s'agissait d'un mammifère autre que le cobaye.

Les faits que je viens de décrire me portent à défendre
l'existence réelle des corps sidérophiles au moins comme *image
équivalente* (Aequivalentbild au sens de Nissl) de la présence,
dans la couche corticale (zone interne de la surrénale du cobaye),
d'une substance probablement de nature adipeuse.

Ces faits sont à rapprocher d'une observation identique que
j'ai faite sur des cellules d'un corps jaune de lapine, que j'ai déjà
signalé en 1901 et qui avait aussi des corps sidérophiles. Cette
question est du reste l'objet d'une communication à cette section
de mon collègue M. le dr. Athias.

Par contre, je ne crois pas qu'on doive rapprocher ces formations sidérophiles de celles dites ergastoplasmiques telles qu'on
les conçoit généralement.

Quant à l'opinion de Mulon, qui pense à une combinaison
d'un acide gras avec de l'adrénaline, je suis de l'avis de Ciaccio
qui ne trouve pas suffisamment prouvée l'existence de ce produit
dans la corticale, malgré ce que disent Abelous, Soulié et Toujan.
Je l'avais déjà affirmé, mais je compte reprendre cette question
dans un travail ultérieur.

III — Ma troisième note concerne les phénomènes de division
nucléaire qu'on observe dans les surrénales.

C'est Mulon qui, dernièrement, a appelé l'attention des histologistes sur la présence de figures de division directe et indirecte
dans la surrénale; l'amitose s'observerait exclusivement au niveau
de la glomérulaire; la caryocinèse, au contraire, est bien plus
fréquente dans les couches superficielles de la fasciculée et ne se
rencontre que rarement dans la glomérulaire.

Mulon conclut de ces faits que la division directe est un
phénomène qui se passe au niveau de la glomérulaire, laquelle
prend ainsi l'importance d'un stratum germinatif; la mitose ne
serait qu'un mode de reproduction accessoire; la genèse des cellules dans la glomérulaire serait la compensation de la destruction qu'on rencontre, d'après lui, au niveau de la réticulée.

Mulon affirme en outre qu'on ne rencontre des figures caryo-
cinétiques chez les cobayes pleines; l'explication de ce fait serait
dans l'antagonisme entre la sécrétion et l'activité cinétique, érigé
en loi par Prenant.

J'ai aussi rencontré des figures mitosiques, non seulement

chez le cobaye, mais aussi chez le chat et le lapin. Elles sont bien plus fréquentes dans la fasciculée et, en général, on peut bien voir le fuseau achromatique et les deux centrosomes. Contrairement à Mulon, c'est dans des surrénales de cobayes enceintes que j'en ai vues en plus grande quantité et, en outre, les cellules qui sont en mitose ont toujours leur protoplasma rempli de gouttelettes graisseuses. Ce fait est, il me semble, de nature à constituer une exception de plus à la loi de Prenant.

Quant aux figures de division directe, on les rencontre, en effet, en assez grand nombre au niveau de la glomérulaire.

L'étude du développement ayant démontré à Gottschau, Soulié, etc. le rôle germinatif de la glomérulaire, on peut, à la rigueur, accepter l'hypothèse de Mulon, sans vouloir toutefois rien préjuger sur le rôle biologique de l'amitose.

Les faits rapportés ci-dessus et d'autres que mes études sur les surrénales m'ont permis d'obtenir me permettent de faire les affirmations suivantes:

1) On ne doit voir dans le cortex surrénal qu'un seul type cellulaire fondamental. La cellule corticale est toujours une cellule à enclaves graisseuses, ce qui donne à son corps cellulaire l'architecture alvéolaire caractéristique.

Les caractères structuraux de la cellule corticale sont au maximum dans la couche moyenne ou fasciculée. Les cellules des couches externe et interne, tout en ayant la même structure fondamentale, ont des caractères propres qui nous font admettre que l'activité cellulaire a des degrés différents suivant la couche du cortex où la cellule est placée.

2) Chez le cobaye, au niveau de la zone interne, le cytoplasme est imprégné d'une substance sidérophile, c'est-à-dire prenant fortement la laque ferrique. Il est de tous points probable qu'il s'agisse d'un stade de l'élaboration du produit de sécrétion définitif (graisse surrénale) et que des conditions de composition chimique, particulières à cette espèce animale, permettent de l'y déceler.

3) La fonction principale de la cellule corticale doit être l'élaboration d'une substance de nature graisseuse (peut-être une lécithine [Halsgren et Anderson, Mulon, Bernard et Bigart, etc.] L'élaboration du pigment est loin d'être constante et, même chez le cobaye, on ne le rencontre pas toujours.

Bien que quelquefois j'aie rencontré une grande quantité de granulations pigmentaires intra-cellulaires au niveau de la réti-

enlée, je ne peux pas accepter la dénomination de zone pigmentaire proposée par Mulon et Delamare pour la couche interne
du cortex du cobaye, car elle me semble trop exclusive.

Quant aux autres granulations intra-cellulaires que les
réactifs décèlent, il ne m'est pas encore possible de décider quelles
sont leur nature et signification. Dans des études ultérieures
je chercherai à établir ce point et d'autres encore concernant la
structure et fonctions du cortex surrénal.

4) De la présence de figures de division nucléaire dans les
cellules corticales on peut conclure qu'il s'agit là d'un phénomène
constant de renouvellement cellulaire. Les faits rapportés par
Nicolas et Bonnamour, Moschini, etc., permettent d'y voir un des
processus de réaction de la surrénale aux intoxications.

Quelques vues sur la structure des cellules glandulaires

Par M. A. Celestino da Costa, Lisbonne.

On connaît les trois grandes théories sur la structure du
protoplasma: celles d'Altmann, Flemming et Bütschli. Elles ont
trouvé dans les cellules glandulaires des faits qui ont servi à les
étayer.

Les cellules glandulaires ont été aussi de très beaux sujets
d'étude pour Altmann, pour la théorie duquel elles ont fourni
les meilleurs documents. Cependant, les granulations que ce savant a rencontrées avec sa méthode peuvent être rattachées en
grande partie à des produits de sécrétion, et non pas à des unités vivantes, à des bioblastes. Nicolas en fit la démonstration
dans un intéressant mémoire [1] où il démontre aussi pour les
éléments étudiés par lui (cellules glandulaires séreuses) la faus-
seté des interprétations de Bütschli et Flemming. En effet, s'il
est souvent parvenu à colorer les grains de sécrétion et à voir
dans le corps cellulaire une composition granulaire, il a reconnu
d'autres fois que des causes d'ordre technique n'avaient pas
conservé ces grains de sécrétion, que la cellule montrait alors
la texture alvéolaire ou spongieuse décrite par Bütschli. Seulement, il considère cette disposition alvéolaire comme tout à fait
secondaire et réalisée seulement quand il y a des grains.

---

[1] Arch. de Physiol., 1891.

Les travaux tout récents de l'École de Nancy sur les cellules glandulaires sont venus remettre la question en discussion.
Les formations que, après Solger et Erik Möller, Garnier et Bouin
ont décrites sous le nom d'ergastoplasmiques ne seraient pour
eux que des épaississements des travées qui composent la charpente du cytoplasme avec des changements de chromaticité, etc.
Ils considèrent le cytoplasme des cellules glandulaires comme
composé d'une charpente filaire avec des microsomes aux points
nodaux du réticulum, et des grains de sécrétion qui y sont
tout d'abord et ne tombent dans les mailles du réseau que plus
tard.

Vers la même époque ont paru les travaux de Benda qui
a décrit sous le nom de *mitochondries* des granulations colorées
par une méthode spéciale, qui pourraient constituer par leur
groupement, des filaments appelés *chondriomites*. Ces constatations ont été faites sur des cellules des organes sexuels, musculaires, rénaux, des glandes salivaires, etc. Il les considère comme
analogues à l'ergastoplasme de Prenant, Bouin, Garnier, mais, contrairement à ceux-ci, il y voit des formations nettement indivi-
dualisées, permanentes, un véritable organe intra-cellulaire.

Laguesse a étudié, avec la méthode de coloration vitale,
après Michaëlis, quelques cellules glandulaires (pancréas de
Salamandre) et il a toujours rencontré des granulations et des
filaments nettement individualisés et isolables du cytoplasme.
Celui-ci aurait une *architecture* (non une *structure*) alvéolaire,
grâce à ses nombreuses enclaves, et ne serait lui-même qu'une
masse homogène non différenciée. Les filaments (bâtonnets tout
petits ou *vermicules*) et les granulations qu'il colore par le vert
Janus comme Michaëlis il les nomme ergastidions.

Les aspects décrits par Mouret-Garnier, Matheus, Launoy,
etc., ne seraient dus qu'à une coagulation du protoplasme par
les réactifs autour du filament.

Dès le commencement de mes études sur les glandes surrénales, je soutiens les mêmes idées que Nicolas et Laguesse [1].
Dans les cellules corticales de la surrénale on rencontre un produit d'élaboration de nature graisseuse (écidique peut-être) sous
la forme de granulations dans les pièces fixées au Flemming et
dans celles qui sont traitées par la méthode de Daddi au Su-

---

[1] Medicina Contemporanea, 1913.

dan III. Ces granulations se dissolvent très facilement et alors il apparaît l'état alvéolaire ou spongieux qui est ainsi une disposition secondaire, et non une structure cytoplasmique. Le cytoplasma est réduit à ce que dans le corps optique nous paraît être des travées d'un réseau et il m'a paru toujours homogène, non différencié, pouvant cependant contenir quelques enclaves, comme des microsomes, etc.

J'ai confirmé ce fait dans d'autres espèces de cellules glandulaires que j'ai étudiées: cellules médullaires des surrénales, cellules du pancréas de Lacerta ocellata, de salamandre et de hérisson, cellules des îlots de Langerhans de ce mammifère, cellules hépatiques de Molge buscaii, Lacerta ocellata, salamandre, cellules des glandes salivaires des mammifères, cellules rénales d'amphibiens et mammifères, cellules du corps jaune et du tissu interstitiel de l'ovaire.

Chez toutes ces cellules les fixations ordinaires dissolvent les produits de sécrétion et d'autres enclaves; c'est ce qui permet de reconnaître la disposition alvéolaire que j'ai rencontrée dans tous ces éléments. On parvient cependant bien des fois à conserver les produits de sécrétion: grains de zymogène du pancréas, gouttelettes graisseuses et d'autres dans les cellules hépatiques, grains *endocrines* (Laguesse) des îlots de Langerhans chez quelques animaux, en particulier les ophidiens; grains des cellules rénales des vertébrés inférieurs, etc.

Je me rattache donc à la conception de Laguesse d'après laquelle le cytoplasme nous paraît homogène et que, seulement, il peut contenir des différenciations de diverse nature, dont les rapports de position avec lui constituent ce qu'on appelle vulgairement les structures du cytoplasme.

Je ne crois pas, au moins pour mes objets d'étude, à l'existence d'un nucléome et d'un suc cellulaire, d'un spongioplasme et d'un hyaloplasme. Du moins, nos méthodes actuelles ne me démontrent comme véritable cytoplasme que ce qui constitue le mitome de Flemming, le spongioplasme de Bütschli ou la substance intermédiaire d'Altmann.

Quant aux différenciations cytoplasmiques, mes faits sont aussi d'accord avec ceux que Laguesse a décrits avec une méthode différente.

J'ai employé les méthodes cytologiques courantes, en me servant surtout, comme coloration, de la méthode d'Heidenhain à l'hématoxyline au fer. J'ai vu des filaments *ergastoplasmiques*

dans les cellules pancréatiques des glandes salivaires et les cellules hépatiques de *Molge buscati* et salamandre. Des formations
analogues avaient été décrites tout récemment par *Koiransky* dans
les cellules hépatiques des amphibiens. Malgré l'emploi des méthodes qui ont servi à l'édification des théories des histologistes
de Nancy et d'autres, mon impression a été qu'il s'agissait toujours de formations indépendantes, isolables du cytoplasme qui
dans les cellules remplies d'enclaves est réduit aux parois des lo-
gettes creusées dans la masse cellulaire. J'ai pu même voir des
cellules fixées au Flemming qui s'étaient rétractées, mais dont
les filaments basaux s'étaient séparés du reste de la masse, d'ailleurs bien conservée. Dans les cellules hépatiques que j'ai étudiées, j'ai rencontré aussi des filaments et des bâtonnets colorés
par l'hématoxyline au fer, par l'éosine en de certaines conditions,
par le bleu de toluidine. Ils rappellent les filaments des cellules
glandulaires séreuses et comme eux ce sont des formations isolées.

Quelquefois les filaments ergastoplasmiques m'ont paru notablement plus trapus. Dans un travail (¹), où presque tous ces
faits ont été relatés, j'ai émis l'hypothèse d'une sorte d'*agglutina-
tion* probablement artificielle de ces filaments, car on peut y reconnaître une fasciculation longitudinale. Étant donné cependant
l'empirisme des méthodes dont nous nous servons pour la fixation
et la coloration, il est très difficile de faire toujours la part des erreurs de technique.

On le voit, mes études confirment les vues de Lagesse. Il
me semble que ces différenciations cytoplasmiques, que j'ai
nommées aussi ergastoplasmiques par commodité d'expression,
sont bien celles que Benda a décrites. Les travaux de Bouin semblent le prouver, au moins pour les cellules des glandes salivaires; Benda partage cette opinion. Je n'ai pas encore essayé la
coloration vitale, ni la méthode de Benda. Je ne peux donc pas
me prononcer définitivement, mais cependant j'incline à penser
que filaments ergastoplasmiques, ergastolines et mitochondries
sont au fond la même chose.

En résumé:

1. Dans les cas que j'ai étudiés, les trois théories de structure du cytoplasme ne sont que de fausses interprétations, le véritable cytoplasme nous paraissant sans structure.

2) On doit considérer: a) les granulations comme des enclaves de diverse natures, en général produits d'élaboration cellulaire; b) les formations filamenteuses et d'autres comme des différentiations cellulaires, en général comme des organes cellulaires ayant des fonctions déterminées (filaments ergastoplasmiques, neurofibrilles des cellules nerveuses, etc.), et la *structure* alvéolaire comme le résultat de la dissolution d'enclaves cellulaires.

3) Je ne peux donc pas confirmer les idées de Garnier sur les rapports de son ergastoplasme avec le cytoplasme et je l'en considère comme indépendant, différencié.

La méthode à l'argent réduit de Ramón y Cajal et les glandes

Par M. CELESTINO DA COSTA, Lisbonne

Laignel-Lavastine a décrit les résultats qu'il a obtenus, à l'aide de la méthode de Ramón y Cajal, sur les cellules médullo-surrénales. Il a vu que l'argent y était réduit sous la forme de granulations très fines, remplissant le protoplasme. Il attribue cette réaction à une action réductrice de l'adrénaline sur le nitrate d'argent.

Je suis parvenu, chez le hérisson, à obtenir des résultats semblables. Les cellules médullaires ou chromaffines de la capsule surrénale sont presque toutes remplies de fines granulations brunes ou noires et, à de faibles grossissements, la substance médullaire tranche fortement en noir sur la couleur jaune du cortex. Au niveau de celui-ci, il y a aussi une réduction du nitrate en granulations de formes et dimensions variables, très irrégulièrement distribuées. Ceci doit être un précipité artificiel qui ne se confond nullement avec la réaction très nette des cellules chromaffines.

J'ai cherché depuis, dans diverses glandes, quelle serait l'action de cette méthode.

Mes recherches ne sont que commencées et je n'ai encore obtenu de résultats satisfaisants que dans un rein de hérisson.

Les tubes rénaux, surtout le segment contourné, se sont montrés remplis de granulations intracellulaires, petites, noires, très irrégulières et très nombreuses, remplissant uniformément toute la cellule. Elles n'ont nullement l'aspect d'un précipité artificiel; mais je ne peux pas encore affirmer quelle est leur nature et me faire une idée de leur signification. Elles seront peut-être à rapprocher des diverses formations qu'on a décrites dans les

cellules rénales et auxquelles on a donné la valeur de produits
de sécrétion.

Ce fait ne s'est pas répété dans des reins de cobaye traités
par la même méthode. Cependant, il m'a semblé utile de rapporter ce fait, qui est de nature, il me semble, à justifier l'intérêt
qu'il y a à essayer la méthode de Cajal sur les glandes.

Notes cytologiques sur les Trypanosomes parasites de la grenouille

(Rana esculenta)

Par MM. C. França et M. Athias, Lisbonne.

Au cours des recherches que nous avons entreprises sur les
Trypanosomes des Amphibiens, nous avons rencontré chez la
Rana esculenta des environs de Lisbonne cinq espèces, les unes
déjà connues, d'autres nouvelles; ces espèces, qui sont décrites en
détail dans un mémoire qui sera bientôt publié dans le N° 1 des
Archives de l'Institut Royal de Bactériologie Camara Pestana
de Lisbonne, sont les suivantes: *Trypanosoma loricatum ou costatum* (Mayer), *T. rotatorium* (Mayer) s. st., *T. undulans* França
et Athias, *T. elegans* França et Athias et *T. inopinatum* (Et.
et Ed. Sergent).

Sauf le *T. inopinatum*, qui ne possède que 13 à 24 μ de long
sur 1 à 2 μ de large, ces espèces sont toutes de grande taille, qui
dépasse presque toujours celle des Trypanosomes des Mammifères; le *T. costatum*, par exemple, mesure 42 à 48 μ de long sur
24 à 26 μ de large; ils se prêtent pour cela à l'étude de la
structure des différentes parties du corps de ces animaux; nous
allons en donner un court résumé dans cette communication. Nous
avons toujours examiné ces Trypanosomes aussi bien à l'état
frais dans une goutte de sang placée entre lame et lamelle, que
sur des préparations fixées et colorées par les méthodes de
Leishman et de Giemsa.

Cytoplasma.—Examiné à l'état vivant, le cytoplasma des
Trypanosomes des Grenouilles se montre, en général, rempli de
granulations réfringentes rondes, bien visibles, ayant des dimensions variables. Elles sont presque toujours disposées sans ordre,
depuis l'extrémité antérieure jusqu'à l'extrémité postérieure du
corps. Chez le *T. costatum*, ces granulations sont plus denses
dans les côtes qui séparent les sillons qui entaillent la surface
du corps, ce qui contribue à donner l'aspect strié de cette espèce.
Dans d'autres espèces, elles forment des rangées longitudinales,

Ces granulations respectent quelquefois une zone excessivement mince à la périphérie du corps, sur toute la portion qui
n'est pas parcourue par la membrane ondulante et qui a un aspect homogène. Cette zone est surtout visible dans les extrémités
du parasite, où les granulations cessent souvent à une certaine
distance de la pointe par laquelle elles finissent d'ordinaire. On
peut alors, dans ces cas, établir une division du cytoplasma en
une *zone ectoplasmique* à la périphérie et une portion centrale,
bien plus considérable, *l'endoplasma*. Cette distinction n'est guère
possible que dans les espèces volumineuses, telles que les *T. costatum*, *undulans* et *rotatorium*; dans les plus petites, nous ne
sommes pas parvenus à voir nettement un ectoplasma étendu à
toute la périphérie du corps.

D'après quelques auteurs (Rose, etc.), la membrane ondulante est une portion très développée de l'ectoplasma, ayant acquis
une grande mobilité. Nos recherches nous font incliner vers cette
façon de voir; nous y reviendrons plus loin lorsque nous par-
lerons de l'appareil de locomotion des Trypanosomes.

Dans les préparations colorées, les granulations prennent une
teinte violette plus ou moins bleuâtre, mais ne sont pas toujours
faciles à apercevoir à cause de la teinte assez foncée que prend
le reste de l'endoplasma. Dans quelques exemplaires de *T. rotatorium* nous avons vu tout le corps rempli de granulations très
foncées, qui étaient bien visibles sur un fond plus pâle que d'habitude; cette abondance de granulations est une des caractéristiques de cette espèce. Laveran et Mesnil donnent à ces granulations le nom de *granulations chromatiques*; nous préférons les
nommer *chromophiles* pour éviter des confusions.

La structure fine de la masse cytoplasmique, où sont inclu-
ses les granulations dont nous venons de parler, est très difficile
à résoudre, malgré l'emploi de forts grossissements. En général,
elle prend une teinte plus ou moins uniforme et a un aspect
homogène; dans certains cas, cependant, on aperçoit par places
une disposition vaguement alvéolaire. Mais il est impossible
d'affirmer s'il s'agit bien réellement d'une structure alvéolaire,
au sens de Bütschli, du protoplasma de ces animacules, ou si ce
n'est pas là un aspect dû à la distribution de granulations foncées plus ou moins rapprochées. La structure alvéolaire est, par
contre, très nette dans les exemplaires dégénérés et en voie de
subir la transformation globuleuse.

Le cytoplasma des Trypanosomes présente fréquemment des

vacuoles qu'on peut voir à l'état vivant sous forme de taches claires, mais qui sont plus nettes chez les exemplaires colorés. Ce sont de petites vacuoles ayant des dimensions variables, distribuées par-ci par-là dans le corps de l'animal; elles sont souvent plus nombreuses vers les extrémités, surtout la postérieure. Nous n'avons jamais pu constater la présence de vacuoles contractiles chez les Trypanosomes que nous avons observés vivants.

En examinant à l'aide d'objectifs puissants (apochromatiques 1.30, 2mm. Zeiss) des Trypanosomes bien fixés et colorés, on remarque assez souvent que leur cytoplasma est parcouru par de fines stries claires, sinueuses, souvent bifurquées, qui cheminent en différents sens et qui semblent se terminer dans de petites vacuoles. Parfois deux ou plusieurs de ces stries convergent vers une même vacuole. Il n'est pas rare de voir des stries semblables se diriger vers la surface du corps qui, à ce niveau, offre une faible dépression. Les caractères que nous venons d'assigner à ces stries nous portent à croire qu'il s'agit là d'un système de canalicules excessivement fins sillonnant le cytoplasma des gros Trypanosomes et servant vraisemblablement à leur nutrition. Ce fait n'est pas nouveau, car il est connu que d'autres Protozoaires (Infusoires) présentent des formations canaliculaires venant s'ouvrir dans des vacuoles ou à la surface du corps.

Noyau — Il occupe le plus souvent le milieu du cytoplasma, présente une forme arrondie ou ovalaire et mesure 2,5 $\times$ 1,7 μ chez l'espèce la plus petite, 4 $\times$ 6 μ et 5 $\times$ 3 μ en moyenne chez les espèces plus grosses. Les méthodes de coloration que nous avons employées ne mettent pas en évidence des détails structuraux bien nombreux. Il prend presque toujours, par ces méthodes, une teinte rose uniforme plus ou moins pâle et ce n'est que dans un petit nombre de cas qu'on peut y constater la présence de quelques granules chromatiques colorés en rouge et disposés presque toujours à la périphérie. Le noyau des Trypanosomes de la grenouille est donc un noyau pauvre en chromatine, notamment chez les *T. costatum*, *undulans* et *rotatorium*; elle est plus abondante chez les *T. inopinatum*, et *elegans*, où elle forme des granules parfois assez gros.

Cette simplicité structurale du noyau des Trypanosomes en général avait déjà frappé Prowazek qui le considère comme le type le plus simple du noyau des Flagellés. Nous pouvons affirmer que ce caractère est encore plus prononcé chez les Trypanosomes que nous décrivons.

La pâleur du noyau et la teinte foncée du cytoplasma rendent souvent difficile à voir nettement ses contours. Il est invisible dans la plupart des exemplaires de *T. rotatorium* ; par contre, chez le *T. costatum* et *elegans* on peut l'apercevoir très nettement.

Le noyau subit, chez les Trypanosomes qui sont en train de prendre la forme en boule qui précède la mort, des modifications assez intéressantes. Dans les gros *T. costatum* on voit dans ces conditions apparaître quelquefois un réseau qui se montre coloré en rouge et qui tranche bien sur le fond pâle du caryoplasma. Ce réseau qui ne se voit jamais chez les individus normaux de ces espèces ressemble à celui qui existe dans le noyau des Trypanosomes de quelques poissons.

Dans d'autres cas, au lieu d'un réseau, il se forme un croissant rouge plus ou moins foncé à la périphérie du noyau. D'autres fois enfin, il y a une zone périphérique étroite plus claire que la partie centrale.

Nous ne sommes pas parvenus à résoudre s'il y a ou non chez les Trypanosomes une *membrane nucléaire* ; en tous cas nous inclinons vers la dernière hypothèse, car nous n'avons jamais rien pu voir qui puisse être considéré comme une véritable membrane nucléaire.

Blépharoplaste — Ce corpuscule, dont la présence est constante et caractéristique de ces Protozoaires, est d'ordinaire assez gros chez les Trypanosomes de la Grenouille. Il est presque toujours de forme allongée, elliptique, arrondie chez le *T. costatum*, il offre des dimensions le plus souvent inférieures à 1 μ et se colore en violet d'une façon si intense qu'il est toujours visible même si le cytoplasma est fortement imprégné de couleur.

Il est toujours placé en arrière du noyau, à une distance variable suivant les espèces ; dans les unes (*T. costatum*) il en est très rapproché, tandis que dans d'autres il en est très éloigné (*T. undulans, elegans* et *inopinatum*) et placé quelquefois à une petite distance de l'extrémité postérieure (*T. rotatorium*).

Le blépharoplaste de ces Trypanosomes n'est jamais entouré d'une auréole claire à limites nettes, comme il arrive chez quelques Tryp. des Mammifères. Ce qu'on peut remarquer assez souvent, c'est que le cytoplasma autour de ce corpuscule est moins dense et moins granuleux et forme une zone un peu plus pâle qui n'est pas bien délimitée ; à la périphérie cette zone se confond insensiblement avec le reste du cytoplasma, et les granulations cytoplasmiques n'affectent jamais une disposition radiée autour d'elle.

Du blépharoplaste part toujours directement un filament qui dans sa partie libre représente le flagelle, duquel il sera bientôt question. Chez les Trypanosomes de Mammifères le filament part souvent de la périphérie de l'auréole claire qui environne le blépharoplaste, et ne va pas jusqu'à celui-ci; c'est là une disposition que nous n'avons jamais rencontrée chez les Trypanosomes de la Grenouille. L'insertion du filament se fait tantôt à l'une des extrémités, tantôt au milieu du blépharoplaste. Dans un exemplaire de *T. rotatorium* il y avait un tout petit corpuscule rond accolé au blépharoplaste, sur lequel s'insérait le filament.

Le blépharoplaste est très résistant; nous l'avons vu persister avec tous ses caractères morphologiques et tinctoriaux chez des Trypanosomes ayant subi des altérations cadavériques très avancées, même après désagrégation du cytoplasma.

De grandes incertitudes règnent encore au sujet de la signification de ce corpuscule. Pour quelques auteurs c'est un *nucléole*, pour d'autres un *micronucleus* identique à celui des Infusoires. D'autres auteurs, en tête desquels Laveran et Mesnil, le considèrent comme un *centrosome* et lui donnent ce nom. Les auteurs allemands le désignent le plus souvent sous les noms de *Blépharoplaste* et *Geisselwurzel*, termes qui rappellent bien ses relations avec le filament, sans rien préjuger de sa signification.

Nous ne saurions nous étendre ici sur la question si débattue de la nature de ce corpuscule, car cela nous entraînerait trop loin et nos observations ne nous fournissent pas assez d'arguments pour nous permettre de nous placer carrément dans l'un ou l'autre camp; disons seulement que, à notre avis, les faits invoqués à l'appui de l'identification du blépharoplaste au centrosome ne sont pas assez démonstratifs. En effet, on compare le blépharoplaste au corpuscule basal des cils vibratils des cellules épithéliales des Métazoaires, corpuscule qui est regardé par plusieurs savants comme étant un centrosome. Or, ceci n'est pas prouvé, et même il y a des observateurs qui ont pu voir dans des cellules ciliées un centrosome indépendant des cils et se comportant comme tel pendant la division mitosique.

On rapproche aussi le blépharoplaste des Trypanosomes du corpuscule central du spermatozoïde. Mais il ne nous semble pas qu'il y ait entre ces deux sortes de formations une analogie morphologique suffisante pour les considérer tous les deux comme ayant une signification absolument identique.

Les Trypanosomes ne se divisent pas mitosiquement, de sorte qu'il nous manque l'un des meilleurs critériums pour déterminer si le blépharoplaste possède bien la signification qu'on lui attribue. Cette question mérite encore des recherches plus approfondies.

Membrane ondulante et flagelle. — La membrane ondulante est insérée sur l'un des bords du Trypanosome, le bord convexe, qu'elle parcourt depuis la région où se trouve le blépharoplaste jusqu'à l'extrémité antérieure du corps. Sa largeur varie beaucoup d'une espèce à l'autre; très étroite chez le petit *T. inopinatum*, étroite aussi chez le *T. undulans*, elle atteint un grand développement chez le *T. costatum* (3 à 5 μ de largeur). Cette membrane est le plus souvent festonnée; plus elle est large plus ses festons sont nombreux et profonds. Elle se colore en rose très pâle et ne montre en général aucun détail structural. Il y a des cas cependant (quelques *T. costatum*) où nous avons vu une traînée de granulations excessivement petites, situées à une petite distance de son bord libre; ces granulations prennent une belle teinte violette par la méthode de Giemsa et semblent identiques à celle de l'entoplasma.

La membrane ondulante n'est pas à proprement parler une membrane; pour nous, d'accord en cela avec d'autres auteurs, parmi lesquels Bosc, cette formation n'est qu'une portion très développée de l'ectoplasma ayant acquis des caractères particuliers en rapport avec la motilité de l'animal. Avant d'en donner les raisons qui nous font incliner vers cette opinion, il faut décrire l'autre partie de l'appareil locomoteur: le *filament* et le *flagelle* qui lui fait suite.

Le filament longe le bord libre de la membrane ondulante à la façon d'un liséré; il prend naissance sur le blépharoplaste, ainsi que nous l'avons déjà dit, et se continue presque toujours au-delà de la membrane en constituant un flagelle dont la longueur est très variable, pouvant être de 1,5 μ (*T. undulans*) à 22-30 μ (*T. rotatorium*). Il est plus gros chez certaines espèces que chez d'autres et se colore toujours en rouge plus ou moins clair par les méthodes que nous avons employées.

Les rapports entre la membrane ondulante et le filament sont, comme on vient de le voir, très intimes; on dirait, en examinant ces flagellés, que la membrane n'est qu'une portion périphérique du cytoplasma qui serait pour ainsi dire soulevée par le filament. Cette hypothèse rend compréhensible la nature ectoplasmatique de la membrane ondulante, ce qui est du reste appuyé par des faits que nous croyons être assez probants.

En effet, l'existence de granulations évidemment cytoplasmiques dans l'épaisseur de la membrane est un fait qui parle en faveur de cette opinion. Il est même des cas où il y a pénétration de portions de l'endoplasma plus ou moins loin dans les festons de la membrane ondulante, ainsi qu'il arrive chez le *T. rotatorium*. Mais c'est à l'état vivant, en suivant la tranformation en boule du parasite, que l'on se convainc que cette formation est bien une partie de l'ectoplasma.

Placés dans les conditions anormales, les *T. costatum* et *rotatorium* présentent, avant de mourir, une série de transformations qui consistent essentiellement en une disparition progressive de la membrane ondulante et du flagelle et une augmentation de volume avec mise en boule du cytoplasma. En observant sous un grossissement assez puissant le mécanisme de ces modifications, on constate que la membrane ondulante se confond peu à peu avec le cytoplasma, par pénétration successive dans son intérieur des granulations endoplasmiques; vers la fin de ce processus, il ne reste de la membrane ondulante qu'une mince bordure en tout identique à la couche d'ectoplasma qui existe parfois tout autour de la masse cytoplasmique, et qui se continue sans aucune ligne de démarcation nette avec l'endoplasma. Le flagelle libre disparaît petit à petit, et le filament se trouve enfin englobé dans le cytoplasma. Cette régression de la membrane ondulante démontre bien, croyons-nous, que cette formation fait partie de l'ectoplasma, dont elle n'est qu'une différenciation qui s'y produit en rapport avec les phénomènes de mouvements si vifs dont sont doués les Flagellés du genre *Trypanosoma*.

Tels sont en résumé les faits d'ordre cytologique général que nous avons constatés chez les Trypanosomes des Grenouilles et que nous avons cru pouvoir intéresser les histologistes (¹).

DISCUSSION

M. Gessna dit qu'il est d'accord avec les auteurs au sujet de la nature du blépharoplaste, qu'il ne peut pas considérer comme un centrosome en se basant

---

(¹) Travail du laboratoire d'histologie et physiologie de l'École de Médecine de Lisbonne.

principalement sur la forte fixation qu'il prend par les méthodes de Giemsa et de Leishmann qui ne colorent pas les centrosomes des leucocytes dans les mêmes préparations. Il se met en désaccord avec eux pour ce qui a trait à la question du corpuscule basal des cils des cellules épithéliales; l'orateur pense que ce corpuscule est bien de nature centrosomique et ne peut pas être identifié avec le blépharoplaste des Trypanosomes. Il refuse à nier les rapports de ce corpuscule et du flagelle chez ces Protozoaires.

M. ATHIAS: Je suis heureux que M. le prof. Benda ait la même opinion que nous relativement au blépharoplaste; le fait que ce corpuscule se colore vivement par des méthodes qui ne teignent pas le centrosome est un argument de plus contre sa nature centrosomique, du moins exclusive.

Si j'ai exprimé quelques doutes sur l'opinion d'après laquelle les corpuscules basaux des cils auraient la valeur de centrosomes, c'est parce qu'elle ne me semble pas suffisamment démontrée et que tout récemment M. Wallengren a décrit dans les cellules ciliées des Najades un centrosome absolument distinct des corpuscules basaux et jouant un rôle actif pendant les phénomènes mitosiques. Si ce fait ne suffit pas à détruire la théorie admise par M. Benda, il n'est pas moins vrai qu'il autorise à avoir des doutes sur la signification attribuée aux corpuscules basaux.

Quant aux rapports du blépharoplaste avec le filament, ils nous semblent indubitables; nous avons pu toujours voir le filament inséré sur ce corpuscule.

DÉMONSTRATIONS

M. RAMÓN y CAJAL démontre une série de belles préparations se rapportant au *développement des éléments nerveux de la moelle et des ganglions de l'embryon de poulet et à la régénération des nerfs sectionnés chez le lapin.*

À 4 heures l'ordre du jour étant épuisé, M. MATTOSO SANTOS reprend la présidence pour déclarer terminés les travaux de la section et remercier les personnes qui ont bien voulu présenter des rapports ou des communications, ainsi que les présidents d'honneur et les autres congressistes qui ont assisté aux séances.

TABLE DES MATIÈRES

Première partie — Rapports officiels

Deuxième partie — Comptes rendus des séances

ERRATA

Page		au lieu de	il faut lire
Page 37		Micramères	Micromères.
» 39		succulaires	sacculaires.
» 41		accessorische Nucleolus	Nucleolen.
» 41		Külle	Hülle.
» 41		Zellleibs	Zellleib.
» 43		Telodendrier	Telodendrien.
» 43		Längsäste	Längsäste.
» 43		untere Längsäste	Queräste.
» 46		festreifte	gestreifte.
» 50		kernhaltiger	kernhaltiges.
» 51 fig. 18		mehrkernige	einkernige.
» 54 » 7		Les termes *Vaisseaux sanguins et récurrents* se rapportent aux muscles striés page 50	
» 56		Tunica der Submucosa	Gefässe der …
» 58		Verzweigten	verzweigten
» 62 » 25		théliale	sous-endothéliale.
» 63 » 10		Ganglien	Ganglien.
» 65		Cellules à hématocytes	… à hématolytes, haematolytenhaltige.
» 69		Pendellilgefässe	Penicilli
» 70		Konzontrische	Konzentrisch.
» 71		Nervenkläuel	Nervenknäuel.
» 73		Cutis-lamellen	Cutislamellen.
» 74		Kleinenschaulippen	kleinen Schaulippen.
» 76		mammillae	mammilore.
» 77		macula	maculosa.
» 78		körniger	körniger.
» 78		onyetogenes	onychogenes.
» 79		äussere Balgepithel	äussere Balgepithelscheide.
» 80		Pigmentkörper	Pigmentkörner.
» 81		gefensterten	gefensterten.
» 81		feinem	feinen.
» 82		Zwiebelregion	Zwiebelregion.
» 83		Nacken	Hacken.
» 85		Stiftchenzellen	Stiftchenzellen.
» 88		remtiens	remtiens.
» 89		Modiolus	Modiolus.
» 90		Corti'schen	Corti'scher.
» 91 » 23		Epitheli	Epithels.
» 91 » 37		tymp	tymp.
» 93		lage	lage.
» 94		Abtheilung	Abtheilung.
» 95		Steigbügel	Steigbügel.
» 95		Muskeln	Muskeln.
» 97		Steigbügel	Steigbügel.
» 97		knöchernen	knöcherner.
» 97		Tuba	Tuba.
» 98		Flimmerepithel	Flimmerepithel.

Page			au lieu de lire	il faut lire ou écrire
»	96			
»	97	fig. 1	cartilce	lecture
»	97	« 9 — d'en bas		
			platte	glatte.
»	101		Zoliwulst	Zellwulst.
»	101		Zapfenzellen	Zapfenzellen
»	101		Scheibenverklärung	Scheibenverklärung.
»	102		Trоnsendrüsen	Talgdrüsen.
»	103		Conjonctiva	Conjunctiva.
»	104	« 41	palpebra	palpebral
»	104		Couche périchoroidale	périchoroidale.
»	105		lacrimale	lacrymale.
»	106		exokrinen Mündung	exogebildter Mündung.
»	107		Heteromorphe	Heteromorphe.
»	108		Lebergänge	Lebere Gänge.
»	109	« 8	Glandes	Glande.
»	110	« 18	Ehrlich	Ehrlich.
»	110	« 25	Nerol	Nerol.
»	111	« 14	nucleole	nucléoles.
»	112	al. 2	cellule-lobulaires	centre-lobulaires.
»	112	fig. 28	Korotkoff	Korotkoff.
»	113	« 19	du colv del	du lobule droit.
»	113	« 33	Lawson	Chinois.
»	118	« 32	Spirlax	Spirlax.
»	119	« 13	corton	corton.
»	115	« 3 — d'en bas		
			Golestramqui	Golestran.
»	124	« 6 — d'en bas		
			algena	algena.

XV Congrès International de Médecine

Lisbonne — 19-26 Avril 1906

Section I

ANATOMIE

2ᵐᵉ FASCICULE

LISBONNE
Imprimerie Adolpho de Mendonça
1906